Digital Addictions

André Luiz Monezi Andrade
Editor

Digital Addictions

An Interdisciplinary Approach to Behavioral Addictions and Digital Media

Springer

Editor
André Luiz Monezi Andrade
Department of Psychology
Pontifícia Universidade Católica de Campinas
Campinas, São Paulo, Brazil

ISBN 978-3-031-87988-3 ISBN 978-3-031-87986-9 (eBook)
https://doi.org/10.1007/978-3-031-87986-9

This Springer imprint is published by the registered company Springer Nature Switzerland AG
The registered company address is: Gewerbestrasse 11, 6330 Cham, Switzerland

Contents

1 **Introduction to Behavioral Addictions and Digital Media** 1
Fernando Ferreira Semolini, Laura Soares da Silva, Amanda Severo Lins Vitta, Evelin Moreira Freires, and André Luiz Monezi Andrade

2 **Internet and Smartphone Addiction: Characteristics, Impacts, Diagnosis, and Treatment** 23
Fernando Ferreira Semolini, Laura Soares da Silva, Amanda Severo Lins Vitta, Evelin Moreira Freires, and André Luiz Monezi Andrade

3 **Binge-Watching and the Digital Era: A New Pattern of Media Consumption** 35
Laura Soares da Silva, Evelin Moreira Freires, Amanda Severo Lins Vitta, Adriana Scatena, Fernando Ferreira Semolini, Denise De Micheli, and André Luiz Monezi Andrade

4 **Gaming Disorder: Neurobiological Foundations, Clinical Features, Psychosocial Impacts, and Evidence-Based Interventions** 47
Manoela Fontelles, Isabela Brasil Correia, Richard Alecsander Reichert, Filipe Reis Teodoro Andrade, Rosa Maria Martins de Almeida, and Denise De Micheli

5 **Exploring the Intersection of Cyberbullying and Digital Addiction** 65
Cláudio Romualdo, Antônio Marcos Neves Esteca, and Wanderlei Abadio de Oliveira

6 **Hazardous Gambling and Online Sports Betting: A New Frontier of Behavioral Addiction—Overview, Clinical Correlates, and Interventions** 83
Richard Alecsander Reichert, Filipe Reis Teodoro Andrade, Manoela Fontelles, Nicoly Camile Mendes Reichert, Rosa Maria Martins de Almeida, and Denise De Micheli

7 **Parental Mediation in the Use of Digital Media by Children and Adolescents** 123
Isabela Brasil Correia, Manoela Fontelles, Victor Hugo Silva Turnes, Natália Minatti de Souza, Weliton da Silva, João Vitor Girardi Turqueti da Rocha, Nicoly Camile Mendes Reichert, Eloísa Medeiros Avancini, Richard Alecsander Reichert, and Denise De Micheli

8 **The Gamblification of Video Games: A Case Study on Loot Boxes** 139
Maya C. Thulin, Lindsey A. Snaychuk, Jenna L. Vieira, Sophie G. Coelho, and Hyoun S. Kim

9 **From Virtual to Real: Considerations on Life Purpose and Media Use in Adolescents** 153
Juliano Porto de Cerqueira Leite and Letícia Lovato Dellazzana-Zanon

10 **Digital Addiction, Depression, and Suicide** 163
Makilim Nunes Baptista, Vithor Rosa Franco, Bruno Bonfá-Araujo, Mateus Eduardo Romão, Giacomo Belli, Silvia Damiana Visonà, Ilaria Setti, and Serena Barello

11 **Transmedia and Digital Addiction** 177
Fernando Ferreira Semolini, Laura Soares da Silva, Amanda Severo Lins Vitta, Evelin Moreira Freires, and André Luiz Monezi Andrade

Index 193

Chapter 1
Introduction to Behavioral Addictions and Digital Media

Fernando Ferreira Semolini, Laura Soares da Silva, Amanda Severo Lins Vitta, Evelin Moreira Freires, and André Luiz Monezi Andrade

Definition and Characteristics of Behavioral Dependencies Related to the Use of Digital Media

To understand how behavioral dependencies relate to the use of digital media, it is necessary first to comprehend the process by which problematic behaviors came to be regarded as dependencies, as well as when and in what context digital media entered this discussion. In this regard, it is important to emphasize that, beyond previous contributions, the study of behavioral dependencies gained significant prominence in the early twentieth century with the advancement of research on human behavior. In this context, behaviorists such as B. F. Skinner and Ivan Pavlov laid the theoretical foundations for understanding how behavior could be conditioned and reinforced, exploring the mechanisms through which repetitive actions could trigger behavioral dependency processes (Skinner, 1938). With the advancement of neuroscience, the influence of the brain's reward system on repetitive behaviors was examined, particularly focusing on the role of the neurotransmitter dopamine in modulating pleasure-seeking behaviors. Thus, the late twentieth century was marked by the expansion of research aimed at understanding compulsive behaviors and dependencies not related to substance consumption, such as gambling addiction, sex addiction, compulsive shopping, and Internet addiction. This effort accumulated enough scientific scope for the Diagnostic and Statistical Manual of Mental Disorders (DSM-III) to include gambling dependencies within impulse-control disorders in 1980.

Continuing this trend, in 1996, Mak Griffiths proposed that some problematic behaviors could lead individuals to develop dependencies through psychobiological

F. F. Semolini · L. S. da Silva · A. S. L. Vitta · E. M. Freires · A. L. M. Andrade (✉)
Pontifical Catholic University of Campinas, Campinas, Brazil
e-mail: fernando.fs4@puccampinas.edu.br; amanda.slv@puccampinas.edu.br; evelin.mf@puccampinas.edu.br; andre.andrade@puc-campinas.edu.br

A. L. M. Andrade (ed.), *Digital Addictions*,
https://doi.org/10.1007/978-3-031-87986-9_1

mechanisms similar to those of chemical dependencies. Accordingly, behavioral dependencies, associated with impulsivity and compulsivity, would follow these stages: (1) Salience, when activities related to addictive behaviors become a priority in the individual's routine; (2) mood alteration, primarily characterized by the euphoria and emotions felt during the problematic behavior; (3) tolerance, referring to the increasing amount of time spent engaging in the behavior in pursuit of sensations; (4) withdrawal, concerning the physiological, psychological, and emotional changes resulting from a period without the addictive behavior; (5) conflicts, which involve familial, social, and occupational problems arising from excessive behavior; (6) and relapse, referring to the loss of control over abstinence, leading the individual to resume the addictive behavior. Thus, establishing a cycle of dependency (Griffiths, 1996).

Given the growing research in this area, the evidence that behavioral addictions activate the same reward circuits and neural mechanisms involved in chemical addictions has enabled the study of these addictions from a biopsychosocial model, aiming to understand the genetic, biological, psychological, and social influences associated with problematic behaviors. The advancement of these studies, along with their similarities to chemical dependencies, contributed to the inclusion of behavioral dependencies (gambling disorder) in the DSM-5 under the category of Substance-Related and Addictive Disorders in 2013.

In this context, behavioral dependencies related to the use of digital media began to be researched in response to the increasing influence that these technologies exerted over individuals' daily lives. More specifically, since the late twentieth century, with the widespread advent of the Internet, researchers began to observe patterns of compulsive behaviors related to computer use and online browsing. In 1995, Ivan Goldberg categorized this problematic behavior as Internet Addiction Disorder, a term later supported by contemporary researchers (Goldberg, 1995). However, research did not remain limited to Internet use. The first decade of the twenty-first century was marked by the advent of smartphones, online gaming, and social media, which, alongside technological advancements, brought new possibilities for compulsive behaviors identified among users. Identifying and categorizing such repetitive behaviors, phenomena such as smartphone addiction, online gaming addiction, and social media addiction have been widely explored to this day, with researchers seeking to understand their psychological, physiological, behavioral, and emotional effects. The scope of these studies has expanded to include repetitive activities on digital media as enablers and reinforcers of the addiction cycle (Allcott et al., 2022). As a result, smartphone addiction was also included in the DSM-5's appendix as a focus for future studies.

Currently, research and studies on digital addictions are significant due to the exponential growth of Internet users and electronic devices, as well as the future trends towards nearly complete globalization of digital media worldwide. According to the "Digital 2024: Global Overview Report," the number of Internet users worldwide exceeded 5.4 billion people in 2024, representing more than 66% of the global population. By comparison, in 2014 this number was 2.7 billion, marking a doubling of users over the span of 10 years. Internet usage is most prevalent in Northern

Europe (97.6%) and North America (96.8%), in contrast to Southeastern Africa (26.7%) and Central Africa (32.1%). Of these users, more than 97% access the Internet via smartphones, with approximately 70% of the global population owning or maintaining contact with mobile phones. In this context, digital media play a significant role in the behavior of individuals on the Internet, such that in 2024, humanity reached the milestone of 5 billion digital media users, nearly three times the 1.8 billion users from 10 years ago (DATAREPORTAL, 2024).

Thus, behavioral dependencies related to the use of digital media can be categorized based on the excessive and uncontrolled use of digital technologies (Allcott et al., 2022). Moreover, given the vast scope of these technologies, which tend to increase as technology evolves, research has focused on the excessive use of the Internet, smartphones, social media, video games, and streaming platforms. These modes of digital media consumption can intensify compulsive behaviors that may lead to significant harm in an individual's personal, professional, and social life (Andrade et al., 2022; Martins et al., 2021; Reichert et al. 2021a).

A deeper understanding of the latent characteristics in digital media addicts highlights (1) constant preoccupation with digital media as an important factor in understanding this addiction. More specifically, this is akin to the craving symptom experienced by individuals with substance addictions, where thoughts about digital media prevail even when these individuals are not engaging with it, potentially affecting daily life domains such as professional productivity, academic performance, and concentration on other daily activities (Hartogsohn & Vudka, 2023). This preoccupation, particularly with digital media, is also associated with the phenomenon of "Fear of Missing Out" (FoMO), which is characterized by the fear of being out of touch with digital matters or missing out on important information and experiences (Gupta & Sharma, 2021). In the case of digital media, this fear is strongly fueled by transmedia strategies, reward mechanisms in online games, and constant real-time updates that unfold at high speed on social media. In this sense, the anxiety generated induces compulsive use of digital media, while also amplifying the desire to remain continuously connected to the digital world (Elhai et al., 2021).

Much of this is related to (2) the uncontrollable need to use digital media. This phenomenon is reflected in the impulses to check social media without any apparent reason, or to turn on the phone without a specific prior purpose. In this context, research indicates that high impulsivity is a key factor in the increase of digital behaviors associated with a low level of self-control regarding the desire to use digital media. Thus, the inability to resist this desire increases vulnerability to compulsive behaviors, a symptom present in digital addictions (Andrade et al., 2024; Augner et al., 2023; Kim et al., 2023).

This excessive use becomes more concerning when it persists (3) despite the negative consequences for the user. In other words, when individuals continue to engage in problematic and compulsive behaviors related to digital media, even after experiencing symptoms of stress, fatigue, and sleep disturbances (common in excessive screen time), as well as greater difficulties in social interactions and deterioration of existing interpersonal relationships (Andrade et al., 2020a; Puukko et al.,

2020; Yang et al., 2020). This cycle of compulsive use despite negative consequences is primarily reinforced by psychobiological mechanisms of dopamine release and activation of brain reward circuits, which, in the case of addicts, become hyperactivated (Small et al., 2020).

Another characteristic of digital addictions is the (4) difficulty in controlling the time spent online. It is common for compulsive users to spend more time in the digital world than they had initially planned, mainly due to the immersive potential of digital media and the constant loss of time awareness while connected to the online universe. In this context, both time loss and temporal immersion are phenomena strongly explored and induced by the interfaces and designs of online games, apps, and social media, enhancing user engagement for extended periods (Allcott et al., 2022; Caroux & Pujol, 2024).

This engagement potential, in the case of digital addictions, is related to (5) neglect of other important activities for the individual. In other words, when the digital world becomes a priority in the user's life, surpassing essential activities such as studying (in the case of young people), work, leisure, or social interactions, these characteristic compromises physical health, mental health, academic performance, and professional career (Han et al., 2023).

Finally, one of the central characteristics of digital media addiction (which can induce the others) is the presence of (6) withdrawal symptoms when there is no access to digital media. These symptoms primarily manifest as increased anxiety, irritability, frustration, and mood changes. They are present in nearly all types of addiction, both chemical and behavioral (Truzoli et al., 2023).

In line with the categorization and identification of these characteristics, some researchers have sought to address the need for standardization and quantification of the intensity of digital addictions, in order to enable assessments of addiction levels and guide interventions and treatments. In this context, the development of scales for digital addiction has been crucial in guiding future research and producing a broad, standardized scientific range (Andrade et al., 2020b, 2020c).

It was with these objectives in mind that Kimberly Young, in 1998, developed the Internet Addiction Test (IAT) in the United States (Young, 1998), one of the first scales created to assess problematic Internet use and one of the most widely used in the world. More specifically, the goal of the IAT is to identify and measure levels of Internet addiction by assessing its excessive use and how it affects an individual's productivity, social life, daily activities, and other involved aspects. Additionally, the test also seeks symptoms of compulsivity and lack of control regarding the time spent using the Internet. Understanding all these elements, the IAT consists of a 20-item questionnaire answered on a Likert scale, ranging from "rarely" to "always," classifying the addiction as mild, moderate, or severe.

Next, delving into the theme of games, in the Netherlands, Lemmens et al. (2009) developed the Game Addiction Scale (GAS) in 2009, with the aim of identifying and measuring online gaming addiction, focusing on video games. The GAS is thus a scale consisting of 21 items, also on a 5-point Likert scale ranging from "never" to "always," so that the final score allows for the evaluation of the level of problematic involvement with video games, helping identify potential addicts. Therefore, the GAS is widely used in research to understand excessive video game use, loss of control over use, withdrawal symptoms, salience, and social and occupational harms resulting from problematic video game use.

In turn, in 2013 in South Korea, Kwon et al. (2013) sought to assess problematic smartphone use through the Smartphone Addiction Scale (SAS), an instrument widely used in the scientific literature related to smartphone addiction. Thus, the SAS is a scale that allows for the differentiation between non-problematic users and smartphone addicts by investigating aspects such as excessive use and compulsivity, as well as social, emotional, and cognitive consequences. These aspects are further elaborated in the 33 items of the scale, divided into 6 factors: (1) control over usage time, (2) disruptions in daily life, (3) withdrawal, (4) tolerance, (5) emotional consequences, and (6) use for pleasure-seeking. Furthermore, the SAS is evaluated on a 6-point Likert scale, ranging from "strongly disagree" to "strongly agree."

Regarding social media, it was only in 2016 in Norway that the Bergen Social Media Addiction Scale (BSMAS) was developed by Andreassen et al. (2016) to identify social media addictions. More specifically, based on the same stages of behavioral addiction proposed by Griffiths (1996), the scale investigates the six factors: (1) salience, (2) mood alteration, (3) tolerance, (4) withdrawal symptoms, (5) conflict, and (6) relapse, adapted to the context of social media use. Thus, the BSMAS consists of only 6 items that vary on a 5-point Likert scale, from "very rarely" to "very frequently." Its final result allows for the identification of the level of behavioral addiction concerning social media.

Prevalence and Social Impact of Digital Addictions in Different Populations

Digital addictions encompass circumstantial factors that significantly influence the way behavior unfolds. In this context, it is essential to clarify how digital addictions affect different populations concerning age groups, in order to understand this phenomenon more comprehensively. Thus, despite the similarities in the addiction process and the observations on how the consequences of these problematic behaviors remain similar across the populations analyzed, cultural, developmental, and occupational differences influence and modify aspects and characteristics of digital addiction.

Within this scope, research on digital addiction among children and adolescents suggests that this group is particularly vulnerable to the effects of digital media and presents a higher risk for developing addiction due to how prolonged exposure to digital media can interfere with emotional well-being and cognitive functions (León Méndez et al., 2024; Ramos et al., 2023; Ricci et al., 2023). Contextualizing this audience, recent surveys point to a significant increase in the use of electronic devices by young children. For example, a study in Japan concluded that 37.5% of 2-year-old children were already using digital devices, rising to 50% among children aged 3–5 years (Nakayama et al., 2020), a trend also observed in other developed countries. In this context, these data are crucial for understanding digital addictions, considering that the earlier the initiation with digital tools, the higher the association with the risks of developing problematic Internet usage (Nakayama et al., 2020).

Entering the adolescent population, scientific literature understands that they exhibit higher prevalences of digital addiction compared to children. Recent studies on problematic Internet use (PIU) have indicated a prevalence of 24.5% among adolescents aged 9–12 years in India (Shanthi et al., 2024), which aligns with studies in Turkey that found higher prevalences of digital addiction among adolescents aged 10–14 years (Oktay & Ozturk, 2024).

Within this context, a crucial factor in understanding the development of digital addictions among children and adolescents is screen time spent with digital media. Studies have shown that levels of digital addiction increased with more screen time (Parlak et al., 2023). However, equally important is the type of usage, which also significantly influences the development of digital addictions. Children and adolescents who use digital media for studying, for example, showed lower levels of addiction compared to those who prioritize online gaming as their main digital activity (Oktay & Ozturk, 2024).

The main concern observed in children and adolescents revolves around the psychobiological impacts caused by digital exposure. Within this theme, it is understood that excessive exposure to the digital environment is associated with alterations in the neurological development of children. Research has demonstrated how modifications in neurotransmitter pathways during childhood development can trigger future mental health and behavioral problems, affecting cognitive control, reward sensitivity, inhibitory control, and anomalies in brain activation. More specifically, MRI studies have shown how digital addiction can cause functional and structural changes in the frontal cortex and structures associated with the dopaminergic system, impairing the development of children and adolescents (Ding et al., 2023; Oktay & Ozturk, 2024). Regarding inhibitory control, weaker activation was observed in the inferior frontal gyrus and striatum during tasks requiring inhibitory control. Additionally, hyperactivity in areas related to reward processing and increased activation in prefrontal regions suggest anomalies in the reward system. Finally, it was noted that the prefrontal lobe is the most affected area among digital addicts, leading to impairments in the development of executive functions, including impulse control, emotional regulation, and decision-making (Ding et al., 2023; Martins et al., 2021; Reichert et al., 2021b).

Despite concerns about digital addiction in children and adolescents, the adult population remains the most affected by digital addictions. In recent decades, this group has seen a significant increase in the prevalence of Internet addiction, smartphone addiction, and video game addiction (Pereira et al., 2021). The higher problematic use may be linked to social and work pressures faced by this population. Many adults turn to digital media and video games as a coping mechanism for personal problems or stress relief in their daily lives. However, problematic and excessive use can compromise professional and occupational productivity, leading to social issues and even mental health problems, such as depression, anxiety, and stress (Andrade et al., 2020a; Kim et al., 2024).

In this context, digital addictions and intensive use of digital media in adults are associated with the phenomenon of "technostress," characterized as stress resulting from the intensive use of digital devices linked to the work environment, which extends into the individual's personal life (Dragano & Lunau, 2020). This excessive stress originates from the constant pressure to remain connected, available, and up-to-date due to technologies, computers, and electronic devices that allow the work environment to spill over into a person's personal life, a situation intensified during the pandemic with the popularization of remote work (Bahamondes-Rosado et al., 2023). As a result, information overload, combined with intensive use of electronic devices, can lead to symptoms such as irritability, mental fatigue, anxiety, and cognitive impairments. These factors, influenced by the social context, can contribute to an increase in burnout symptoms as well as depressive and anxious symptoms, highlighting the importance of new strategies and adaptations to the emerging work models that increasingly rely on technology and digital media (Andrade et al., 2023a; Gonçalves et al., 2022; Marsh et al., 2024).

Although less studied, the elderly population is also affected by digital addictions, facing greater risks of social isolation and the development of depressive disorders intensified by the improper use of digital media. Regarding the prevalences observed, in developed countries, more than 50% of seniors aged 64–75 use digital media and the Internet, with nearly 40% of seniors over 75 actively using the Internet, websites, and social networks (Győrffy et al., 2023). In this regard, recent research shows how problematic use of digital media in older populations can aggravate depressive symptoms and grief, as well as increase or decrease the sense of social isolation depending on how it is used. Digital media can both help maintain social connections (especially due to distance or mobility difficulties), but when misused, they are associated with a lack of engagement in physical and social activities, hindering in-person contact (Lee & Bae, 2023; Wang et al., 2024a). Furthermore, problematic use of digital media can be linked to difficulties in managing screen time, as well as risks arising from excessive exposure to harmful content. Therefore, while digital media can serve as an emerging support factor for maintaining family and friend connections, excessive and intensive use can exacerbate emotional and mental health problems, especially in vulnerable elderly individuals (Xu et al., 2023).

Regarding the social impacts of digital addictions, it is understood not only as the consequences for the individual engaging in the problematic behavior but also the impacts that affect interpersonal relationships, family dynamics, as well as educational and professional spheres (Cilligol Karabey et al., 2024).

In this context, significant harm has been observed in the academic performance of children and adolescents and in the professional performance of adults among digital dependents. Specifically, intensive use of digital devices, particularly concerning digital media and gaming, has been associated with learning difficulties, poor academic performance, and concentration and attention issues (Dresp-Langley, 2020). Studies have found associations between screen time spent on digital media by youth and issues including limitations in working memory, difficulty concentrating, less time dedicated to studying, and lower engagement in physical activities—factors that negatively impact academic performance (Adelantado-Renau et al., 2019; Andrade et al., 2021).

On the other hand, adults with digital addictions and excessive use of digital media and electronic devices face higher risks of reduced productivity and efficiency at work. In this context, prolonged smartphone use can impair concentration and task performance, while Fear of Missing Out (FoMO) is associated with the constant need to check social media, further compromising attention (Marsh et al., 2024; Qutishat & Abu Sharour, 2019).

Another analyzed impact of digital addiction is the increased difficulty in interpersonal relationships. Studies on this issue have concluded that digital dependence can predict up to 25% of an individual's social connections, particularly related to feelings of loneliness and social dissatisfaction in adolescents (Parlak et al., 2023). Additionally, digital dependence can harm interpersonal relationships when associated with increased isolation, limiting the quality of face-to-face interactions. In this sense, the constant presence of smartphones during in-person conversations has been linked in some studies to a decrease in satisfaction with social interactions, compromising the formation of social bonds (Cilligol Karabey et al., 2024). Alongside this dissatisfaction, excessive use of social media is also associated with the construction of unrealistic expectations and distorted comparisons, which can hinder the establishment of real-world connections. For example, it was found that digital game addicts had higher levels of loneliness and social dissatisfaction (Parlak et al., 2023). In this context, the replacement of face-to-face interactions with virtual ones also contributes to higher risks of social isolation and loneliness, reinforcing problematic gaming behaviors as a form of escapism.

Health issues, both physical and mental, remain some of the most studied impacts of digital addiction. In terms of physical health, it has been observed that the increase in screen time among dependents is linked to the rise of myopia in children (one of the leading causes of blindness worldwide). Excessive use of digital technologies partly explains the higher prevalence of myopia in children and young adults (Dresp-Langley, 2020). Another factor associated with problematic behavior regarding digital media is the increase in obesity among children and adolescents due to greater consumption of unhealthy foods during device use (Zhou et al., 2022). Additionally, there has been an increase in sleep disturbances, as the large number of hours spent in front of screens (particularly at night) can disrupt sleep patterns, leading to issues such as daytime drowsiness, shorter overall sleep duration, and delays in bedtime (Cilligol Karabey et al., 2024). Related to sleep disturbances, prolonged exposure to digital environments is also associated with a decrease in natural sunlight exposure, increasing the risk of vitamin D and melatonin deficiencies, which impair both serotonin neural pathways and the individual's circadian rhythm (Oktay & Ozturk, 2024).

Regarding mental health impacts, it is crucial to highlight the increased risks for psychiatric disorders such as depression, anxiety, and stress. Additionally, cognitive development deficiencies—particularly in children and adolescents—along with compromised neural system functionality are prominent consequences of problematic behavior. These issues can affect inhibitory, emotional, and cognitive systems (Dresp-Langley, 2020).

Finally, it is essential to emphasize the relationship between the rise in digital dependencies and increased risks for accidents. Digital dependencies are associated with higher risks for accidents at work or on the road due to their potential for distraction and impairment of attention, as well as a noticeable decrease in reaction time (Ortega et al., 2021; Zatezalo et al., 2018). Moreover, research indicates that nomophobia, as well as "Fear of Missing Out" (FoMO), contributes to the development of impulsive behaviors, such as constantly checking electronic devices in inappropriate or dangerous situations (Notara et al., 2021), thereby increasing the risk of traffic accidents due to smartphone use while driving, and work-related accidents when operating machinery.

Connection Between Digital Dependencies and Other Mental Health Disorders

Following the trend of expected harms in any type of addiction, whether chemical or behavioral, digital addictions are associated with various psychiatric disorders such as anxiety, depression, and ADHD.

In relation to anxiety, the increase in the use of digital media can be understood, in part, as a way to escape anxious symptoms (Dresp-Langley, 2020). In this sense, excessive use can become an attempt to relieve situations that evoke negative emotions or anxiety. This is largely due to how digital media, games, and social networks offer constant reinforcements (such as notifications and likes) that create a sense of immediate gratification, temporarily alleviating anxious symptoms and encouraging continued use of digital media. However, the vicious cycle created around digital media can lead the individual to experience severe anxiety symptoms in the eventual situation where they have no access to digital media (Andrade et al., 2023b; Saikia et al., 2019).

Similarly, the intensive use of digital media can worsen symptoms of depression. In this sense, individuals with depressive symptoms often abuse digital media as a coping strategy for negative feelings (Marzilli et al., 2020). However, some studies indicate that excessive use of digital media can have the opposite effect, exacerbating depressive symptoms when individuals explore digital content that reinforces negative emotions. The impacts of social media are also linked to depressive symptoms due to distortions caused by the continuous display of positive moments, leading to a skewed view of reality that worsens isolation and dissatisfaction in depressed individuals. This isolation can intensify feelings of loneliness, often amplified by excessive use of digital media, worsening depressive symptoms (Karakose et al., 2023).

Regarding ADHD, it is understood that difficulties in controlling screen time and impulsivity can increase the risk of digital addiction within this population (Wang et al., 2024b). Studies have found correlations between ADHD and digital addictions due to the loss of impulse control. Equally important is understanding how attention deficits are associated with intensive use of digital media. The immediate reinforcement and rewards found in games and digital media can worsen ADHD symptoms, especially due to difficulties in concentration and the constant search for stimuli (Thorell et al., 2024).

Risk and Protective Factors for the Development of Digital Addictions

Due to the growing prominence and relevance in modern society, the study of digital addictions has not been limited to describing their characteristics and aspects. It has also expanded to understanding their psychobiological alterations and possible associations with psychological disorders. Beyond this, following prophylactic objectives in the health field, researchers have sought to understand the risk and protective factors related to the development of digital addictions.

Among the risk factors, genetic predisposition can be a significant factor in the relationship between the individual and digital media. Studies have shown that genetic polymorphisms related to the reward system and dopaminergic pathways may be associated with an increased vulnerability to problematic use of digital media and electronic devices. Similarly, individuals with a family history of behavioral addiction have significantly higher risks of developing similar behaviors (Hahn et al., 2017; Rył et al., 2024).

As already mentioned, factors surrounding the individual's personality also impact the risks for digital addiction. More specifically, personality traits such as higher impulsivity and low self-esteem are correlated with greater risks for digital addictions associated with problematic use of digital media. In this context, it is observed that individuals with high sensitivity to rewards and alterations in inhibitory control are more likely to engage in behaviors that provide immediate gratification, such as gaming and social media use (Diotaiuti et al., 2022).

Equally relevant is the influence of family factors in the development of digital addictions, especially in the case of children and adolescents. More specifically, it has been observed that children and adolescents in families with low levels of parental supervision, permissive parenting, or constant internal conflicts are at higher risk of developing problematic use of digital media and digital addiction (Cilligol Karabey et al., 2024; Yamada et al., 2021). Similarly, the constant exposure of children to family members who exhibit excessive use of digital media can serve as a model and behavioral example, increasing the likelihood that they will replicate the same digital behavior patterns (Li et al., 2024).

Another risk factor is the difficulty in managing one's emotions, which is associated with the development of digital addiction as a maladaptive way of coping with negative emotions. In this context, research shows positive correlations between emotional dysregulation and excessive use of digital media. This association is largely due to the way games and social media offer mechanisms of coping and escapism for negative emotions. The immediate rewards and high engagement potential also contribute to the dependency process, offering a distraction mechanism that allows individuals to temporarily forget their emotional distress (Yan et al., 2022).

In children and young people, the absence of extracurricular activities also allows individuals to spend more time on the excessive use of digital media (Sayılı et al., 2021; Yamada et al., 2021). This behavior pattern is due to the need to seek entertainment, often associated with online social interactions, but also to cope with boredom resulting from the absence of other extracurricular activities. In this context, research points to how encouraging involvement in sports, arts, or other in-person activities during the school period helps the young individual as a protective factor against digital addictions.

Finally, the ease of access to digital media has also proven to be a risk factor for digital addictions. In this sense, the significant increase in access to digital devices, as well as the greater availability of online content, has led to greater risks of problematic use of digital media. More specifically, developed countries with widespread access to technology are among those with the highest prevalence of digital addiction cases. Likewise, research with youth and children reveals a higher risk of problematic behaviors among those who have personal smartphones or easy access to electronic devices without parental restrictions (Nakayama et al., 2020).

Turning now to the protective factors against the development of digital addiction, it is possible to understand, in contrast to what has been presented in risk factors, how family support and parental control play a crucial role in this process. In this regard, research shows that the presence of a supportive family environment that meets the various needs of the young person (emotional, social, and cognitive) is essential to prevent excessive use of digital media. More specifically, the establishment of healthy digital boundaries, digital supervision, setting limits, monitoring screen time, selecting healthy digital content, as well as reducing isolation and creating safe spaces for emotional expression, all contribute as protective factors against digital addiction (Dresp-Langley, 2020; Li et al., 2024; Parlak et al., 2023).

From the individual's perspective, regarding personality, studies show that high self-esteem remains a significant protective factor against problematic digital media use (Ketata et al., 2021). This phenomenon can be explained by the reduced need for constant validation or social comparison within social networks. Achieving extraordinary feats in games or status in digital platforms is also relevant factors contributing to excessive use, especially when the same achievements are not attainable in reality. Therefore, elevated self-esteem helps the individual cope with challenges without resorting to escapism through digital media (Chettiar & Malik, 2022). In a similar context, the presence or development of social skills is essential to reduce dependence on virtual interactions, thereby promoting and facilitating the formation of healthy social relationships. Research indicates that individuals who find it easy to establish and maintain interpersonal connections are less likely to seek digital media to fill social gaps.

Furthermore, education about the risks of excessive digital media use has potential benefits for protecting individuals. Through education, it is possible to develop critical understanding of the impacts of digital media on social relationships, as well as physical and mental health. In this way, it is understood that awareness of the symptoms of problematic digital media use, along with adaptive strategies and healthy habits, become protective factors for both young people and adults (Dresp-Langley, 2020).

Differences and Similarities Between Behavioral Addictions and Substance Use Disorder

The study of behavioral addictions followed the already established scientific literature on chemical dependencies and the processes involved. In this sense, it can be said that behavioral addictions began to consolidate as a new form of addiction once sufficient evidence was gathered showing that they went through similar processes to those observed in chemical addictions and were also associated with significant harm in the individual's life. However, it is crucial to understand behavioral addictions as a separate dependency process from chemical addictions in several ways, even though there are many similarities.

In this context, the main difference between chemical and behavioral addictions is that the latter does not involve the use of chemical substances. That is, chemical addictions involve a direct alteration in the brain's chemical composition due to the action of neurotransmitters on physiological processes. As a result, addiction becomes an adaptation of the organism to the neurochemical effects of the substance, generating withdrawal symptoms when use is interrupted. On the other hand, behavioral addictions act on the organism indirectly, through the activation of the dopaminergic system without the presence of external chemical substances, triggering internal responses that reinforce the reward cycle, leading to the repetition of the behavior and creating a behavioral and psychological relationship with the problematic activity. In short, the main difference is that while chemical addiction involves the participation of an external substance that alters the body's chemistry, behavioral addiction involves external stimuli that induce internal reactions (Zou et al., 2017).

Another important point is that the withdrawal symptoms in behavioral addictions may differ from those observed in chemical addictions. In chemical addictions, the person develops a physiological adaptation to the substances, resulting in intense reactions when consumption is interrupted, leading to physical symptoms such as seizures, sweating, tremors, and nausea (De Micheli et al., 2021; Oliveira et al., 2016). In contrast, in behavioral addictions, withdrawal symptoms tend to be more psychological and emotional, such as anxiety, irritability, insomnia, restlessness, and emptiness, not causing as severe physiological reactions as those seen in chemical addictions (Rosenberg, 2014).

Another difference lies in the treatments for chemical and behavioral addictions, which primarily differ due to the involvement of external substances and the physiological effects associated with them. In chemical addictions, treatment necessarily includes a phase of detoxification and readaptation of the organism, requiring the use of medications to assist in detoxification and alleviate withdrawal symptoms (De Micheli et al., 2021). In contrast, in behavioral addictions, treatment does not include a detoxification phase, and the use of medications specifically for withdrawal symptoms is rare. However, antidepressants and anxiolytics are often used to treat symptoms related to anxiety and depression, which are commonly found in individuals with behavioral addictions (Rosenberg, 2014).

As for the similarities, it is widely observed that both chemical and behavioral addictions can lead to significant impairments in the individual's life. Several similar aspects are also noted in the psychobiology behind chemical and behavioral addictions. Addictions, in general, are associated with feelings of pleasure and euphoria triggered by neural systems responsible for maintaining and worsening the addiction (Abrahao et al., 2017; Andrade & De Micheli, 2016). In this sense, digital addictions resemble chemical addictions in that they share similar neural systems (Ding et al., 2023). In this context, drugs, in general, can activate dopaminergic neurons in the ventral tegmental area (VTA), releasing the neurotransmitter dopamine to the nucleus accumbens (NAc), amygdala, and other limbic structures through the mesolimbic pathway (Koob & Volkow, 2016). Thus, the NAc is responsible for the brain's reward system, which manages the pleasurable sensations caused by the ingestion of chemical substances. Meanwhile, the amygdala manages the emotional content associated with the substance, which can evoke negative feelings and distress in the absence of the drug, reinforcing the dependent behavior. Alongside the mesolimbic pathway's action, the VTA also releases dopamine through the mesocortical pathway, affecting, for example, regions of the frontal cortex, orbitofrontal cortex, and striatum (Koob & Volkow, 2016; Yang et al., 2018).

In this context, the etiology of digital addictions can be understood through quantitative and qualitative alterations in the central nervous system via neuroplastic processes. Research has been demonstrating the similarities between chemical and behavioral addictions in relation to anomalies in the reward systems, mesolimbic and mesocortical pathways, as well as hyperactivation of the amygdala, hypoactivation of the prefrontal cortex (PFC), reduced monoamines in the nucleus accumbens (NAc), and lower connectivity between cortical and limbic regions. Accordingly, studies show that psychobiological changes resulting from Internet Gaming Disorder (IGD) are primarily observed in the domains of the reward system, cognitive control, and decision-making (Niu et al., 2022; Yao et al., 2017). Similarly, problematic smartphone use and AI are associated with reduced gray/white matter in regions responsible for executive functions and reward processing in motor activities, such as the cerebellum and caudate nucleus, demonstrating the need for greater effort to execute cognitive functions related to the inhibition of motor behaviors that intensify the addiction (Ding et al., 2023).

This highlights that individuals with digital addictions exhibit structural and functional changes in the brain's reward circuits and regions (Ding et al., 2023; Yao et al., 2017; Qiu et al., 2023). Studies in this area demonstrate the particularities of dysfunctions in dopaminergic pathways (Ko et al., 2023), with a significant reduction in the availability of dopamine D2 receptors and transporters in the regions linked to the reward system. Additionally, there is decreased functional connectivity between the ventral tegmental area (VTA) with the NAc and the orbitofrontal cortex (OFC) in situations that do not involve digital behaviors, such that the more severe the addiction, the weaker this connectivity becomes (Wang et al., 2019; Wen et al., 2021). Similar alterations are observed between the NAc and regions of the hippocampus, as well as between the supplementary motor area (SMA) and the left middle temporal gyrus (Niu et al., 2023; Qiu et al., 2023). Therefore, given the importance of dopaminergic pathways in addiction processes, there is evidence that the severity of IGD, AI, and smartphone addiction (SA) is linked to neuropathological changes in the functional connectivity of the VTA circuits and other structures involved in reward pathways (Qiu et al., 2022; Wang et al., 2019; Wen et al., 2021; Yao et al., 2017). In this sense, the abnormal functioning of the amygdala is responsible for difficulties in self-control and regulation of desires, thus enhancing the maintenance of compulsive behaviors (León Méndez et al., 2024). Similarly, anomalies in frontostriatal circuits and executive functions, with a focus on the insula (responsible for establishing meaning and relationships between sensations of reward and emotions), amplify the aforementioned alterations. The reduced functional connectivity of this structure during rest states explains the heightened sensitivity to rewards (Kim et al., 2017; von Deneen et al., 2022).

Regarding the role of cortical regions and executive function in the neural processes associated with the reward system, individuals with digital addictions exhibit changes in the intensity of activation of these regions. Thus, hyperactivations and hypoactivations in frontostriatal and frontocingulate circuits, particularly in the OFC, dorsolateral prefrontal cortex (DLPFC), anterior cingulate cortex (ACC), supplementary motor area (SMA), and inferior frontal gyrus, are associated with dysregulation of reward responses in the reinforcing effects of games, series, and digital media, potentiating addictive behaviors through hyperactivation of the reward system (Ding et al., 2023; Kim et al., 2017). In addition, individuals with digital addictions present a smaller volume of gray matter in cortical regions involved in processing and managing the value of rewards, such as the OFC and ACC, which weakens behavioral control, associated with the calculation of risks and rewards, thus potentiating impulsive addictive behaviors (Lee et al., 2018; Niu et al., 2022). These structural and functional changes in reward circuits are also present in individuals with chemical dependencies, suggesting similarities in addiction processes (Ding et al., 2023). In this sense, withdrawal symptoms, compulsive behavior, craving, and intense desire, as well as deficits in cognitive control, affect individuals with digital addictions similarly to those with chemical dependencies (Qiu et al., 2023; von Deneen et al., 2022; Wen et al., 2021).

Cognitive control capacities, which involve the regulation and management of emotions, thoughts, and actions, also exhibit anomalies that manifest as reduced efficiency in cognitive control among individuals with problematic digital media behaviors (Marciano et al., 2021; Yao et al., 2017). Thus, adolescents with digital addictions display changes in connectivity in regions responsible for cognitive functions, such as low functional connectivity between thalamic structures and somatosensory cortex, as well as in frontostriatal circuits. This necessitates greater effort from the individual to perform activities requiring inhibitory control, attention, and planning (Ding et al., 2023; Marciano et al., 2021; Niu et al., 2023; von Deneen et al., 2022). Similarly, thinning of the cortex, especially in the OFC, is related to higher levels of cognitive impulsivity (Lee et al., 2018). Digital addiction also causes neuroplastic changes in the prefrontal lobe, particularly the OFC, DLPFC, cingulate gyrus, and SMA (Ding et al., 2023; Liu et al., 2023; Montag & Becker, 2023; Sun et al., 2023). In this context, research shows reductions in gray/white matter volume in these regions linked to cognitive control (Hutton et al., 2024; Pan et al., 2018). Moreover, changes in the volume of gray matter in the ventromedial PFC, superior frontal gyrus, ACC, and dorsal striatum may be associated with cognitive control problems in relation to addictive gaming behaviors (Niu et al., 2022; Yao et al., 2017). Similarly, recent studies demonstrated that reduced ACC activity was related to difficulties in cognitive control of rewards in digital addicts (León Méndez et al., 2024; Sun et al., 2023).

Both digital addicts and binge-watchers exhibit dysfunctions in inhibitory control systems (Dieterich et al., 2021; Kilian et al., 2020). Thus, the central role of the OFC is understood, as it also contributes to decision-making and emotional processing. Its dysfunction in digital addictions, impacted by reduced volume, is associated with behavioral discontrol that facilitates the execution of desires related to technology use, such as gaming and Internet browsing (Ding et al., 2023; Tseng et al., 2024). Studies have also shown reduced cortical thickness in this region in digital addicts, a phenomenon associated with greater impulsivity towards short-term rewards, such as the uncontrolled consumption of games, due to difficulties in decision-making related to reward processing. Moreover, this behavioral discontrol is also linked to changes in the connections between the PFC and the basal ganglia (León Méndez et al., 2024; Liu et al., 2023; Montag & Becker, 2023). Likewise, difficulties in utilizing inhibition systems are compounded by lower activation in the striatum and inferior frontal gyrus in situations requiring inhibitory control. Therefore, the hyperactivation of prefrontal regions, such as the OFC and inferior frontal gyrus, along with limbic regions like the amygdala, insula, and hippocampal gyrus, suggests that digital addicts need to exert greater effort to inhibit responses (Ding et al., 2023).

The reduction in the volume of the SMA is linked to repetitive motor actions, which, in the case of gaming or internet addiction, manifest in standardized finger movements or clicks, commonly observed in IGD. This is also seen in social media platforms like Instagram and TikTok, where repetitive actions like swiping down in search of new content occur (Kim et al., 2017; Niu et al., 2023). These changes in the sensorimotor cortex, related to compulsive behaviors, resemble those found in addicts to stimulant drugs, such as smoking, and influence inhibitory control over motor behaviors (Ding et al., 2023).

The maintenance of digital addictions and relapse processes are also linked to anomalies in neural systems involved in decision-making (Kim et al., 2017).

Research indicates decreased activation in cortical regions such as the PFC, inferior frontal gyrus, middle frontal gyrus, and lingual gyrus during situations requiring executive control to manage impulsive behaviors and emotional dysregulation in decision-making (Niu et al., 2022; Qiu et al., 2022; Yao et al., 2017). This may be related to increased cortical thinning, as well as reduced gray matter volume in frontoparietal areas responsible for managing and controlling behavior during decision-making processes (Lee et al., 2018). Furthermore, structural changes in frontostriatal circuits enhance difficulties related to impulsivity in decision-making (von Deneen et al., 2022).

References

Abrahao, K. P., Salinas, A. G., & Lovinger, D. M. (2017). Alcohol and the brain: Neuronal molecular targets, synapses, and circuits. *Neuron, 96*(6), 1223–1238. https://doi.org/10.1016/j.neuron.2017.10.032

Adelantado-Renau, M., Moliner-Urdiales, D., Cavero-Redondo, I., Beltran-Valls, M. R., Martínez-Vizcaíno, V., & Álvarez-Bueno, C. (2019). Association between screen media use and academic performance among children and adolescents: A systematic review and meta-analysis. *JAMA Pediatrics, 173*(11), 1058–1067. https://doi.org/10.1001/jamapediatrics.2019.3176

Allcott, H., Gentzkow, M., & Song, L. (2022). Digital addiction. *American Economic Review, 112*(7), 2424–2463. https://doi.org/10.1257/aer.20210867

Andrade, A. L. M., & De Micheli, D. (2016). *Innovations in the treatment of substance addiction* (1st ed.). Springer. https://doi.org/10.1007/978-3-319-43172-7

Andrade, A. L. M., Scatena, A., Bedendo, A., Enumo, S. R. F., Dellazzana-Zanon, L. L., Prebianchi, H. B., Macgado, W. L., et al. (2020a). Findings on the relationship between internet addiction and psychological symptoms in Brazilian adults. *International Journal of Psychology, 55*(6), 941–950. https://doi.org/10.1002/ijop.12670

Andrade, A. L. M., Kim, D. J., Caricati, V. V., Martins, G. D. G., Kirihara, I. K., Barbugli, B. C., Enumo, S. R. F., et al. (2020b). Validity and reliability of the Brazilian version of the smartphone addiction scale-short version for university students and adult population. *Estudos de Psicologia (Campinas), 37*, e190117. https://doi.org/10.1590/1982-0275202037e190117

Andrade, A. L. M., Scatena, A., Martins, G. D. G., de Oliveira Pinheiro, B., da Silva, A. B., Enes, C. C., Oliveira, W. A., et al. (2020c). Validation of smartphone addiction scale-short version (SAS-SV) in Brazilian adolescents. *Addictive Behaviors, 110*, 106540. https://doi.org/10.1016/j.addbeh.2020.106540

Andrade, A. L. M., Enumo, S. R. F., Passos, M. A. Z., Vellozo, E. P., Shoen, T. H., Kulik, M. A., Niskier, S. R., et al. (2021). Problematic internet use, emotional problems and quality of life among adolescents. *Psico-USF, 26*(1), 41–51. https://doi.org/10.1590/1413-82712021260104

Andrade, A. L. M., Di Girolamo Martins, G., Scatena, A., Lopes, F. M., de Oliveira, W. A., Kim, H. S., & De Micheli, D. (2022). The effect of psychosocial interventions for reducing co-occurring symptoms of depression and anxiety in individuals with problematic internet use: A systematic review and Meta-analysis. *International Journal of Mental Health and Addiction*, 1–22. https://doi.org/10.1007/s11469-022-00846-6

Andrade, A. L. M., Scatena, A., Bedendo, A., Machado, W. L., Oliveira, W. A. D., Lopes, F. M., & De Micheli, D. (2023a). Excessive internet and smartphone use and emotional problems in students of psychology and psychologists. *Estudos de Psicologia, 40*, e210010. https://doi.org/10.1590/1982-0275202340e210010en

Andrade, A. L. M., Scatena, A., Bedendo, A., Machado, W. L., Oliveira, W. A., Lopes, F. M., & Micheli, D. D. (2023b). Uso excessivo de internet e smartphone e problemas emocionais em estudantes de psicologia e psicólogos. *Estudos De Psicologia (campinas), 40*, e210010. https://doi.org/10.1590/1982-0275202340e210010

Andrade, A. L. M., Lobato, F. B. H., Stange, N., Scatena, A., Oliveira, W. A. D., Kim, H. S., & Lopes, F. M. (2024). The association between gaming disorder and impulsivity: A systematic review. *Estudos de Psicologia (Campinas), 41*, e220032. https://doi.org/10.1590/1982-0275202441e220032

Andreassen, C. S., Pallesen, S., & Griffiths, M. D. (2016). The relationship between addictive use of social media, narcissism, and self-esteem: Findings from a large national survey. *Addictive Behaviors, 64*, 287–293. https://doi.org/10.1016/j.addbeh.2016.03.006

Augner, C., Vlasak, T., & Barth, A. (2023). The relationship between problematic internet use and attention deficit, hyperactivity and impulsivity: A meta-analysis. *Journal of Psychiatric Research, 168*, 1–12. https://doi.org/10.1016/j.jpsychires.2023.10.032

Bahamondes-Rosado, M. E., Cerdá-Suárez, L. M., Ortiz, D., de Zevallos, G. F., & Espinosa-Cristia, J. F. (2023). Technostress at work during the COVID-19 lockdown phase (2020-2021): A systematic review of the literature. *Frontiers in Psychology, 14*, 1173425. https://doi.org/10.3389/fpsyg.2023.1173425

Caroux, L., & Pujol, M. (2024). Player enjoyment in video games: A systematic review and meta-analysis of the effects of game design choices. *International Journal of Human-Computer Interaction, 40*, 4227–4238. https://doi.org/10.1080/10447318.2023.2210880

Chettiar, C., & Malik, A. (2022). Impact of internet addiction on self-esteem and social anxiety. *Research Horizon, 12*, 153–164.

Cilligol Karabey, S., Palanci, A., & Turan, Z. (2024). How does smartphone addiction affect the lives of adolescents socially and academically?: A systematic review study. *Psychology, Health & Medicine, 29*(3), 631–654. https://doi.org/10.1080/13548506.2023.2229241

DATAREPORTAL. (2024). *Digital 2024: Global overview report*. https://datareportal.com/reports/digital-2024-global-overview-report

De Micheli, D., Andrade, A. L. M., Reichert, R. A., Pinheiro, B. O., da Silva, E. A., & Lopes, F. M. (2021). *Aspectos comportamentais, neurobiológicos e psicossociais do uso e dependência de drogas*. Editora CRV.

Dieterich, R., Wüllhorst, V., Berghäuser, J., Overmeyer, R., & Endrass, T. (2021). Electrocortical correlates of impaired motor inhibition and outcome processing are related in high binge-watching. *Psychophysiology, 58*(6), e13814. https://doi.org/10.1111/psyp.13814

Ding, K., Shen, Y., Liu, Q., & Li, H. (2023). The effects of digital addiction on brain function and structure of children and adolescents: A scoping review. *Healthcare, 12*(1), 15. https://doi.org/10.3390/healthcare12010015

Diotaiuti, P., Mancone, S., Corrado, S., De Risio, A., Cavicchiolo, E., Girelli, L., & Chirico, A. (2022). Internet addiction in young adults: The role of impulsivity and codependency. *Frontiers in Psychiatry, 13*, 893861. https://doi.org/10.3389/fpsyt.2022.893861

Dragano, N., & Lunau, T. (2020). Technostress at work and mental health: Concepts and research results. *Current Opinion in Psychiatry, 33*(4), 407–413. https://doi.org/10.1097/YCO.0000000000000613

Dresp-Langley, B. (2020). Children's health in the digital age. *International Journal of Environmental Research and Public Health, 17*(9), 3240. https://doi.org/10.3390/ijerph17093240

Elhai, J. D., Yang, H., & Montag, C. (2021). Fear of missing out (FOMO): Overview, theoretical underpinnings, and literature review on relations with severity of negative affectivity and problematic technology use. *Revista brasileira de psiquiatria, 43*(2), 203–209. https://doi.org/10.1590/1516-4446-2020-0870

Goldberg, I. (1995). *Internet addiction disorder un fenomeno sociale in espansione*. In Cinti M. E. (a cura di) (pp. 6–7).

Gonçalves, L. L., Nardi, A. E., Bortolanza, S., King, M., Santos, H., Rodrigues, D., & King, A. L. S. (2022). Evaluation of digital dependence of employees in the organizational environment. *Inquiry: A Journal of Medical Care Organization, Provision and Financing, 59*, 469580211055582. https://doi.org/10.1177/00469580211055582

Griffiths, M. D. (1996). Behavioural addiction: An issue for everybody? *Employee Counselling Today, 8*(3), 19–25. https://doi.org/10.1108/13665629610116872

Gupta, M., & Sharma, A. (2021). Fear of missing out: A brief overview of origin, theoretical underpinnings and relationship with mental health. *World Journal of Clinical Cases, 9*(19), 4881–4889. https://doi.org/10.12998/wjcc.v9.i19.4881

Győrffy, Z., Boros, J., Döbrössy, B., & Girasek, E. (2023). Older adults in the digital health era: Insights on the digital health related knowledge, habits and attitudes of the 65 year and older population. *BMC Geriatrics, 23*(1), 779. https://doi.org/10.1186/s12877-023-04437-5

Hahn, E., Reuter, M., Spinath, F. M., & Montag, C. (2017). Internet addiction and its facets: The role of genetics and the relation to self-directedness. *Addictive Behaviors, 65*, 137–146. https://doi.org/10.1016/j.addbeh.2016.10.018

Han, S. J., Nagduar, S., & Yu, H. J. (2023). Digital addiction and related factors among college students. *Healthcare (Basel, Switzerland), 11*(22), 2943. https://doi.org/10.3390/healthcare11222943

Hartogsohn, I., & Vudka, A. (2023). Technology and addiction: What drugs can teach us about digital media. *Transcultural Psychiatry, 60*(4), 651–661. https://doi.org/10.1177/13634615221105116

Hutton, J. S., Piotrowski, J. T., Bagot, K., Blumberg, F., Canli, T., Chein, J., Christakis, D. A., Grafman, J., Griffin, J. A., Hummer, T., Kuss, D. J., Lerner, M., Marcovitch, S., Paulus, M. P., Perlman, G., Romeo, R., Thomason, M. E., Turel, O., Weinstein, A., … Potenza, M. N. (2024). Digital media and developing brains: Concerns and opportunities. *Current Addiction Reports, 11*(2), 287–298. https://doi.org/10.1007/s40429-024-00545-3

Karakose, T., Yıldırım, B., Tülübaş, T., & Kardas, A. (2023). A comprehensive review on emerging trends in the dynamic evolution of digital addiction and depression. *Frontiers in Psychology, 14*, 1126815. https://doi.org/10.3389/fpsyg.2023.1126815

Ketata, N., Ben Ayed, H., Ben Jmeaa, M., Maamri, H., Baklouti, M., Yaich, S., Jedidi, J., Feki, H., & Damak, J. (2021). Is internet addiction related to self-esteem and insomnia among engineering students? *European Journal of Public Health, 31*(3). https://doi.org/10.1093/eurpub/ckab165.404

Kilian, C., Bröckel, K. L., Overmeyer, R., Dieterich, R., & Endrass, T. (2020). Neural correlates of response inhibition and performance monitoring in binge watching. *International Journal of Psychophysiology: Official Journal of the International Organization of Psychophysiology, 158*, 1–8. https://doi.org/10.1016/j.ijpsycho.2020.09.003

Kim, Y. J., Kim, D. J., & Choi, J. S. (2017). The cognitive dysregulation of internet addiction and its neurobiological correlates. *Frontiers in Bioscience (Elite Edition), 9*(2), 307–320. https://doi.org/10.2741/e804

Kim, H. S., Leslie, R. D., Stewart, S. H., King, D. L., Demetrovics, Z., Andrade, A. L. M., Choi, J. S., Tavares, H., Almeida, B., & Hodgins, D. C. (2023). A scoping review of the association between loot boxes, esports, skin betting, and token wagering with gambling and video gaming behaviors. *Journal of Behavioral Addictions, 12*, 309–351. https://doi.org/10.1556/2006.2023.00013

Kim, S. H., Kim, Y. H., Lee, C.-H., & Lee, Y. (2024). Smartphone usage and overdependence risk among middle-aged and older adults: A cross-sectional study. *BMC Public Health, 24*(1), 413. https://doi.org/10.1186/s12889-024-17873-8

Ko, M., Chi, S. H., Lee, J. H., Suh, S. I., & Lee, M. S. (2023). Altered functional connectivity of the nucleus accumbens and amygdala in cyber addiction: A resting state functional magnetic resonance imaging study. *Clinical Psychopharmacology and Neuroscience: The Official Scientific Journal of the Korean College of Neuropsychopharmacology, 21*(2), 304–312. https://doi.org/10.9758/cpn.2023.21.2.304

Koob, G. F., & Volkow, N. D. (2016). Neurobiology of addiction: A neurocircuitry analysis. *The Lancet Psychiatry, 3*(8), 760–773. https://doi.org/10.1016/S2215-0366(16)00104-8

Kwon, M., Kim, D. J., Cho, H., & Yang, S. (2013). The smartphone addiction scale: Development and validation of a short version for adolescents. *PLoS One, 8*(12), e83558. https://doi.org/10.1371/journal.pone.0083558

Lee, J. H., & Bae, S. M. (2023). The relationship between smartphone use motives, social capital, digital literacy, and life satisfaction in elderly Koreans. *Iranian Journal of Public Health, 52*(12), 2554–2562. https://doi.org/10.18502/ijph.v52i12.14316

Lee, D., Park, J., Namkoong, K., Kim, I. Y., & Jung, Y. C. (2018). Gray matter differences in the anterior cingulate and orbitofrontal cortex of young adults with internet gaming disorder: Surface-based morphometry. *Journal of Behavioral Addictions, 7*(1), 21–30. https://doi.org/10.1556/2006.7.2018.20

Lemmens, J. S., Valkenburg, P. M., & Peter, J. (2009). Development and validation of a game addiction scale for adolescents. *Media Psychology, 12*(1), 77–95.

León Méndez, M., Padrón, I., Fumero, A., & Marrero, R. J. (2024). Effects of internet and smartphone addiction on cognitive control in adolescents and young adults: A systematic review of fMRI studies. *Neuroscience and Biobehavioral Reviews, 159*, 105572. https://doi.org/10.1016/j.neubiorev.2024.105572

Li, H., Luo, M., Duan, B., Kawulia, A., Su, M., & Di, H. (2024). Family socioeconomic status and young children digital addiction: A moderated mediation model. *Frontiers in Psychology, 15*, 1435575. https://doi.org/10.3389/fpsyg.2024.1435575

Liu, J. L., Sun, J. T., Hu, H. L., Wang, H. Y., Kang, Y. X., Chen, T. Q., Chen, Z. H., Shang, Y. X., Li, Y. T., Hu, B., & Liu, R. (2023). Structural and functional neural alterations in internet addiction: A study protocol for systematic review and meta-analysis. *Psychiatry Investigation, 20*(1), 69–74. https://doi.org/10.30773/pi.2021.0383

Marciano, L., Camerini, A. L., & Morese, R. (2021). The developing brain in the digital era: A scoping review of structural and functional correlates of screen time in adolescence. *Frontiers in Psychology, 12*, 671817. https://doi.org/10.3389/fpsyg.2021.671817

Marsh, E., Perez Vallejos, E., & Spence, A. (2024). Overloaded by information or worried about missing out on it: A quantitative study of stress, burnout, and mental health implications in the digital workplace. *SAGE Open, 14*(3). https://doi.org/10.1177/21582440241268830

Martins, G. D. G., Caricati, V. V., Barbugli, B. C., Silva Ribeiro, C. M. D., Lobato, F. B. H., Scatena, A., et al. (2021). The biopsychosocial impact of abusive use of digital media. In *Drugs and human behavior* (pp. 459–468). Springer.

Marzilli, E., Cerniglia, L., Ballarotto, G., & Cimino, S. (2020). Internet addiction among young adult university students: The complex interplay between family functioning, impulsivity, depression, and anxiety. *International Journal of Environmental Research and Public Health, 17*(21), 8231. https://doi.org/10.3390/ijerph17218231

Montag, C., & Becker, B. (2023). Neuroimaging the effects of smartphone (over-)use on brain function and structure—A review on the current state of MRI-based findings and a roadmap for future research. *Psychoradiology, 3*. https://doi.org/10.1093/psyrad/kkad001

Nakayama, H., Ueno, F., Mihara, S., Kitayuguchi, T., & Higuchi, S. (2020). Relationship between problematic internet use and age at initial weekly internet use. *Journal of Behavioral Addictions, 9*(1), 129–139. https://doi.org/10.1556/2006.2020.00009

Niu, X., Gao, X., Zhang, M., Yang, Z., Yu, M., Wang, W., Wei, Y., Cheng, J., Han, S., & Zhang, Y. (2022). Meta-analysis of structural and functional brain alterations in internet gaming disorder. *Frontiers in Psychiatry, 13*, 1029344. https://doi.org/10.3389/fpsyt.2022.1029344

Niu, X., Gao, X., Zhang, M., Dang, J., Sun, J., Lang, Y., Wang, W., Wei, Y., Cheng, J., Han, S., & Zhang, Y. (2023). Static and dynamic changes of intrinsic brain local connectivity in internet gaming disorder. *BMC Psychiatry, 23*(1), 578. https://doi.org/10.1186/s12888-023-05009-y

Notara, V., Vagka, E., Gnardellis, C., & Lagiou, A. (2021). The emerging phenomenon of nomophobia in young adults: A systematic review study. *Addiction & Health, 13*(2), 120–136. https://doi.org/10.22122/ahj.v13i2.309

Oktay, D., & Ozturk, C. (2024). Digital addiction in children and affecting factors. *Children (Basel, Switzerland), 11*(4), 417. https://doi.org/10.3390/children11040417

Oliveira, B. P., Andrade, A. L. M., & De Micheli, D. (2016). Relationship between levels of physical activity and quality of life in drug use in teenagers. *SMAD. Revista eletrônica saúde mental álcool e drogas, 12*(3), 178–187. https://doi.org/10.11606/issn.1806-6976.v12i3p178-187

Ortega, C. A. C., Mariscal, M. A., Boulagouas, W., Herrera, S., Espinosa, J. M., & García-Herrero, S. (2021). Effects of mobile phone use on driving performance: An experimental study of workload and traffic violations. *International Journal of Environmental Research and Public Health, 18*(13), 7101. https://doi.org/10.3390/ijerph18137101

Pan, N., Yang, Y., Du, X., Qi, X., Du, G., Zhang, Y., Li, X., & Zhang, Q. (2018). Brain structures associated with internet addiction tendency in adolescent online game players. *Frontiers in Psychiatry, 9*, 67. https://doi.org/10.3389/fpsyt.2018.00067

Parlak, M. E., Öz, E., Ener, D., Kurt, F., Küçükkelepçe, O., & Kapıcı, Y. (2023). The relationship between digital game addiction and loneliness and social dissatisfaction in adolescents. *Cureus, 15*(2), e34604. https://doi.org/10.7759/cureus.34604

Pereira, H., Fehér, G., Tibold, A., Esgalhado, G., Costa, V., & Monteiro, S. (2021). The impact of internet addiction and job satisfaction on mental health symptoms among a sample of Portuguese workers. *International Journal of Environmental Research and Public Health, 18*(13), 6943. https://doi.org/10.3390/ijerph18136943

Puukko, K., Hietajärvi, L., Maksniemi, E., Alho, K., & Salmela-Aro, K. (2020). Social media use and depressive symptoms—A longitudinal study from early to late adolescence. *International Journal of Environmental Research and Public Health, 17*(16), 5921. https://doi.org/10.3390/ijerph17165921

Qiu, X., Han, X., Wang, Y., Ding, W., Sun, Y., Lei, H., Zhou, Y., & Lin, F. (2022). Reciprocal modulation between cigarette smoking and internet gaming disorder on participation coefficient within functional brain networks. *Brain Imaging and Behavior, 16*(5), 2011–2020. https://doi.org/10.1007/s11682-022-00671-4

Qiu, X., Han, X., Wang, Y., Ding, W., Sun, Y., Lei, H., Zhou, Y., & Lin, F. (2023). Interaction effects between smoking and internet gaming disorder on resting-state functional connectivity of the ventral tegmental area and hippocampus. *Frontiers in Neuroscience, 17*, 1270014. https://doi.org/10.3389/fnins.2023.1270014

Qutishat, M., & Abu Sharour, L. (2019). Relationship between fear of missing out and academic performance among Omani University students: A descriptive correlation study. *Oman Medical Journal, 34*(5), 404–411. https://doi.org/10.5001/omj.2019.75

Ramos, R. F. S., Scatena, A., Kim, H. S., de Oliveira, W. A., & Andrade, A. L. M. (2023). Brazilian digital warriors: Unraveling the nexus of adolescent cyber aggressors, problematic internet & smartphone use, emotional struggles, and parental mediation. *Trends in Psychology*, 1–17. https://doi.org/10.1007/s43076-023-00338-z

Reichert, R. A., Martins, G. D. G., Silva, A. M. B. D., Scatena, A., Barbugli, B. C., Micheli, D. D., & Andrade, A. L. M. (2021a). New forms of addiction: Digital media. In *Psychology of substance abuse* (pp. 43–53). Springer.

Reichert, R. A., Calixto, F., Silva, A. M. B. D., Martins, G. D. G., Barbugli, B. C., Scatena, A., et al. (2021b). Digital games, shopping, sex, and other addictions: Neuropsychological and behavioral correlates. In *Drugs and human behavior* (pp. 443–458). Springer.

Ricci, R. C., Paulo, A. S. C., Freitas, A. K. P. B., Ribeiro, I. C., Pires, L. S. A., Facina, M. E. L., Cabral, M. B., Parduci, N. V., Spegiorin, R. C., Bogado, S. S. G., Chociay Junior, S., Carachesti, T. N., & Larroque, M. M. (2023). Impacts of technology on children's health: A systematic review. *Revista Paulista de Pediatria, 41*, e2020504. https://doi.org/10.1590/1984-0462/2023/41/2020504

Rosenberg, K. P. (Ed.). (2014). *Behavioral addictions: Criteria, evidence, and treatment*. Academic Press.

Rył, A., Tomska, N., Jakubowska, A., Ogrodniczak, A., Palma, J., & Rotter, I. (2024). Genetic aspects of problematic and risky internet use in young men-analysis of ANKK1, DRD2 and NTRK3 gene polymorphism. *Genes, 15*(2), 169. https://doi.org/10.3390/genes15020169

Saikia, A. M., Das, J., Barman, P., & Bharali, M. D. (2019). Internet addiction and its relationships with depression, anxiety, and stress in urban adolescents of Kamrup district, Assam. *Journal of Family & Community Medicine, 26*(2), 108–112. https://doi.org/10.4103/jfcm.JFCM_93_18

Sayılı, U., Vehid, S., & Erginöz, E. (2021). Problematic internet use in Turkish high school students: Prevalence and related factors. *American Journal of Health Behavior, 45*(1), 31–43. https://doi.org/10.5993/AJHB.45.1.3

Shanthi, L., Ashwath, J., Raju, M. K., & Ramalingam, S. (2024). Problematic internet use among adolescent school attendees: A school-based study from Tamil Nadu, India. *Indian Pediatrics, 61*(10), 973–977.

Skinner, B. F. (1938). *The behavior of organisms: An experimental analysis*. Appleton-Century.

Small, G. W., Lee, J., Kaufman, A., Jalil, J., Siddarth, P., Gaddipati, H., Moody, T. D., & Bookheimer, S. Y. (2020). Brain health consequences of digital technology use. *Dialogues in Clinical Neuroscience, 22*(2), 179–187. https://doi.org/10.31887/DCNS.2020.22.2/gsmall

Sun, J. T., Hu, B., Chen, T. Q., Chen, Z. H., Shang, Y. X., Li, Y. T., Wang, R., & Wang, W. (2023). Internet addiction-induced brain structure and function alterations: A systematic review and meta-analysis of voxel-based morphometry and resting-state functional connectivity studies. *Brain Imaging and Behavior, 17*(3), 329–342. https://doi.org/10.1007/s11682-023-00762-w

Thorell, L. B., Burén, J., Ström Wiman, J., Sandberg, D., & Nutley, S. B. (2024). Longitudinal associations between digital media use and ADHD symptoms in children and adolescents: A systematic literature review. *European Child & Adolescent Psychiatry, 33*(8), 2503–2526. https://doi.org/10.1007/s00787-022-02130-3

Truzoli, R., Magistrati, L., Viganò, C., Conte, S., Osborne, L. A., & Reed, P. (2023). Social media users potentially experience different withdrawal symptoms to non-social media users. *International Journal of Mental Health and Addiction, 21*(1), 411–417. https://doi.org/10.1007/s11469-021-00602-2

Tseng, Y. L., Su, Y. K., Chou, W. J., Miyakoshi, M., Tsai, C. S., Li, C. J., Lee, S. Y., & Wang, L. J. (2024). Neural network dynamics and brain oscillations underlying aberrant inhibitory control in internet addiction. IEEE transactions on neural systems and rehabilitation engineering. *IEEE Engineering in Medicine and Biology Society, 32*, 946–955. https://doi.org/10.1109/TNSRE.2024.3363756

von Deneen, K. M., Hussain, H., Waheed, J., Xinwen, W., Yu, D., & Yuan, K. (2022). Comparison of frontostriatal circuits in adolescent nicotine addiction and internet gaming disorder. *Journal of Behavioral Addictions, 11*(1), 26–39. https://doi.org/10.1556/2006.2021.00086

Wang, R., Li, M., Zhao, M., Yu, D., Hu, Y., Wiers, C. E., Wang, G. J., Volkow, N. D., & Yuan, K. (2019). Internet gaming disorder: Deficits in functional and structural connectivity in the ventral tegmental area-Accumbens pathway. *Brain Imaging and Behavior, 13*(4), 1172–1181. https://doi.org/10.1007/s11682-018-9929-6

Wang, D., Liu, X., Chen, K., Gu, C., Zhao, H., Zhang, Y., & Luo, Y. (2024a). Risks and protection: A qualitative study on the factors for internet addiction among elderly residents in Southwest China communities. *BMC Public Health, 24*(1), 531. https://doi.org/10.1186/s12889-024-17980-6

Wang, J. L., Yin, X. Q., Wang, H. Z., King, D. L., & Rost, D. H. (2024b). The longitudinal associations between internet addiction and ADHD symptoms among adolescents. *Journal of Behavioral Addictions, 13*(1), 191–204. https://doi.org/10.1556/2006.2023.00080

Wen, X., Sun, Y., Hu, Y., Yu, D., Zhou, Y., & Yuan, K. (2021). Identification of internet gaming disorder individuals based on ventral tegmental area resting-state functional connectivity. *Brain Imaging and Behavior, 15*(4), 1977–1985. https://doi.org/10.1007/s11682-020-00391-7

Xu, Y., Zeng, K., Dong, L., Zheng, X., & Si, Y. (2023). Understanding older adults' smartphone addiction in the digital age: Empirical evidence from China. *Frontiers in Public Health, 11*, 1136494. https://doi.org/10.3389/fpubh.2023.1136494

Yamada, M., Sekine, M., Tatsuse, T., & Asaka, Y. (2021). Prevalence and associated factors of pathological internet use and online risky behaviors among Japanese elementary school children. *Journal of Epidemiology, 31*(10), 537–544. https://doi.org/10.2188/jea.JE20200214

Yan, X., Gao, W., Yang, J., & Yuan, J. (2022). Emotion regulation choice in internet addiction: Less reappraisal, lower frontal alpha asymmetry. *Clinical EEG and Neuroscience, 53*(4), 278–286. https://doi.org/10.1177/15500594211056433

Yang, H., de Jong, J. W., Tak, Y., Peck, J., Bateup, H. S., & Lammel, S. (2018). Nucleus accumbens subnuclei regulate motivated behavior via direct inhibition and disinhibition of VTA dopamine subpopulations. *Neuron, 97*(2), 434–449.e4. https://doi.org/10.1016/j.neuron.2017.12.022

Yang, J., Fu, X., Liao, X., & Li, Y. (2020). Association of problematic smartphone use with poor sleep quality, depression, and anxiety: A systematic review and meta-analysis. *Psychiatry Research, 284*, 112686. https://doi.org/10.1016/j.psychres.2019.112686

Yao, Y. W., Liu, L., Ma, S. S., Shi, X. H., Zhou, N., Zhang, J. T., & Potenza, M. N. (2017). Functional and structural neural alterations in internet gaming disorder: A systematic review and meta-analysis. *Neuroscience and Biobehavioral Reviews, 83*, 313–324. https://doi.org/10.1016/j.neubiorev.2017.10.029

Young, K. S. (1998). Internet addiction: The emergence of a new clinical disorder. *Cyber Psychology & Behavior, 1*(3), 237–244. https://doi.org/10.1089/cpb.1998.1.237

Zatezalo, N., Erdogan, M., & Green, R. S. (2018). Road traffic injuries and fatalities among drivers distracted by mobile devices. *Journal of Emergencies, Trauma, and Shock, 11*(3), 175–182. https://doi.org/10.4103/JETS.JETS_24_18

Zhou, M., Zhu, W., Sun, X., & Huang, L. (2022). Internet addiction and child physical and mental health: Evidence from panel dataset in China. *Journal of Affective Disorders, 309*, 52–62. https://doi.org/10.1016/j.jad.2022.04.115

Zou, Z., Wang, H., d'Oleire Uquillas, F., Wang, X., Ding, J., & Chen, H. (2017). Definition of substance and non-substance addiction. *Advances in Experimental Eedicine and Biology, 1010*, 21–41. https://doi.org/10.1007/978-981-10-5562-1_2

Chapter 2
Internet and Smartphone Addiction: Characteristics, Impacts, Diagnosis, and Treatment

Fernando Ferreira Semolini, Laura Soares da Silva, Amanda Severo Lins Vitta, Evelin Moreira Freires, and André Luiz Monezi Andrade

Main Characteristics of Internet and Smartphone Addiction

Internet addiction was initially characterized as a disturbance in the impulse control mechanisms associated with behaviors involving technology and the Internet (Griffiths, 1996). Two years later, in 1998, Kimberly Young developed the Internet Addiction Test (IAT), the most widely used tool to assess Internet addiction globally (Moon et al., 2018). The IAT was theoretically grounded in the behavioral addiction criteria of the DSM-IV for Gambling Disorder, which, like Internet addiction, involves impulse control issues not related to chemical substances (Young, 1998). Today, Internet addiction is primarily characterized by excessive and uncontrolled use of the Internet, significantly impairing individuals' well-being and quality of life.

Recent surveys report varying results across studies but generally indicate an average global prevalence of 8.23% for Internet addiction (Meng et al., 2022). Adolescents and university students are the most affected groups, with a study among young students reporting a 12.5% prevalence of Internet addiction (Andrade et al., 2021a) and up to 70% showing moderate levels of dependence (Cruz et al., 2018). Additionally, studies have found that the prevalence of Internet addiction tends to be higher in developed countries, such as a recent survey in Spain, which reported a 33% prevalence among Spanish adolescents (Nogueira-López et al., 2023). Furthermore, research suggests that Internet addiction is on the rise as access to technology becomes more widespread (Pan et al., 2020).

Subsequent research on Internet addiction has sought to understand this behavior through specific methods of accessing the Internet and the digital world. In this

---

F. F. Semolini · L. S. da Silva · A. S. L. Vitta · E. M. Freires · A. L. M. Andrade (✉)
Pontifical Catholic University of Campinas, Campinas, Brazil
e-mail: fernando.fs4@puccampinas.edu.br; laura.ss2@puccampinas.edu.br; amanda.slv@puccampinas.edu.br; evelin.mf@puccampinas.edu.br; andre.andrade@puc-campinas.edu.br

A. L. M. Andrade (ed.), *Digital Addictions*,
https://doi.org/10.1007/978-3-031-87986-9_2

context, smartphone addiction, which is characterized by the compulsive behavior of excessive smartphone use despite the negative consequences of such use (Lin et al., 2014), has been distinguished from Internet addiction and other digital addictions. Smartphones allow individuals to remain continuously connected to the Internet anywhere due to their portability, ease of use, and the vast range of mobile applications available. Consequently, although study results vary, the average prevalence of smartphone addiction is 17.42%, and similar to other digital addictions, it tends to rise as mobile device access becomes more widespread (Meng et al., 2022). Among adolescents, studies have shown that the average daily smartphone usage can reach up to 5 h (Andrade et al., 2023).

Thus, Internet and smartphone addiction are contemporary phenomena with significant implications for research, mainly due to their impact on individuals' physical and mental health and the psychobiological changes resulting from the societal changes brought about by these technologies (Reichert et al., 2021). More recent studies reveal that this compulsive behavior presents various characteristics that can be identified at different levels among Internet users and smartphones. The primary characteristics include constant preoccupation with the Internet and smartphones, an uncontrollable need to check and use the device, excessive use despite negative consequences, difficulty controlling time spent online, withdrawal symptoms when access to the Internet or smartphone is unavailable, and neglect of other important life activities.

About constant preoccupation with the Internet and smartphones, studies suggest that individuals with smartphone addiction may exhibit obsessive behaviors toward their device, frequently thinking about it even in everyday situations unrelated to its use. This excessive concern is often accompanied by increased symptoms of anxiety, as well as the constant feeling of missing out on important information, a phenomenon known as Fear of Missing Out (FoMO) (Guan et al., 2023; Shahidin et al., 2022). As such, FoMO remains a predictor of reduced productivity, fear of negative evaluation, and heightened social anxiety among Internet and smartphone addicts, particularly among younger individuals (Tao et al., 2024).

This preoccupation is closely related to the uncontrollable need to check and use the device, which stems from an almost irresistible impulse to constantly access the Internet or smartphone, even without an apparent justification for the need. This impulsive behavior is most notably observed in repeatedly checking the device, messages, apps, or social media within short periods. Recent studies have identified significant correlations between Internet and smartphone addiction and higher levels of impulsivity (Li et al., 2020; Sánchez-Kuhn et al., 2024).

Despite negative consequences, excessive use occurs when individuals continue to use the Internet or electronic devices even when this leads to harmful outcomes. These consequences include academic difficulties, decreased work performance, interpersonal relationship problems, and compromised physical and mental health (Paterna et al., 2024; Ratan et al., 2021; Shi et al., 2023).

Difficulty controlling time spent online is another central characteristic of Internet and smartphone addiction, mainly characterized by the individual's inability or great difficulty in limiting usage. Studies have shown that individuals with

Internet or smartphone addiction tend to spend more time using these technologies than they initially planned (Rajguru et al., 2024). As a result, this behavior contributes to previously noted issues, such as reducing time available for other essential daily activities. Consequently, neglect of other important life activities is more frequent among Internet and smartphone addicts. This neglect may manifest disregard for personal responsibilities, face-to-face social interactions, hobbies, or leisure activities, as well as neglecting basic bodily needs, such as sleep (Alimoradi et al., 2019; Nikolic et al., 2023).

Finally, withdrawal symptoms when access to the Internet or smartphone is unavailable primarily manifest as increased irritability, anxiety, concentration difficulties, and restlessness when the individual is without their smartphone or Internet connection. In this context, studies focusing on the withdrawal period for individuals who excessively use smartphones and the Internet have observed similarities with withdrawal processes seen in other behavioral and chemical addictions. Specifically, a significant increase has been observed in the scores on the "Smartphone Withdrawal Scale" and "Fear of Missing Out Scale," suggesting a more pronounced presence of withdrawal symptoms, such as inattention, irritability, anxiety, and a compulsion to check the device (Eide et al., 2018).

Impacts of Internet and Smartphone Addiction

Extensive research conducted globally on excessive Internet and smartphone use has identified and assessed how these problematic behaviors adversely affect various aspects of individuals' lives. In this context, significant impacts are observed in personal, professional, and social spheres, as well as in physical and mental health.

About the personal and social lives of individuals who engage in excessive Internet and smartphone use, studies have highlighted potential impacts on interpersonal relationships, social skill deterioration, and a reduction in face-to-face interactions. These factors increase the likelihood of social isolation and neglect of personal responsibilities (Small et al., 2020; Tateno et al., 2019). These social challenges are often exacerbated in individuals with psychiatric conditions such as ADHD (Chou et al., 2017). Additionally, smartphone addiction has been positively correlated with heightened social appearance anxiety, which further contributes to increased isolation and a sense of loneliness (Karaoglan Yilmaz et al., 2024). In this context, compulsive use of these technologies can cause individuals to invest more time in the online world at the expense of real-world interactions, such as spending time with family and engaging in in-person contact with friends. This trend can lead to emotional distancing in relationships, frequently exacerbating social isolation.

In the professional and academic domains, individuals who engage in excessive Internet and smartphone use exhibit declines in both performance and productivity (Guclu et al., 2024). A meta-analysis concluded that higher levels of smartphone overuse were associated with poorer academic performance among students. While these associations were moderated by factors such as age, gender, and education level, aspects of smartphone and Internet addiction, such as increased distraction, reduced self-control, and less study time in favor of electronic devices, were identified as contributors to academic decline (Paterna et al., 2024).

While these factors are significant, the most critical impacts highlighted in research focus on the physical and mental health of Internet and smartphone addicts. Regarding physical health, studies have shown higher rates of sedentary behavior, weight gain, and eating disorders among individuals who use more electronic devices or engage in excessive Internet and smartphone use (Wang et al., 2023). Moreover, other health-related consequences of compulsive behavior include increased eye problems (Mylona et al., 2020), sleep disturbances (Guclu et al., 2024), and problematic substance use (Andrade et al., 2022a; Silveira et al., 2021).

Research linking problematic smartphone and Internet use to sleep disturbances has found a positive correlation between these variables (Lin et al., 2023). These sleep issues and insomnia are closely related to "Bedtime Procrastination," where individuals delay bedtime to stay engaged with electronic devices. The screen brightness interferes with melatonin production, disrupting sleep and, as a result, increasing stress and anxiety symptoms (Geng et al., 2021).

The heightened involvement of this group in risky behaviors should also be considered an indirect factor affecting physical and mental health. In this regard, problematic Internet use has been associated with virtual aggression as a mechanism to escape negative emotions and reality. Research on cyberaggression and cyberbullying has identified a significant prevalence of Internet addiction among perpetrators, suggesting that issues related to excessive Internet use correlate with higher levels of aggression (Ramos et al., 2023; Wang et al., 2024a).

Specifically, in the domain of mental health, excessive Internet and smartphone use can elevate levels of depression, anxiety, stress, low self-esteem, and emotional dysregulation (Andrade et al., 2021b; Wang et al., 2024a; Shahidin et al., 2022). Recent studies indicate that high negative affect and low positive affect, such as depression, anxiety, and stress, along with lower life satisfaction and emotional regulation capacity, are some of the strongest predictors of Internet and smartphone addiction (Andrade et al., 2021a, 2023; Wang et al., 2023).

In this context, anxiety and depression are the most associated psychiatric conditions with smartphone and Internet addiction (Andrade et al., 2022a; Passos et al., 2022). A recent meta-analysis confirmed that depression is positively correlated with Internet addiction, with adolescents addicted to the Internet at higher risk for developing depression (Andrade et al., 2020; Ye et al., 2023). Another study suggests that anxiety may mediate the relationship between Internet addiction and depression (Zhao et al., 2023), while other research indicates that loneliness mediates the link between smartphone addiction and depression (Shi et al., 2023). In this context, both greater depression and higher anxiety in individuals with smartphone addiction were associated with increased suicidal ideation (Noel et al., 2023). Furthermore, research has shown that symptoms of anxiety and depression are particularly prominent during periods of technology withdrawal, with higher levels of restlessness and concentration difficulties being identified (Guo et al., 2023). Associated with withdrawal symptoms, it was also observed that individuals at risk of smartphone addiction with higher self-control exhibited lower levels of depression and anxiety compared to those with low self-control (Geng et al., 2021).

Regarding emotional issues, a recent meta-analysis identified a positive correlation between problematic smartphone use and emotional dysregulation (Shahidin et al., 2022). Studies on this topic also demonstrate that excessive smartphone and Internet use is often employed to cope with daily problems and challenges. In this coping process, escapism and boredom avoidance emerged as significant factors motivating smartphone addiction. Moreover, using devices was shown to be a maladaptive strategy for managing emotional distress (Lin et al., 2023).

Symptoms and Diagnostic Criteria for Internet and Smartphone Addiction

In the early twenty-first century, the China Youth Association for Network Development (CYAND) introduced a standardized method for assessing Internet addiction. Beyond the prerequisite that problematic Internet use must significantly impair an individual's functioning in social or functional contexts, three key criteria for addiction were established: (1) self-actualization, where the Internet serves as a means to achieve things that are difficult to attain in real life; (2) withdrawal symptoms, referring to the discomfort or dysphoria experienced when Internet access is unavailable; and (3) concealing Internet usage, where individuals hide the actual amount of time spent online from family members (CYAND, 2005).

Furthermore, Chinese researchers extensively explored the motivations behind the behaviors leading to Internet addiction and defined the neuropsychological process of addiction through the following stages: (1) primitive impulse, reflecting the innate drive to seek pleasure and avoid discomfort, expressed through the impulse to use the Internet; (2) Internet use, where the primitive impulse is fulfilled; (3) euphoric experience, when the individual feels pleasure and satisfaction due to the effects of Internet use on the central nervous system; (4) repeated use, where the individual continues to use the Internet to seek euphoric experiences, eventually transforming it into a numbing habit; (5) tolerance, when the sensory threshold for euphoria decreases, leading the individual to increase Internet usage to achieve the same level of satisfaction; (6) withdrawal reaction, where psychological and physical symptoms occur during a period of Internet absence, such as emotional distress, insomnia, irritability, anxiety, and dysphoria; (7) passive coping, when accumulated frustrations and emotional distress are suppressed maladaptively, often leading to relapse as a means of escapism through Internet use (Tao et al., 2007).

Building on this model, another study proposed a diagnostic criterion for Internet addiction based on seven symptoms: (1) constant preoccupation with the Internet, (2) withdrawal symptoms, (3) tolerance, (4) lack of control, (5) continued use despite negative consequences, (6) loss of interest in other activities, and (7) use of the Internet as an escape from negative emotions. To establish a diagnosis, at least three of these symptoms must be present, with the constant preoccupation with the Internet and withdrawal symptoms being mandatory (Tao et al., 2010).

However, while DSM-5 does not directly recognize Internet and smartphone addiction as formal disorders, researchers suggest that the diagnostic criteria for these addictions may be similar to those for Internet Gaming Disorder (IGD), as outlined in the DSM-5, sharing several standard features. Similar to the IGD criteria, the DSM-5 includes the following symptoms for Internet and smartphone addiction: (1) excessive preoccupation, (2) withdrawal symptoms, (3) increasing use over time to achieve satisfaction, (4) frustrated attempts to reduce usage time, (5) loss of interest in other activities, (6) continued use despite negative consequences, (7) deception about the time spent online, (8) use as an escape from negative emotions, and (9) impairment in social, academic, or professional functioning. A diagnosis requires the presence of five or more of these symptoms over the past 12 months, evidence of significant impairment in major life areas, and the exclusion of other possible causes for the symptoms presented (APA, 2022; Chadha et al., 2024).

Prevention and Treatment Strategies for Internet and Smartphone Addiction

As cases of Internet and smartphone addiction have steadily increased over the past few decades, it has become essential to develop and promote measures aimed at fostering protective factors against excessive use of these technologies, as well as more effective coping strategies. In this context, key preventive measures explored and studied include education on the risks of excessive use, the establishment of limits, the creation of a healthy family environment, the development of parental strategies, encouragement of physical activity, and the availability of psychological support or counseling (Andrade et al., 2022b; Efrati et al., 2024; Ke et al., 2024; Theopilus et al., 2024).

Education on the risks of excessive use involves interventions designed to educate children and adolescents about appropriate and inappropriate online behaviors while promoting digital skills that facilitate safer and healthier engagement in the digital world. In this context, using smartphones or the Internet to search for information has been negatively correlated with addiction, underscoring the importance of educating users on proper technology use (Jeong & Bae, 2022). Furthermore, studies have shown that this preventive strategy can benefit children by raising awareness about Internet and smartphone use and improving their understanding of associated risks. Interventions that promote online skills have proven more effective than restricting screen time (Theopilus et al., 2024).

Developing parental strategies and establishing limits also play a key role in preventing risky behaviors and Internet and smartphone addiction by reinforcing rules and enhancing parenting skills that help regulate children's and adolescents' technology use (de Oliveira Pinheiro et al., 2022). Risk factors for Internet addiction include low parental involvement, emotional unavailability, and insufficient monitoring of online activities. Adolescents with Internet addiction tend to have less social and parental support and lower levels of parental supervision (Karaer & Akdemir, 2019). A study found that parental strategies—such as communication about smartphone use, consistent parental support, and joint use of devices—can help reduce problematic smartphone use (Efrati et al., 2024). In this context, intervention programs like the "Positive Parenting Program" have shown significant effectiveness in reducing screen time and improving cases involving psychiatric conditions. However, challenges persist, such as parents' difficulty implementing or maintaining such strategies (Theopilus et al., 2024).

Promoting physical activity is a preventive strategy to reduce leisure time spent on online activities. Studies have found a significant negative correlation between physical activity and the development of smartphone addiction, with impacts on self-esteem and self-assessment (Gong et al., 2023; Ke et al., 2024). Other research highlighted how physical activity can reduce the effects of loneliness, a significant risk factor associated with Internet and smartphone addiction (Zhang et al., 2024). Additionally, physical exercise has shown a significant regulatory effect on the relationship between smartphone addiction and sleep quality (Zhu et al., 2024). By shifting children's focus from online activities to real-world experiences, compulsive behaviors related to the Internet and smartphones can be mitigated. Physical activity also positively influences factors indirectly related to digital addiction, such as promoting social interactions, improving physical and motor conditioning, and enhancing executive functions and self-regulation (Theopilus et al., 2024).

When it comes to treatments for Internet and smartphone addiction, Cognitive Behavioral Therapy (CBT), family therapy, and pharmacological treatments stand out (Goslar et al., 2020; Martins et al., 2021; Wang et al., 2024b). A recent meta-analysis aimed at evaluating the efficacy of various treatments for Internet addiction concluded that the most effective treatments involve combining CBT with repetitive Transcranial Magnetic Stimulation (rTMS), followed by treatments combining medications and rTMS combined with electroacupuncture and CBT (Zhu et al., 2023). Another study indicated that the most effective treatment for Internet addiction in children and adolescents was the combination of CBT with pharmacological treatment (Chang et al., 2022). These findings support other research suggesting that combined treatments for Internet and smartphone addiction are more effective than monotherapies (Goslar et al., 2020).

Family therapies are notable for involving the family in the therapeutic process. Family involvement is particularly effective for adolescents, aiming to strengthen family and emotional support, improve family dynamics, and develop coping strategies that engage all family members. Research suggests that the severity of Internet and smartphone addiction significantly decreases in family therapy groups. Additionally, the effectiveness of family therapy increases when combined with other treatments and medications (Wang et al., 2024b).

Finally, in cases where psychiatric conditions accompany Internet and smartphone addiction, pharmacological treatments are essential. In situations where excessive technology use is associated with anxiety, stress, or depression, significant improvements in the reduction of compulsive behaviors have been observed in the short term when psychological treatments are combined with pharmacological interventions (Goslar et al., 2020).

Conclusions

Internet and smartphone addiction is a serious condition that must be effectively addressed. By understanding its characteristics, impacts, symptoms, and diagnostic criteria, it is possible to prevent and treat this addiction consciously and responsibly. Therefore, ongoing investigation into the psychological, physiological, social, and emotional aspects of this phenomenon is essential in order to understand better the spectrum of behaviors and tendencies associated with Internet and smartphone addiction. Future research should carefully examine the criteria and boundaries between frequent and problematic use to avoid the pathologization of common behaviors. Finally, considering the current trend of technological globalization, it is crucial to deepen our understanding of Internet and smartphone addiction, including its characteristics, impacts, symptoms, diagnostic criteria, prevention strategies, and potential treatments.

References

Alimoradi, Z., Lin, C. Y., Broström, A., Bülow, P. H., Bajalan, Z., Griffiths, M. D., Ohayon, M. M., & Pakpour, A. H. (2019). Internet addiction and sleep problems: A systematic review and meta-analysis. *Sleep Medicine Reviews, 47*, 51–61. https://doi.org/10.1016/j.smrv.2019.06.004

American Psychiatric Association (APA). (2022). *DSM-5-TR: Diagnostic and statistical manual of mental disorders* (text revision).

Andrade, A. L. M., Scatena, A., Bedendo, A., Enumo, S. R. F., Dellazzana-Zanon, L. L., Prebianchi, H. B., de Lara Machado, W., & de Micheli, D. (2020). Findings on the relationship between internet addiction and psychological symptoms in Brazilian adults. *International Journal of Psychology: Journal International De Psychologie, 55*(6), 941–950. https://doi.org/10.1002/ijop.12670

Andrade, A. L. M., Scatena, A., Bedendo, A., Enumo, S. R. F., Dellazzana-Zanon, L. L., Prebianchi, H. B., & De Micheli, D. (2021a). Internet addiction among Brazilan students: Prevalence and association with emotional problems. *Universitas Psychologica, 20*, 1–15. https://doi.org/10.11144/Javeriana.upsy20.iabs

Andrade, A. L. M., Enumo, S. R. F., Passos, M. A. Z., Vellozo, E. P., Schoen, T. H., Kulik, M. A., Niskier, S. R., & Vitalle, M. S. S. (2021b). Problematic internet use, emotional problems and quality of life among adolescents. *Psico-USF, 26*, 41–51. https://doi.org/10.1590/1413-82712021260104

Andrade, A. L. M., Passos, M. A. Z., Vellozo, E. P., Schoen, T. H., Kulik, M. A., Niskier, S. R., & Vitalle, M. S. S. (2022a). The contextual factors associated with co-occurring substance and problematic internet use in adolescence: A network approach. *Trends in Psychology, 32*, 1252. https://doi.org/10.1007/s43076-022-00232-0

Andrade, A. L. M., Di Girolamo Martins, G., Scatena, A., Lopes, F. M., de Oliveira, W. A., Kim, H. S., & De Micheli, D. (2022b). The effect of psychosocial interventions for reducing co-occurring symptoms of depression and anxiety in individuals with problematic internet use: A systematic review and meta-analysis. *International Journal of Mental Health and Addiction*, 1–22. https://doi.org/10.1007/s11469-022-00846-6

Andrade, A. L. M., Scatena, A., Bedendo, A., Machado, W. L., Oliveira, W. A., Lopes, F. M., & De Micheli, D. (2023). Excessive internet and smartphone use and emotional problems in students of psychology and psychologists. *Estudos de Psicologia (Campinas), 40*, e210010. https://doi.org/10.1590/1982-0275202340e210010

Chadha, Y., Patil, R., Toshniwal, S., & Sinha, N. (2024). Internet addiction management: A comprehensive review of clinical interventions and modalities. *Cureus, 16*(3), e55466. https://doi.org/10.7759/cureus.55466

Chang, C. H., Chang, Y. C., Yang, L., & Tzang, R. F. (2022). The comparative efficacy of treatments for children and young adults with internet addiction/internet gaming disorder: An updated meta-analysis. *International Journal of Environmental Research and Public Health, 19*(5), 2612. https://doi.org/10.3390/ijerph19052612

China Youth Association for Network Development (CYAND). (2005). *Report of China teenagers' internet addiction information 2005*.

Chou, W. J., Huang, M. F., Chang, Y. P., Chen, Y. M., Hu, H. F., & Yen, C. F. (2017). Social skills deficits and their association with internet addiction and activities in adolescents with attention-deficit/hyperactivity disorder. *Journal of Behavioral Addictions, 6*(1), 42–50. https://doi.org/10.1556/2006.6.2017.005

Cruz, F. A. D., Scatena, A., Andrade, A. L. M., & Micheli, D. (2018). Evaluation of internet addiction and the quality of life of Brazilian adolescents from public and private schools. *Estudos de Psicologia (Campinas), 35*, 193–204. https://doi.org/10.1590/1982-02752018000200008

de Oliveira Pinheiro, B., Monezi Andrade, A. L., Lopes, F. M., Reichert, R. A., de Oliveira, W. A., da Silva, A. M. B., & De Micheli, D. (2022). Association between quality of life and risk behaviors in Brazilian adolescents: An exploratory study. *Journal of Health Psychology, 27*(2), 341–351. https://doi.org/10.1177/1359105320953472

Efrati, Y., Rosenberg, H., & Ophir, Y. (2024). Effective parental strategies against problematic smartphone use among adolescents: A 6-month prospective study. *Addictive Behaviors, 154*, 108024. https://doi.org/10.1016/j.addbeh.2024.108024

Eide, T. A., Aarestad, S. H., Andreassen, C. S., Bilder, R. M., & Pallesen, S. (2018). Smartphone restriction and its effect on subjective withdrawal related scores. *Frontiers in Psychology, 9*, 1444. https://doi.org/10.3389/fpsyg.2018.01444

Geng, Y., Gu, J., Wang, J., & Zhang, R. (2021). Smartphone addiction and depression, anxiety: The role of bedtime procrastination and self-control. *Journal of Affective Disorders, 293*, 415–421. https://doi.org/10.1016/j.jad.2021.06.062

Gong, Y., Yang, H., Bai, X., Wang, Y., & An, J. (2023). The relationship between physical exercise and smartphone addiction among Chinese college students: The mediating effect of core self-evaluation. *Behavioral Sciences (Basel, Switzerland), 13*(8), 647. https://doi.org/10.3390/bs13080647

Goslar, M., Leibetseder, M., Muench, H. M., Hofmann, S. G., & Laireiter, A.-R. (2020). Treatments for internet addiction, sex addiction and compulsive buying: A meta-analysis. *Journal of Behavioral Addictions, 9*(1), 14–43. https://doi.org/10.1556/2006.2020.00005

Griffiths, M. D. (1996). Behavioural addiction: An issue for everybody? *Employee Counselling Today, 8*(3), 19–25. https://doi.org/10.1108/13665629610116872

Guan, J., Ma, W., & Liu, C. (2023). Fear of missing out and problematic smartphone use among Chinese college students: The roles of positive and negative metacognitions about smartphone use and optimism. *PLoS One, 18*(11), e0294505. https://doi.org/10.1371/journal.pone.0294505

Guclu, Y., Guclu, O. A., & Demirci, H. (2024). Relationships between internet addiction, smartphone addiction, sleep quality, and academic performance among high-school students. *Revista Da Associacao Medica Brasileira (1992), 70*(3), e20230868. https://doi.org/10.1590/1806-9282.20230868

Guo, Z., Yang, T., Qiu, R., Qiu, H., Ren, L., Liu, X., Han, Z., & Zhu, X. (2023). Network analysis of the relationships between problematic smartphone use and anxiety, and depression in a sample of Chinese college students. *Frontiers in Psychiatry, 14*, 1097301. https://doi.org/10.3389/fpsyt.2023.1097301

Jeong, J. H., & Bae, S. M. (2022). The relationship between types of smartphone use, digital literacy, and smartphone addiction in the elderly. *Psychiatry Investigation, 19*(10), 832–839. https://doi.org/10.30773/pi.2021.0400

Karaer, Y., & Akdemir, D. (2019). Parenting styles, perceived social support and emotion regulation in adolescents with internet addiction. *Comprehensive Psychiatry, 92*, 22–27. https://doi.org/10.1016/j.comppsych.2019.03.003

Karaoglan Yilmaz, F. G., Ustun, A. B., Zhang, K., & Yilmaz, R. (2024). Smartphone addiction, nomophobia, depression, and social appearance anxiety among college students: A correlational study. *Journal of Rational-Emotive & Cognitive-Behavior Therapy, 42*(2), 305–321. https://doi.org/10.1007/s10942-023-00516-z

Ke, Y., Liu, X., Xu, X., He, B., Wang, J., Zuo, L., Wang, H., & Yang, G. (2024). Self-esteem mediates the relationship between physical activity and smartphone addiction of Chinese college students: A cross-sectional study. *Frontiers in Psychology, 14*, 1256743. https://doi.org/10.3389/fpsyg.2023.1256743

Li, Y., Li, G., Liu, L., & Wu, H. (2020). Correlations between mobile phone addiction and anxiety, depression, impulsivity, and poor sleep quality among college students: A systematic review and meta-analysis. *Journal of Behavioral Addictions, 9*(3), 551–571. https://doi.org/10.1556/2006.2020.00057

Lin, Y. H., Chang, L. R., Lee, Y. H., Tseng, H. W., Kuo, T. B., & Chen, S. H. (2014). Development and validation of the Smartphone Addiction Inventory (SPAI). *PLoS One, 9*(6), e98312. https://doi.org/10.1371/journal.pone.0098312

Lin, C. Y., Ratan, Z. A., & Pakpour, A. H. (2023). Collection of smartphone and internet addiction. *BMC Psychiatry, 23*(1), 427. https://doi.org/10.1186/s12888-023-04915-5

Martins, G. D. G., Caricati, V. V., Barbugli, B. C., da Silva Ribeiro, C. M., Lobato, F. B. H., Scatena, A., Lessa, R. T., De Micheli, D., & Andrade, A. L. M. (2021). The biopsychosocial impact of abusive use of digital media. In D. De Micheli, A. L. M. Andrade, R. A. Reichert, E. A. da Silva, B. O. Pinheiro, & F. M. Lopes (Eds.), *Drugs and human behavior: Biopsychosocial aspects of psychotropic substances use* (pp. 459–468). Springer. https://doi.org/10.1007/978-3-030-62855-0_33

Meng, S. Q., Cheng, J. L., Li, Y. Y., Yang, X. Q., Zheng, J. W., Chang, X. W., Shi, Y., Chen, Y., Lu, L., Sun, Y., Bao, Y. P., & Shi, J. (2022). Global prevalence of digital addiction in general population: A systematic review and meta-analysis. *Clinical Psychology Review, 92*, 102128. https://doi.org/10.1016/j.cpr.2022.102128

Moon, S. J., Hwang, J. S., Kim, J. Y., Shin, A. L., Bae, S. M., & Kim, J. W. (2018). Psychometric properties of the internet addiction test: A systematic review and meta-analysis. *Cyberpsychology, Behavior, and Social Networking, 21*(8), 473–484. https://doi.org/10.1089/cyber.2018.0154

Mylona, I., Deres, E. S., Dere, G. S., Tsinopoulos, I., & Glynatsis, M. (2020). The impact of internet and videogaming addiction on adolescent vision: A review of the literature. *Frontiers in Public Health, 8*, 63. https://doi.org/10.3389/fpubh.2020.00063

Nikolic, A., Bukurov, B., Kocic, I., Vukovic, M., Ladjevic, N., Vrhovac, M., Pavlović, Z., Grujicic, J., Kisic, D., & Sipetic, S. (2023). Smartphone addiction, sleep quality, depression, anxiety, and stress among medical students. *Frontiers in Public Health, 11*, 1252371. https://doi.org/10.3389/fpubh.2023.1252371

Noel, J. K., Sammartino, C. J., Johnson, M., Swanberg, J., & Rosenthal, S. R. (2023). Smartphone addiction and mental illness in Rhode Island young adults. *Rhode Island Medical Journal, 106*(3), 35–41.

Nogueira-López, A., Rial-Boubeta, A., Guadix-García, I., Villanueva-Blasco, V. J., & Billieux, J. (2023). Prevalence of problematic internet use and problematic gaming in Spanish adolescents. *Psychiatry Research, 326*, 115317. https://doi.org/10.1016/j.psychres.2023.115317

Pan, Y. C., Chiu, Y. C., & Lin, Y. H. (2020). Systematic review and meta-analysis of epidemiology of internet addiction. *Neuroscience and Biobehavioral Reviews, 118*, 612–622. https://doi.org/10.1016/j.neubiorev.2020.08.013

Passos, M. A. Z., Vellozo, E. P., Hall, P. R., Andrade, A. L. M., Schoen, T. H., Niskier, S. R., & Vitalle, M. S. S. (2022). Identificação do perfil demográfico, maturação sexual, estado nutricional, saúde comportamental e dependência de internet entre estudantes. *Research, Society and Development, 11*(8), 8. https://doi.org/10.33448/rsd-v11i8.30863

Paterna, A., Alcaraz-Ibáñez, M., Aguilar-Parra, J. M., Salavera, C., Demetrovics, Z., & Griffiths, M. D. (2024). Problematic smartphone use and academic achievement: A systematic review and meta-analysis. *Journal of Behavioral Addictions, 13*(2), 313–326. https://doi.org/10.1556/2006.2024.00014

Rajguru, A. J., Mishra, A. K., Bhargava, R., Sarkar, S., & Balhara, Y. P. S. (2024). Exploring risk factors and determinants: A scoping review of factors associated with nomophobia. *Indian Journal of Psychiatry, 66*(7), 591–602. https://doi.org/10.4103/indianjpsychiatry.indianjpsychiatry_244_24

Ramos, R. F. S., Scatena, A., Kim, H. S., Oliveira, W. A., & Andrade, A. L. M. (2023). Brazilian digital warriors: Unraveling the nexus of adolescent cyber aggressors, problematic internet & smartphone use, emotional struggles, and parental mediation. *Trends in Psychology*. https://doi.org/10.1007/s43076-023-00338-z

Ratan, Z. A., Parrish, A.-M., Zaman, S. B., Alotaibi, M. S., & Hosseinzadeh, H. (2021). Smartphone addiction and associated health outcomes in adult populations: A systematic review. *International Journal of Environmental Research and Public Health, 18*(22), 12257. https://doi.org/10.3390/ijerph182212257

Reichert, R. A., Martins, G. D. G., da Silva, A. M. B., Scatena, A., Barbugli, B. C., De Micheli, D., & Andrade, A. L. M. (2021). New forms of addiction: Digital media. In A. L. M. Andrade, D. De Micheli, E. A. da Silva, F. M. Lopes, B. O. Pinheiro, & R. A. Reichert (Eds.), *Psychology of substance abuse: Psychotherapy, clinical management and social intervention* (pp. 43–53). Springer. https://doi.org/10.1007/978-3-030-62106-3_3

Sánchez-Kuhn, A., Puga, L. J., Flores, P., & Ruiz-Ruano, A. M. (2024). From non-problematic smartphone use to smartphone addiction: Impulsivity-based profiles. Del uso no problemático a la adicción al móvil: Perfiles de impulsividad. *Adicciones, 36*(3), 287–298. https://doi.org/10.20882/adicciones.1847

Shahidin, S. H., Midin, M., Sidi, H., Choy, C. L., Nik Jaafar, N. R., Mohd Salleh Sahimi, H., & Che Roos, N. A. (2022). The relationship between emotion regulation (ER) and problematic smartphone use (PSU): A systematic review and meta-analyses. *International Journal of Environmental Research and Public Health, 19*(23), 15848. https://doi.org/10.3390/ijerph192315848

Shi, X., Wang, A., & Zhu, Y. (2023). Longitudinal associations among smartphone addiction, loneliness, and depressive symptoms in college students: Disentangling between- and within-person associations. *Addictive Behaviors, 142*, 107676. https://doi.org/10.1016/j.addbeh.2023.107676

Silveira, K. M., Assumpção, F., Andrade, A. L. M., De Micheli, D., & Lopes, F. M. (2021). Relação das Dependências Física, Psicológica e Comportamental na Cessação do Tabagismo. *Contextos Clínicos, 14*(2). https://doi.org/10.4013/ctc.2021.142.08

Small, G. W., Lee, J., Kaufman, A., Jalil, J., Siddarth, P., Gaddipati, H., Moody, T. D., & Bookheimer, S. Y. (2020). Brain health consequences of digital technology use. *Dialogues in Clinical Neuroscience, 22*(2), 179–187. https://doi.org/10.31887/DCNS.2020.22.2/gsmall

Tao, R., Ying, L., Yue, X. D., & Hao, X. (2007). *Internet addiction: Exploration and intervention* (p. 12). Shanghai People's Press.

Tao, R., Huang, X., Wang, J., Zhang, H., Zhang, Y., & Li, M. (2010). Proposed diagnostic criteria for internet addiction. *Addiction (Abingdon, England), 105*(3), 556–564. https://doi.org/10.1111/j.1360-0443.2009.02828.x

Tao, Y., Tang, Q., Wang, S., Zou, X., Ma, Z., Zhang, L., Liu, G., & Liu, X. (2024). The impact of long-term online learning on social anxiety and problematic smartphone use symptoms among secondary school students with different levels of fear of missing out: Evidence from a symptom network and longitudinal panel network analysis. *Journal of Behavioral Addictions, 13*(1), 102–119. https://doi.org/10.1556/2006.2023.00081

Tateno, M., Teo, A. R., Ukai, W., Kanazawa, J., Katsuki, R., Kubo, H., & Kato, T. A. (2019). Internet addiction, smartphone addiction, and hikikomori trait in Japanese young adult: Social isolation and social network. *Frontiers in Psychiatry, 10*, 455. https://doi.org/10.3389/fpsyt.2019.00455

Theopilus, Y., Al Mahmud, A., Davis, H., & Octavia, J. R. (2024). Preventive interventions for internet addiction in young children: Systematic review. *JMIR Mental Health, 11*, e56896. https://doi.org/10.2196/56896

Wang, J., Hao, Q.-H., Peng, W., Tu, Y., Zhang, L., & Zhu, T.-M. (2023). Relationship between smartphone addiction and eating disorders and lifestyle among Chinese college students. *Frontiers in Public Health, 11*, 1111477. https://doi.org/10.3389/fpubh.2023.1111477

Wang, J., Chen, J., Wang, P., Zhang, S., Li, Q., Lu, S., & Xiao, J. (2024a). Identifying internet addiction profiles among adolescents using latent profile analysis: Relations to aggression, depression, and anxiety. *Journal of Affective Disorders, 359*, 78–85. https://doi.org/10.1016/j.jad.2024.05.082

Wang, H., Li, X., Lok, G. K. I., Meng, C., Tan, Y., Lee, U. M., Lei, L. S. M., & Chan, N. (2024b). Family-based therapy for internet addiction among adolescents and young adults: A meta-analysis. *Journal of Behavioral Addictions, 13*(2), 295–312. https://doi.org/10.1556/2006.2024.00015

Ye, X.-L., Zhang, W., & Zhao, F.-F. (2023). Depression and internet addiction among adolescents: A meta-analysis. *Psychiatry Research, 326*, 115311. https://doi.org/10.1016/j.psychres.2023.115311

Young, K. S. (1998). Internet addiction: The emergence of new ceical disorder. *Cyberpsychology & Behavior, 1*, 237–244. https://doi.org/10.1089/cpb.1998.1.237

Zhang, R., Jiang, Q., Cheng, M., & Rhim, Y. T. (2024). The effect of smartphone addiction on adolescent health: The moderating effect of leisure physical activities. *Psicologia, reflexao e critica : Revista semestral do Departamento de Psicologia da UFRGS, 37*(1), 23. https://doi.org/10.1186/s41155-024-00308-z

Zhao, M., Huang, Y., Wang, J., Feng, J., & Zhou, B. (2023). Internet addiction and depression among Chinese adolescents: Anxiety as a mediator and social support as a moderator. *Psychology, Health & Medicine, 28*(8), 2315–2328. https://doi.org/10.1080/13548506.2023.2224041

Zhu, Y., Chen, H., Li, J., Mei, X., & Wang, W. (2023). Effects of different interventions on internet addiction: A systematic review and network meta-analysis. *BMC Psychiatry, 23*(1), 921. https://doi.org/10.1186/s12888-023-05400-9

Zhu, W., Liu, J., Lou, H., Mu, F., & Li, B. (2024). Influence of smartphone addiction on sleep quality of college students: The regulatory effect of physical exercise behavior. *PLoS One, 19*(7), e0307162. https://doi.org/10.1371/journal.pone.0307162

Chapter 3
Binge-Watching and the Digital Era: A New Pattern of Media Consumption

Laura Soares da Silva, Evelin Moreira Freires, Amanda Severo Lins Vitta, Adriana Scatena, Fernando Ferreira Semolini, Denise De Micheli, and André Luiz Monezi Andrade

Streaming and the Internet: Redefining Media Consumption

The pursuit of entertainment through media is a defining feature of the digital era, evolving alongside technological advancements. In the twentieth century, television underwent a transformative process, from its creation in the 1920s to its widespread distribution and popularization. It became a standard household fixture by the end of the century and served as a crucial tool for consumption and communication (Lesage & Natale, 2019). However, with the advent of the Internet, significant changes in television content consumption have occurred, mainly due to the emergence of streaming services like Netflix, Amazon Prime Video, and Disney+ (Lull, 2021).

These platforms have revolutionized access to and consumption of films and series previously dictated by television programming schedules. Traditionally, channels with programming rights to specific series released new weekly or monthly episodes at predetermined dates and times (Viens & Farrar, 2021). With the rise of streaming services, these media acquired a new consumption dynamic, simultaneously offering entire seasons and episodes on the platforms (Pittman & Sheehan, 2015).

This shift allows consumers to watch content on demand without purchasing physical media like DVDs and through various devices such as smartphones, tablets, and computers, free from temporal and geographical constraints (Ahmed,

L. S. da Silva · E. M. Freires · A. S. L. Vitta · F. F. Semolini · A. L. M. Andrade (✉)
Pontifical Catholic University of Campinas, Campinas, Brazil
e-mail: laura.ss2@puccampinas.edu.br; evelin.mf@puccampinas.edu.br; amanda.slv@puccampinas.edu.br; fernando.fs4@puccampinas.edu.br; andre.andrade@puc-campinas.edu.br

A. Scatena · D. De Micheli
Universidade Federal de São Paulo, São Paulo, Brazil

A. L. M. Andrade (ed.), *Digital Addictions*,
https://doi.org/10.1007/978-3-031-87986-9_3

2019). These developments have given rise to new phenomena, such as "binge-watching" (BW), characterized by the consecutive and continuous viewing of series episodes. This behavior has become increasingly common, normalized, and even encouraged by the platforms themselves (Tukachinsky & Eyal, 2018).

Understanding Binge-Watching: A Conceptual Perspective

Many authors consider the time spent watching an additional criterion alongside the number of episodes. Many authors specify that consumption must occur "in one sitting" (Starosta & Izydorczyk, 2020), but other variations are described in the literature. This addition arises from the risk of limiting the concept to the number of episodes, as durations can vary significantly between series. Thus, discrepancies in total viewing time may occur, as there is a notable difference between watching three 20-min episodes versus three 60-min episodes. Therefore, the variation in episode durations complicates the standardization of this phenomenon's definition (Viens & Farrar, 2021).

To address this challenge, some researchers have developed instruments to assess the occurrence of BW, aiming to reduce measurement difficulties. The General Binge Watching Scale (GBWS) (Viens & Farrar, 2021), for example, aims to establish an overall assessment of BW behavior, classifying individuals as "binge-watchers" or not. Other scales, such as the Problematic Series Watching Scale (PSWS) (Orosz et al., 2016), Binge-Watching Engagement and Symptoms (BWESQ) (Flayelle et al., 2019a), Questionnaire of Excessive Binge-Watching Behaviors (Starosta et al., 2019), and Binge-Watching Addiction Questionnaire (BWAQ) (Forte et al., 2021), seek to assess excessive and problematic BW practices.

In general, BW is described by some authors as a phenomenon that manifests in various forms, depending on the viewer's consumption pattern, which can be more active or passive (Steiner & Xu, 2018). Active consumption involves more significant attention to the series content, planning viewing sessions, increased social interactions stemming from the series content, and a pleasurable experience (Flayelle et al., 2020; Pittman & Steiner, 2021). Passive consumption is characterized by automaticity and loss of time awareness while watching, as well as greater isolation, lower attentional focus (often associated with the use of a second screen), excessive consumption, and significant relationships with mental health problems (Pittman & Steiner, 2021; Starosta & Izydorczyk, 2020).

Beyond conceptual issues, BW has been extensively researched in various aspects, such as the motivations behind this form of consumption, dependency risks, health-related issues, and even personality traits (Alimoradi et al., 2022; Flayelle et al., 2020; Merikivi et al., 2018). Understanding all these dimensions of such a recent phenomenon is crucial, as it represents a facet of a new consumption pattern in contemporary society (Juli et al., 2020) (Table 3.1).

Table 3.1 Description of different quantitative definitions of binge-watching based on number of episodes and time

Criterion	Quantity	Authors
Number of episodes	Multiple episodes	Conlin et al. (2016), Exelmans and Van den Bulck (2017), Granow et al. (2018), Shim et al. (2018)
Number of episodes	One or more episodes	Ahmed (2017), Flayelle et al. (2019a), Merikivi et al. (2018), Shim and Kim (2018)
Number of episodes	Two or more episodes	Panda and Pandey (2017), Walton-Pattison et al. (2018), Spruance et al. (2017), Sung et al. (2018), Starosta et al. (2019)
Number of episodes	Three or more episodes	Horvath et al. (2017), Riddle et al. (2018), Rubenking and Bracken (2018), Rubenking et al. (2018), Pittman and Steiner (2019)
Number of episodes	One entire season	Shim et al. (2018). Tefertiller and Maxwell (2018)
Consumption time	At once/In one session	Conlin et al. (2016), Ahmed (2017), Exelmans and Van den Bulck (2017)
Consumption time	At least 1 h	Panda and Pandey (2017)
Consumption time	In 1 day	Starosta et al. (2019)
Consumption time	Within a few days	Shim et al. (2018)
Consumption time	Within a week	Pittman and Steiner (2019)

Why We Binge-Watch: Emotional and Social Factors

The reasons for binge-watching multiple series episodes are extensively explored in the literature. Some authors highlight emotional aspects, while others point to simply enjoying immersing in a storyline (Castro et al., 2021). "Hedonic motivation" is directly linked to the pursuit of gratifying experiences that elicit positive emotions (Flayelle et al., 2019b). This aligns with the Uses and Gratifications Theory (U&G), which posits that viewers have psychological needs that media consumption can satisfy, triggering sensations of pleasure (Elliott & Quattlebaum, 1979; Panda & Pandey, 2017).

In addition to positive gratifications, negative gratifications are cited as motivations for BW behavior (Vaterlaus et al., 2018). In this context, series consumption can serve as a strategy for avoiding and escaping negative emotions, acting as escapism (Flayelle et al., 2019a). However, BW sessions motivated by this are more frequently associated with losing control over viewing time (Panda & Pandey, 2017). Another motivation frequently reported is the social benefits derived from BW behavior, as knowledge of popular series facilitates participation in conversations and discussions (Starosta et al., 2019). By engaging in and understanding common interests, individuals experience a sense of belonging and the opportunity to interact more with others, comment on social media posts about the show, and more (Umesh & Bose, 2019).

This motivation can be explained by the Fear of Missing Out (FOMO), which refers to the anxiety of not participating in enjoyable events that others are experiencing (Holte, 2023; Przybylski et al., 2013). FOMO drives a need to engage with trending sociocultural items, primarily due to the desire to maintain a social repertoire that enables interpersonal connections fueled by social media (Gupta & Sharma, 2021). Anghelcev et al. (2020) found higher levels of FOMO in people who binge-watched four or more times per week. Additionally, according to U&G Theory, social interactions stemming from series consumption also serve as an element of gratification (Ramayan et al., 2018).

Moreover, some research points to emotional involvement with the plot as a significant motivator for the desire to continue watching episodes without breaks, considering immersion in the content and narrative (Panda & Pandey, 2017). This is related to "flow," characterized by deep attentional engagement in an activity driven by pleasure, which alters the perception of time spent (Hoffman & Novak, 1996). Flow is frequently reported in suspense and drama genres, which generates a desire to uncover subsequent developments (Rubenking et al., 2018).

These motivations can also be influenced by advertising and strategic elements, mainly by the platforms themselves, which create a virtual environment conducive to successive episode consumption (Song et al., 2022). An example is the autoplay functionality, allowing viewers to continue watching without physical effort (Godinho de Matos & Ferreira, 2020). Additionally, releasing new series seasons at specific intervals creates urgency among viewers to access the storyline's development, amplified by social media marketing campaigns (Schweidel & Moe, 2016).

Finally, concerning sociocultural issues, trending titles become part of socially relevant discussions, especially on social media, and are debated among different groups (Anghelcev et al., 2020). An example is the creation of fan pages that produce content about specific programs where people can discuss and comment on the plot and character development (Steiner & Xu, 2018). Thus, the social aspect of BW is evident, as consumption fosters connections with others. At the same time, interaction with networks generates a desire for consumption, creating a sense of belonging and cultural participation (Starosta & Izydorczyk, 2020).

Emotional Influences on Binge-Watching

Beyond mental health issues, the literature explores the relationship between binge-watching (BW) behavior and emotional traits such as impulsivity and emotional regulation. An individual's reactivity to their emotions and ability to self-regulate play crucial roles in their behavior (Naragon-Gainey et al., 2017). Digital media and technology tools have been identified as effective strategies for mediating emotional regulation by providing instant gratifications and positive responses (Verma et al., 2023).

BW, often associated with the pursuit of pleasure, is seen by many consumers as an activity that promotes relaxation, relief, and distraction from negative emotional states (Vaterlaus et al., 2018). However, emotional regulation difficulties, characterized by mood swings and a lack of resources to manage unpleasant emotions, are regularly cited as predictors of BW behavior (Starosta et al., 2021). Moreover, individuals who use series consumption as a self-regulation tool tend to engage in it more frequently and intensely, leading to a loss of control over the time and number of episodes watched and patterns of Internet dependency (Flayelle et al., 2019b).

Impulsivity, the tendency to act without prior planning and without considering potential consequences, is directly related to compulsive behaviors (Grant & Chamberlain, 2014; Kim et al., 2023; Tóth-Király et al., 2017). In this context, impulsivity is prevalent among individuals who exhibit intense and excessive media use (such as gaming, social media, movies, and series) as a risk factor for technology addiction (Lopes et al., 2022; Shin et al., 2020). Regarding BW, impulsivity is linked to unplanned viewing sessions and more problematic manifestations, such as loss of control and neglect of responsibilities (Andrade et al., 2020b; Riddle et al., 2018).

These two emotional characteristics are also interrelated, as individuals with emotional regulation difficulties are prone to impulsive actions to alleviate adverse effects (Panek, 2014). These issues significantly increase the risk of problematic social media use and BW, considering this behavior's potential maintenance and intensification through negative reinforcement, i.e., the interruption of the individual's focus on their negative thoughts and emotions (Flayelle et al., 2022). In this sense, the lack of self-regulation tools may render BW a maladaptive coping strategy, as it reduces the individual's contact with their effects (Starosta et al., 2021).

Binge-Watching: A Mental Health Issue?

With advancements in technology and the increasing use of the Internet and digital media, the literature indicates negative impacts on individuals' mental and physical health and even the risk of developing behavioral addictions (Andrade et al., 2020a, 2021a, 2021b, 2022a, 2022b, 2023; Chen et al., 2023; Martins et al., 2021; Spritzer et al., 2022; Yamauchi et al., 2019). This is due to the activation of the Brain Reward System (BRS) by media, a central nervous system area responsible for sensations of pleasure and motivation (Moraes et al., 2022; Reichert et al., 2021a, 2021b, 2021c). These responses are triggered by the neurotransmitter dopamine, which activates different areas through dopaminergic pathways (Baik, 2020; De Micheli et al., 2016, 2021; Koob & Volkow, 2016; Lopes et al., 2020).

However, recurrent activation of the BRS through repetitive activity can lead to neurobiological changes, conditioning individuals to seek the reinforcing behavior or substance (Uhl et al., 2019). This can result in excessive use, tolerance, social impairment, and loss of control over consumption (Antons et al., 2020). These adverse outcomes occur because the brain adapts to dopamine levels by reducing the number of neurotransmitter receptors, leading to a need for increasing use. This process underlies both substance use disorders and behavioral dependencies (Méndez-Díaz et al., 2010). An example of this imminent risk related to technology use is the inclusion of Internet Gaming Disorder in the Diagnostic and Statistical Manual of Mental Disorders – Revised Edition, which establishes online gaming dependence as a potential diagnostic category (APA, 2022).

Regarding BW, some authors also highlight the risk of this behavior becoming a dependency. A study comparing a control group and a BW group using an electroencephalogram found decreased inhibitory control and lower prefrontal cortex activation, responsible for evaluating consequences. Although this research is the only one using neurological tools, excessive BW is widely reported in systematic reviews as a behavioral dependency risk with adverse effects on mental, physical, and social health (Forte et al., 2021; Riddle et al., 2018; Starosta & Izydorczyk, 2020).

Beyond addiction issues, BW is also frequently associated with mental health problems such as anxiety, depression, stress, and loneliness (Alimoradi et al., 2022). Regarding depression, significant numbers of individuals with this disorder frequently engage in BW (Ahmed, 2017; Raza et al., 2021; Steins-Loeber et al., 2020). Hypotheses to explain this relationship suggest that individuals seek distracting media elements to avoid contact with negative emotions and depressive symptoms (Ahmed, 2017). Additionally, these individuals often exhibit more behavioral problems related to procrastination and social isolation (Steins-Loeber et al., 2020).

Regarding the relationship between BW and anxiety, it is proposed that series consumption can serve as a form of symptom relief and, primarily, as a tool for obtaining instant gratification (Rubenking & Bracken, 2018). However, anxiety can also be a predictor of frequent BW behavior, particularly regarding the loss of control over the number of episodes watched to quickly uncover narrative developments (Starosta et al., 2021). Furthermore, some studies have found an association between BW and feelings of loneliness, especially among individuals who watch long sessions alone (Ahmed, 2017; Alimoradi et al., 2022; Raza et al., 2021).

Conclusions

The evolution and popularization of technology have transformed contemporary society's daily life, accelerating and enhancing new forms of consumption through the ease and accessibility of a wide variety of digital content. Amid this new pattern of excessive media consumption, manifesting in various ways (online gaming addiction, smartphone dependency, online shopping compulsion, etc.), binge-watching (BW) has become increasingly common. This behavior is facilitated and encouraged not only by streaming platforms themselves but also by sociocultural factors that elevate trending series to cultural phenomena and recurring topics, a process amplified by social media and advertising content.

Therefore, it is crucial to investigate this dynamic's social and emotional aspects, particularly to identify the different facets of its manifestation. Regarding the inference of BW as a potential behavioral dependency, more research is needed to focus on this phenomenon's problematic and compulsive expression to establish thresholds that reduce the risk of pathologizing a typical behavior. Given the current trend of intense media consumption in the society, understanding BW and other phenomena related to excessive technology use enables the identification of risk factors and the development of intervention and prevention strategies.

References

Ahmed, A. (2017). A new era of TV watching behavior: Binge-watching and its psychological effects. *Media Watch, 8*(2), 192–207. https://doi.org/10.15655/mw/2017/v8i2/49006

Ahmed, A. (2019). *Marathon TV watching among emiratis in the interactive media environment* (p. 27). Arab Media & Society. https://www.arabmediasociety.com/marathon-tv-watching-among-emiratis-in-the-interactive-media-environment/

Alimoradi, Z., Jafari, E., Potenza, M. N., Lin, C.-Y., Wu, C.-Y., & Pakpour, A. H. (2022). Binge-watching and mental health problems: A systematic review and meta-analysis. *International Journal of Environmental Research and Public Health, 19*(15), 9707. https://doi.org/10.3390/ijerph19159707

American Psychiatric Association [APA]. (2022). *Diagnostic and statistical manual of mental disorders* (5th ed., text revision). American Psychiatric Association.

Andrade, A. L. M., Scatena, A., Bedendo, A., Enumo, S. R. F., Dellazzana-Zanon, L. L., Prebianchi, H. B., Macgado, W. L., et al. (2020a). Findings on the relationship between internet addiction and psychological symptoms in Brazilian adults. *International Journal of Psychology, 55*(6), 941–950. https://doi.org/10.1002/ijop.12670

Andrade, A. L. M., Scatena, A., Martins, G. D. G., de Oliveira Pinheiro, B., da Silva, A. B., Enes, C. C., Oliveira, W. A., et al. (2020b). Validation of Smartphone Addiction Scale-Short version (SAS-SV) in Brazilian adolescents. *Addictive Behaviors, 110*, 106540. https://doi.org/10.1016/j.addbeh.2020.106540

Andrade, A. L. M., Kim, D. J., Scatena, A., Enes, C. C., Enumo, S. R. F., & De Micheli, D. (2021a). Validity and reliability of the Brazilian version of the Smartphone Addiction Scale-Long version (SAS-LV). *Trends in Psychology, 29*(2), 302–319. https://doi.org/10.1007/s43076-020-00046-y

Andrade, A. L. M., Scatena, A., Bedendo, A., Enumo, S. R. F., Dellazzana-Zanon, L. L., Prebianchi, H. B., & De Micheli, D. (2021b). Internet addiction among Brazilian students: Prevalence and association with emotional problems. *Universitas Psychologica, 20*, 1–15. https://doi.org/10.11144/Javeriana.upsy20.iabs

Andrade, A. L. M., Passos, M. A. Z., Vellozo, E. P., Schoen, T. H., Kulik, M. A., Niskier, S. R., & de Souza Vitalle, M. S. (2022a). The contextual factors associated with co-occurring substance and problematic internet use in adolescence: A network approach. *Trends in Psychology*, 1–16. https://doi.org/10.1007/s43076-022-00232-0

Andrade, A. L. M., Scatena, A., de Oliveira Pinheiro, B., de Oliveira, W. A., Lopes, F. M., & De Micheli, D. (2022b). Psychometric properties of the Smartphone Addiction Inventory (SPAI-BR) in Brazilian adolescents. *International Journal of Mental Health and Addiction, 20*(5), 2690–2705. https://doi.org/10.1007/s11469-021-00542-x

Andrade, A. L. M., Spritzer, D. T., Scatena, A., Pinheiro, B. O., da Silva, G. T., Kim, H. S., Breda, V., de Oliveira, W. A., & De Micheli, D. (2023). Psychometric properties of the Smartphone

Addiction Inventory-Short form (SPAI-SF) in Brazilian adolescents. *Psychiatry Research, 319*, 115001. https://doi.org/10.1016/j.psychres.2022.115001

Anghelcev, G., Sar, S., Martin, J., & Moultrie, J. L. (2020). Is heavy binge-watching a socially driven behaviour? Exploring differences between heavy, regular and non-binge-watchers. *Journal of Digital Media & Policy, 11*(3). https://doi.org/10.1386/jdmp_00026_1

Antons, S., Brand, M., & Potenza, M. N. (2020). Neurobiology of cue-reactivity, craving, and inhibitory control in non-substance addictive behaviors. *Journal of the Neurological Sciences, 415*, 116952. https://doi.org/10.1016/j.jns.2020.116952

Baik, J. H. (2020). Stress and the dopaminergic reward system. *Experimental & Molecular Medicine, 52*(12), 1879–1890. https://doi.org/10.1038/s12276-020-00532-4

Castro, D., Rigby, J. M., Cabral, D., & Nisi, V. (2021). The binge-watcher's journey: Investigating motivations, contexts, and affective states surrounding Netflix viewing. *Convergence, 27*(1), 3–20. https://doi.org/10.1177/1354856519890856

Chen, H., Dong, G., & Li, K. (2023). Overview on brain function enhancement of internet addicts through exercise intervention: Based on reward-execution decision cycle. *Frontiers in Psychiatry, 14*, 1094583. https://doi.org/10.3389/fpsyt.2023.1094583

Conlin, L., Billings, A. C., & Averset, L. (2016). Time-shifting vs. appointment viewing: The role of fear of missing out within TV consumption behaviors. *Communications Society, 29*(4), 151–164. https://doi.org/10.15581/003.29.4.151-164

De Micheli, D., Andrade, A. L. M., Silva, E. A., & Souza-Formigoni, M. L. O. (2016). *Drug abuse in adolescence* (1st ed.). Springer. https://doi.org/10.1007/978-3-319-17795-3

De Micheli, D., Andrade, A. L. M., Reichert, R. A., Pinheiro, B. O., da Silva, E. A., & Lopes, F. M. (2021). *Aspectos comportamentais, neurobiológicos e psicossociais do uso e dependência de drogas*. Editora CRV.

Elliott, W. R., & Quattlebaum, C. P. (1979). Similarities in patterns of media use: A cluster analysis of media gratifications. *Western Journal of Speech Communication, 43*(1), 61–72. https://doi.org/10.1080/10570317909373954

Exelmans, L., & Van den Bulck, J. (2017). Binge viewing, sleep, and the role of pre-sleep arousal. *Journal of Clinical Sleep Medicine, 13*(8), 1001–1008. https://doi.org/10.5664/jcsm.6704

Flayelle, M., Canale, N., Vögele, C., Karila, L., Maurage, P., & Billieux, J. (2019a). Assessing binge-watching behaviors: Development and validation of the "Watching TV Series Motives" and "Binge-watching Engagement and Symptoms" questionnaires. *Computers in Human Behavior, 90*, 26–36. https://doi.org/10.1016/j.chb.2018.08.022

Flayelle, M., Maurage, P., Karila, L., Vögele, C., & Billieux, J. (2019b). Overcoming the unitary exploration of binge-watching: A cluster analytical approach. *Journal of Behavioral Addictions, 8*(3), 586–602. https://doi.org/10.1556/2006.8.2019.53

Flayelle, M., Maurage, P., Di Lorenzo, K. R., et al. (2020). Binge-watching: What do we know so far? A first systematic review of the evidence. *Current Addiction Reports, 7*, 44–60. https://doi.org/10.1007/s40429-020-00299-8

Flayelle, M., Elhai, J., Maurage, P., Vögele, C., Brevers, D., Baggio, S., & Billieux, J. (2022). Identifying the psychological processes delineating non-harmful from problematic binge-watching: A machine learning analytical approach. *Telematics and Informatics, 74*, 101880. https://doi.org/10.1016/j.tele.2022.101880

Forte, G., Favieri, F., Tedeschi, D., & Casagrande, M. (2021). Binge-watching: Development and validation of the Binge-Watching Addiction Questionnaire. *Behavioral Sciences, 11*(2), 27. https://doi.org/10.3390/bs11020027

Godinho de Matos, M., & Ferreira, P. (2020). The effect of binge-watching on the subscription of video on demand: Results from randomized experiments. *Information Systems Research, 31*(4). https://doi.org/10.1287/isre.2020.0948

Granow, V., Reinecke, L., & Ziegele, M. (2018). Binge-watching & psychological wellbeing: Media use between lack of control and perceived autonomy. *Community Research Report, 35*, 392–401. https://doi.org/10.1080/08824096.2018.1525347

Grant, J. E., & Chamberlain, S. R. (2014). Impulsive action and impulsive choice across substance and behavioral addictions: Cause or consequence? *Addictive Behaviors, 39*(11), 1632–1639. https://doi.org/10.1016/j.addbeh.2014.04.022

Gupta, M., & Sharma, A. (2021). Fear of missing out: A brief overview of origin, theoretical underpinnings and relationship with mental health. *World Journal of Clinical Cases, 9*(19), 4881–4889. https://doi.org/10.12998/wjcc.v9.i19.4881

Hoffman, D. L., & Novak, T. P. (1996). Marketing in hypermedia computer-mediated environments: Conceptual foundations. *Journal of Marketing, 60*(3), 50. https://doi.org/10.2307/1251841

Holte, A. J. (2023). The State Fear of Missing Out Inventory: Development and validation. *Telematics and Informatics Reports, 10*, 100055. https://doi.org/10.1016/j.teler.2023.100055

Horvath, J. C., Horton, A. J., Lodge, J. M., & Hattie, J. A. (2017). The impact of binge watching on memory and perceived comprehension. *First Monday, 22*(9). https://doi.org/10.5210/fm.v22i9.7729

Juli, G., Juli, R., & Juli, L. (2020). Is internet changing our mind? *Psychiatria Danubina, 32*(1), 79–82. https://pubmed.ncbi.nlm.nih.gov/32890368/

Kim, H. S., Leslie, R. D., Stewart, S. H., King, D. L., Demetrovics, Z., Andrade, A. L. M., Choi, J. S., Tavares, H., Almeida, B., & Hodgins, D. C. (2023). A scoping review of the association between loot boxes, esports, skin betting, and token wagering with gambling and video gaming behaviors. *Journal of Behavioral Addictions, 12*, 309–351. https://doi.org/10.1556/2006.2023.00013

Koob, G. F., & Volkow, N. D. (2016). Neurobiology of addiction: A neurocircuitry analysis. *The Lancet Psychiatry, 3*(8), 760–773. https://doi.org/10.1016/s2215-0366(16)00104-8

Lesage, F., & Natale, S. (2019). Rethinking the distinctions between old and new media: Introduction. *Convergence: The International Journal of Research into New Media Technologies, 25*, 135485651986336. https://doi.org/10.1177/1354856519863364

Lopes, F. M., Dias, N. M., Mendonça, B. T., Coelho, D. M. V., Andrade, A. L. M., & Micheli, D. D. (2020). What do we know about neurosciences? Concepts and misunderstandings between the general public and between educators. *Revista Psicopedagogia, 37*(113), 129–143. https://doi.org/10.5935/0103-8486.20200011

Lopes, F. M., Coelho, D. M. V., Andrade, A. L. M., da Silva, A. M. B., de Carvalho, C. F., & De Micheli, D. (2022). Differences in attitudes and perceptions between educators with or without knowledge in neuroscience. *Trends in Psychology, 30*, 1–16. https://doi.org/10.1007/s43076-022-00169-4

Lull, J. (2021). Living with television and the internet. *New Media & Society, 23*(7), 1850–1862. https://doi.org/10.1177/14614448211019322

Martins, G. D. G., Caricati, V. V., Barbugli, B. C., Silva Ribeiro, C. M. D., Lobato, F. B. H., Scatena, A., et al. (2021). The biopsychosocial impact of abusive use of digital media. In *Drugs and human behavior* (pp. 459–468). Springer. https://doi.org/10.1007/978-3-030-62855-0_33

Méndez-Díaz, M., Ruiz, C. A. E., Prieto, G. B., et al. (2010). El cerebro y las drogas, sus mecanismos neurobiológicos. *Salud Mental, 33*(5), 451–456. https://www.medigraphic.com/cgi-bin/new/resumen.cgi?IDARTICULO=27169

Merikivi, J., Salovaara, A., Mäntymäki, M., & Zhang, L. (2018). On the way to understanding binge watching behavior: The over-estimated role of involvement. *Electronic Markets, 28*(1), 111–122. https://doi.org/10.1007/s12525-017-0271-4

Moraes, R. L., Nobusa, T. K., Lima, D. K. H., & Souza, J. C. (2022). Neurobiologia do Sistema de Recompensa Cerebral. *Caderno Brasileiro de Medicina, 35*, 52–58. https://www.cadbrasmed.com.br/_files/ugd/c181a5_01e7a938eade4f9b8ee14682f597dc0e.pdf

Naragon-Gainey, K., McMahon, T. P., & Chacko, T. P. (2017). The structure of common emotion regulation strategies: A meta-analytic examination. *Psychological Bulletin, 143*(4), 384–427. https://doi.org/10.1037/bul0000093

Orosz, G., Bőthe, B., & Tóth-Király, I. (2016). The development of the problematic series watching scale (PSWS). *Journal of Behavioral Addictions, 5*, 144–150. https://doi.org/10.1556/2006.5.2016.011

Panda, S., & Pandey, S. (2017). Binge watching and college students: Motivations and outcomes. *Young Consumers, 18*(4), 425–438. https://doi.org/10.1108/YC-07-2017-00707

Panek, E. (2014). Left to their own devices: College students' "guilty pleasure" media use and time management. *Community Research, 41*, 561–577. https://doi.org/10.1177/0093650213499657

Pittman, M., & Sheehan, K. (2015). Sprinting a media marathon: Uses and gratifications of binge-watching television through Netflix. *First Monday, 20*(10). https://doi.org/10.5210/fm.v20i10.6138

Pittman, M., & Steiner, E. (2019). Transportation or narrative completion? Attentiveness during binge-watching moderates regret. *Social Sciences, 8*(3), 1–14. https://doi.org/10.3390/socsci8030099

Pittman, M., & Steiner, E. (2021). Distinguishing feast-watching from cringe-watching: Planned, social, and attentive binge-watching predicts increased well-being and decreased regret. *Convergence, 27*(5), 1507–1524. https://doi.org/10.1177/1354856521999183

Przybylski, A. K., Murayama, K., DeHaan, C. R., & Gladwell, V. (2013). Motivational, emotional, and behavioural correlates of fear of missing out. *Computers in Human Behavior, 29*(4), 1841–1848. https://doi.org/10.1016/j.chb.2013.02.014

Ramayan, S., Estella, A. L. M., & Bakar, I. A. A. (2018). The effects of binge watching on interpersonal communication among Department of Communication and Liberal Arts (DCLA) students. *Idealogy, 3*(3), 127–143. https://ir.uitm.edu.my/30470/1/30470.pdf

Raza, S. H., Yousaf, M., Sohail, F., Munawar, R., Ogadimma, E. C., & Siang, J. M. L. D. (2021). Investigating binge-watching adverse mental health outcomes during covid-19 pandemic: Moderating role of screen time for web series using online streaming. *Psychology Research and Behavior Management, 14*, 1615–1629. https://doi.org/10.2147/PRBM.S328416

Reichert, R. A., Lopes, F. M., Silva, E. A. D., Scatena, A., Andrade, A. L. M., & Micheli, D. D. (2021a). Psychological trauma: Biological and psychosocial aspects of substance use disorders. In *Drugs and human behavior* (pp. 243–260). Springer.

Reichert, R. A., Calixto, F., Silva, A. M. B. D., Martins, G. D. G., Barbugli, B. C., Scatena, A., et al. (2021b). Digital games, shopping, sex, and other addictions: Neuropsychological and behavioral correlates. In *Drugs and human behavior* (pp. 443–458). Springer.

Reichert, R. A., Martins, G. D. G., Silva, A. M. B. D., Scatena, A., Barbugli, B. C., Micheli, D. D., & Andrade, A. L. M. (2021c). New forms of addiction: Digital media. In *Psychology of substance abuse* (pp. 43–53). Springer.

Riddle, K., Peebles, A., Davis, C., Xu, F., & Schroeder, E. (2018). The addictive potential of television binge watching: Comparing intentional and unintentional binges. *Psychology of Popular Media, 7*(4), 589–604. https://doi.org/10.1037/ppm0000167

Rubenking, B., & Bracken, C. C. (2018). Binge-watching: A suspenseful, emotional, habit. *Communication Research Reports, 35*(5), 381–391. https://doi.org/10.1080/08824096.2018.1525346

Rubenking, B., Bracken, C. C., Sandoval, J., & Rister, A. (2018). Defining new viewing behaviours: What makes and motivates TV binge-watching? *International Journal of Digital Television, 9*(1), 69–85. https://doi.org/10.1386/jdtv.9.1.69_1

Schweidel, D. A., & Moe, W. W. (2016). Binge watching and advertising. *Journal of Marketing, 80*(5), 1–19. https://doi.org/10.1509/jm.15.0258

Shim, H., & Kim, K. J. (2018). An exploration of the motivations for binge-watching and the role of individual differences. *Computers in Human Behavior, 82*, 94–100. https://doi.org/10.1016/j.chb.2017.12.032

Shim, H., Lim, S., Jung, E. E., & Shin, E. (2018). I hate binge-watching but I can't help doing it: The moderating effect of immediate gratification and need for cognition on binge-watching attitude-behavior relation. *Telematics and Informatics, 35*, 1971–1979. https://doi.org/10.1016/j.tele.2018.07.001

Shin, Y., Kim, H., Kim, S., & Kim, J. (2020). A neural mechanism of the relationship between impulsivity and emotion dysregulation in patients with internet gaming disorder. *Addiction Biology, 26*, e12916. https://doi.org/10.1111/adb.12916

Song, L., Zhang, Q., Hu, B., & Mou, J. (2022). To resist or to purchase: The causal mechanism of binge-watching and program purchase. *Journal of Retailing and Consumer Services, 68*. https://doi.org/10.1016/j.jretconser.2022.103021

Spritzer, D. T., Andrade, A. L. M., Xavier, A. Z., da Silva, G. T., Kim, H. S., Kaliszewska-Czeremska, K., et al. (2022). The Self-perception of Text message Dependence Scale (STDS): A Brazilian-Portuguese validation and expansion of its psychometric properties. *Current Psychology, 42*, 1–12. https://doi.org/10.1007/s12144-022-02957-8

Spruance, L. A., Karmakar, M., Kruger, J. S., & Vaterlaus, J. M. (2017). "Are you still watching?" Correlations between binge TV watching, diet and physical activity. *Journal of Obesity & Weight Management*, 1–8. https://www.researchgate.net/publication/323200056_Are_you_still_watching_Correlations_between_binge_TV_watching_diet_and_physical_activity

Starosta, J. A., & Izydorczyk, B. (2020). Understanding the phenomenon of binge-watching—A systematic review. *International Journal of Environmental Research and Public Health, 17*(12), 4469. https://doi.org/10.3390/ijerph17124469

Starosta, J., Izydorczyk, B., & Lizińczyk, S. (2019). Characteristics of people's binge-watching behavior in the "entering into early adulthood" period of life. *Health Psychology Report, 7*(2), 149–164. https://doi.org/10.5114/hpr.2019.83025

Starosta, J., Izydorczyk, B., Sitnik-Warchulska, K., & Lizinczyk, S. (2021). Impulsivity and difficulties in emotional regulation as predictors of binge-watching behaviours. *Frontiers in Psychiatry, 12*, 743870. https://doi.org/10.3389/fpsyt.2021.743870

Steiner, E., & Xu, K. (2018). Binge-watching motivates change. *Convergence: The International Journal of Research into New Media Technologies, 26*, 135485651775036. https://doi.org/10.1177/1354856517750365

Steins-Loeber, S., Reiter, T., Averbeck, H., Harbarth, L., & Brand, M. (2020). Binge-watching behaviour: The role of impulsivity and depressive symptoms. *European Addiction Research, 26*, 141–150. https://doi.org/10.1159/000506307

Sung, Y. H., Kang, E. Y., & Lee, W. (2018). Why do we indulge? Exploring motivations for binge watching. *Journal of Broadcasting & Electronic Media, 62*(3), 408–426. https://doi.org/10.1080/08838151.2018.1451851

Tefertiller, A. C., & Maxwell, L. C. (2018). Depression, emotional states, and the experience of binge-watching narrative television. *Atlantic Journal of Communication, 26*, 278–290. https://doi.org/10.1080/15456870.2018.1517765

Tóth-Király, I., Böthe, B., Tóth-Fáber, E., Gyözö, H., & Orosz, G. (2017). Connected to TV series: Quantifying series watching engagement. *Journal of Behavioral Addictions, 6*, 472–489. https://doi.org/10.1556/2006.6.2017.083

Tukachinsky, R., & Eyal, K. (2018). The psychology of marathon television viewing: Antecedents and viewer involvement. *Mass Community and Society, 21*, 275–295. https://doi.org/10.1080/15205436.2017.1422765

Uhl, G. R., Koob, G. F., & Cable, J. (2019). The neurobiology of addiction. *Annals of the New York Academy of Sciences, 1451*, 5–28. https://doi.org/10.1111/nyas.13989

Umesh, S., & Bose, S. (2019). Binge-watching: A matter of concern? *Indian Journal of Psychological Medicine, 41*, 182–184. https://doi.org/10.4103/IJPSYM.IJPSYM_279_18

Vaterlaus, J. M., Spruance, L. A., Frantz, K., & Kruger, J. S. (2018). College student televisión binge watching: Conceptualization, gratifications, and perceived consequences. *The Social Science Journal, 56*(4). https://doi.org/10.1016/j.soscij.2018.10.004

Verma, A., Islam, S., Moghaddam, V., & Anwar, A. (2023). Digital emotion regulation on social media. a*rXivpreprint*. https://doi.org/10.48550/arXiv.2307.13187

Viens, A., & Farrar, K. M. (2021). Conceptualizing and measuring binge watching. *Communication Studies, 72*(3), 267–284. https://doi.org/10.1080/10510974.2021.1876748

Walton-Pattison, E., Dombrowski, S. U., & Presseau, J. (2018). 'Just one more episode': Frequency and theoretical correlates of television binge watching. *Journal of Health Psychology, 23*(1), 17–24. https://doi.org/10.1177/1359105316643379

Yamauchi, L. M., Andrade, A. L. M., Pinheiro, B. O., Enumo, S. R. F., & De Micheli, D. (2019). Evaluation of the social representation of the use of alcoholic beverages by adolescents. *Estudos de Psicologia (Campinas), 36*, e180098. https://doi.org/10.1590/1982-0275201936e180098

Chapter 4
Gaming Disorder: Neurobiological Foundations, Clinical Features, Psychosocial Impacts, and Evidence-Based Interventions

Manoela Fontelles, Isabela Brasil Correia, Richard Alecsander Reichert, Filipe Reis Teodoro Andrade, Rosa Maria Martins de Almeida, and Denise De Micheli

Electronic Games

Technological advancements and the growing expansion of digital reach have enabled the electronic gaming industry to become one of the most lucrative sectors, with a substantial user base, particularly among younger individuals. It is estimated that the popularization of video games became evident in 2014 when the number of players reached 1.8 billion. Within just 5 years, this figure surged to 2 billion (Limone et al., 2023). This growth has raised concerns regarding excessive or problematic video game use, prompting the inclusion of gaming-related disorders in medical classifications, such as the *International Classification of Diseases* (ICD; World Health Organization [WHO], 2018) and the fifth edition of the *Diagnostic and Statistical Manual of Mental Disorders* (DSM-5), along with its revised version, the DSM-5-TR (American Psychiatric Association [APA], 2013, 2022; King et al., 2020).

Electronic games, or video games, are entertainment activities using electronic devices such as consoles, computers, smartphones, and tablets to interact in a virtual environment. These games vary in genre, including adventure, sports, strategy, and online multiplayer (Imakata et al., 2024). While evidence suggests that balanced

M. Fontelles · I. B. Correia
Universidade do Vale do Itajaí, Itajaí, SC, Brazil

R. A. Reichert · D. De Micheli (✉)
Universidade Federal de São Paulo, São Paulo, SP, Brazil
e-mail: reichert@unifesp.br

F. R. T. Andrade
Zentralinstitut für seelische Gesundheit, Mannheim, Germany

R. M. M. de Almeida
Universidade Federal do Rio Grande do Sul, Porto Alegre, RS, Brazil

A. L. M. Andrade (ed.), *Digital Addictions*,
https://doi.org/10.1007/978-3-031-87986-9_4

and healthy video game use may provide cognitive and social benefits, problems arise when gaming occupies a significant portion of individuals' time (Santos et al., 2021). This behavior can impair family, academic, professional, and social domains. Despite these observed challenges, gaming addiction has shown a continuous increase and is likely to grow exponentially with the intensification of access to digital platforms (Nielsen et al., 2021; Reichert et al., 2021a).

In addition to their visually and audibly appealing features, video games offer social rewards such as a sense of belonging, recognition, and opportunities to form friendships. This combination, coupled with the pursuit of pleasure and, in some cases, the use of experiential avoidance strategies to cope with aversive environmental contingencies, can lead to behavioral excesses or deficits associated with gaming (Bonner et al., 2022; Borsato et al., 2020; Cepni et al., 2019; Gentile et al., 2009; Liao et al., 2020; Li et al., 2023; Lorenz et al., 2015; Mohammad et al., 2023; Reichert et al., 2021a; Zhang et al., 2023).

Characteristics of Electronic Games

Games have been part of human history for centuries, understood as playful manifestations that simulate real-life situations with the purpose of entertainment, appearing in various forms across different cultures over time. With the emergence of electronic games in the 1980s, they became popularized through video game consoles and portable devices. Currently, due to technological advancements, many games are available on mobile platforms via smartphone applications or in desktop versions, accessible online for computers in both paid and free models (Bowman & Wulf, 2023; Imakata et al., 2024; Mardon, 2021; Wang et al., 2023; Wardle, 2021).

Today, various factors make electronic games highly engaging, attracting new players and sustaining the interest of those already involved. These factors include the following (Bonner et al., 2022; Borsato et al., 2020; Cepni et al., 2019; Gentile et al., 2009; Lorenz et al., 2015; Mohammad et al., 2023):

- **Interactivity:** Players interact directly with the game environment, responding to stimuli in real-time.
- **Rewards and progression:** Games offer reward systems, such as unlocking new levels, items, or skills, encouraging continued engagement.
- **Competition and cooperation:** Many games feature multiplayer modes, which foster competition or group cooperation and enhance the social experience.
- **Engaging narratives:** Captivating storylines in many games maintains player interest and deepens engagement with the plot.
- **Accessibility:** Games are available across various platforms, such as computers, consoles, and mobile devices, enabling play at different times of the day and encouraging repetitive behavior.
- **Augmented/virtual reality:** Advanced technologies are employed to create more immersive and realistic experiences.

- **Diverse genres:** The variety of game types, such as action, adventure, sports, strategy, and role-playing games (RPGs), appeals to distinct audiences.

It is also essential to consider the age groups associated with games, as different games attract audiences of specific ages. Players often identify with particular game classifications, such as action, adventure, strategy, sports, racing, or role-playing game (RPG, a genre in which players assume fictional roles and interact in virtual or in-person environments with other participants), which are closely related to social interests outside the gaming context. In this scenario, sustained engagement with games can also be viewed as a form of social identification, fostering communities and a sense of belonging to a specific space. For some, this can serve as a protective factor against challenges encountered in "real life" (Borsato et al., 2020).

Gaming Disorder

Gaming addiction was first introduced in nosological manuals in 1980, when the DSM included "pathological gambling" in its third edition, classifying it as one of the five types of "Impulse Control Disorders." The DSM-III diagnostic criteria for "pathological gambling" emphasized the progressive loss of control over gambling and its adverse impacts on various life domains, such as family, work, and finances. The diagnosis was based on several criteria, including difficulty resisting the urge to gamble, constant pursuit of gambling-related excitement, and the impairments caused by this activity (APA, 1980).

In the fourth edition of the DSM, published in 1994, the criteria for "pathological gambling" were revised to align more closely with the criteria for substance addiction. One additional diagnostic criterion that gained prominence was "repeated and unsuccessful attempts to control, reduce, or stop gambling" (APA, 1994).

With the publication of the fifth edition of the DSM in 2013 and its revised version in 2022 (DSM-5-TR), "pathological gambling" was reclassified. Considering the similarities between "pathological gambling" and substance use disorders—such as underlying neurobiological mechanisms, clinical characteristics, and genetic predisposition—the disorder was relocated from the category of "Impulse Control Disorders" to "Substance-Related and Addictive Disorders." Moreover, its designation was updated to "Gaming Disorder." For a diagnosis, individuals must present at least five of the nine diagnostic criteria listed below over a 12-month period, with these criteria resulting in clinically significant impairments (APA, 2022):

1. A compelling need to play video games
2. Experiencing unpleasant symptoms when gaming is interrupted
3. Feeling the need to spend more time gaming
4. Difficulty controlling the time spent on gaming
5. Loss of interest in activities unrelated to video games, feeling drawn to gaming
6. Continuing to game despite awareness of associated psychosocial issues

7. Concealing the amount of time spent gaming by family members and healthcare professionals
8. Using video games as a means of escaping or managing negative emotions (experiential avoidance)
9. Damaging or losing relationships, professional, or educational opportunities due to gaming

The WHO has also emphasized the importance of recognizing Internet Gaming Disorder as potentially harmful behavior when associated with psychosocial dysfunction and clinically significant distress for affected individuals. For the behavior to be considered a disorder, the pattern must be severe enough to result in substantial impairments across personal, familial, social, educational, occupational, or other vital areas of life and typically persist continuously for at least 12 months (Király et al., 2018). Additionally, common symptoms include decreased self-esteem, reduced social competence, and feelings of loneliness, indicating that Gaming Disorder can exacerbate mood and anxiety disorders. Conversely, mood and anxiety disorders can predispose individuals to Gaming Disorder (Northrup & Shumway, 2024).

The frequency of gaming, the time devoted to these activities, neglect of other responsibilities and priorities, engagement in risky behaviors associated with gaming, and its adverse effects can increase the risk of developing Gaming Disorder. These factors may also elevate the risk of physical or psychological harm to individuals and/or those close to them (Király et al., 2018). In this context, assessment and diagnosis are conducted by mental health professionals, taking into account the severity and impact of these behaviors on individuals' lives (Imakata et al., 2024).

Furthermore, it is important to discuss the diagnostic criteria for Gaming Disorder through the lens of the transdiagnostic approach, which represents a significant shift in the understanding of mental disorders. Instead of focusing exclusively on the specific symptoms of each disorder, this approach seeks to identify common underlying processes across various clinical presentations. Integrating the transdiagnostic approach with the current diagnostic criteria for Gaming Disorder could provide a more comprehensive understanding of the factors contributing to the development and maintenance of this condition, offering a more robust foundation for planning individualized, tailored, and effective intervention strategies (Sandín et al., 2012).

Neurobiology of Gaming Disorder

Brain Regions Associated with Gaming Disorder

Neuroimaging studies have identified several brain regions implicated in Gaming Disorder, similar to those observed in substance dependencies. Functional magnetic resonance imaging (fMRI) studies show significant alterations in the prefrontal cortex, striatum, amygdala, and hippocampus, suggesting dysregulation in inhibitory control and emotional processing (Dong et al., 2011; Han et al., 2012). The prefrontal cortex is responsible for impulse control and decision-making, and deficits in this region contribute to the difficulty that players experience in stopping gaming, even when aware of the negative impacts (Ko et al., 2014; Kuss & Griffiths, 2018).

Reward System and Dopamine

The dopaminergic system plays a central role in understanding Gaming Disorder. The nucleus accumbens and the ventral tegmental area are key regions in the reward circuit that regulate dopamine release in response to unpredictable rewards, such as those in games (Kühn et al., 2011). Repeated exposure to these stimuli can lead to sensitization of the reward system and increased response to game-related cues, while non-related stimuli become less relevant, promoting a cycle of game-seeking behavior (Kuss, 2013; Weinstein, 2017). Additionally, prolonged involvement in gaming is associated with reduced activation of the natural reward system, making other activities less enjoyable (Han et al., 2012).

Inhibitory Control and Decision-Making

Individuals with Gaming Disorder frequently exhibit impairments in inhibitory control, regulated by the dorsolateral prefrontal cortex and striatum. Again, fMRI studies show reduced activation in these areas and decreased connectivity between the prefrontal cortex and striatum, indicating disruptions in circuits involved in impulse control and decision-making (Ko et al., 2014). These patterns are similar to those observed in substance dependencies, suggesting that excessive gaming can reconfigure neural circuits similarly to other forms of addiction (Kuss & Griffiths, 2018; Reichert et al., 2021a, 2021b). Studies on problematic alcohol use, for instance, indicate that high levels of impulsivity and lack of inhibitory control are critical factors in the development and maintenance of addictive behaviors, which may also apply to Gaming Disorder (Andrade et al., 2022; Marin et al., 2021).

Plasticity and Structural Changes

In addition to functional changes, Gaming Disorder is also associated with alterations in brain morphology. Studies using voxel-based morphometry (VBM) have observed volume reductions in regions such as the anterior cingulate cortex and the orbitofrontal cortex, responsible for emotional processing and motivational behavior (Zhou et al., 2011). These structural alterations may be long-lasting and indicate that Gaming Disorder can lead to permanent changes in brain architecture.

Brain plasticity changes and structural reorganization are significant features in individuals with Gaming Disorder. Neuroimaging studies prove that excessive gaming is associated with white and gray matter modifications, reflecting changes in cognitive functions such as inhibitory control and emotional processing (Yuan et al., 2013a). Such neurological changes can have long-term effects, impacting cognitive flexibility and behavioral control.

Structural Evidence

Research by Yuan et al. (2016) and other studies on the disorder have revealed volume reductions in the striatum and prefrontal cortex, indicating adaptive or pathological plasticity due to repeated exposure to gaming stimuli (Yuan et al., 2016). This is relevant because it suggests that Gaming Disorder is not just a dysregulation of existing circuits but also a significant structural reconfiguration of the brain.

Specifically, the decrease in cortical thickness in prefrontal areas and the anterior cingulate cortex suggests impairments in executive control, leading to difficulties in suppressing impulses and making adaptive decisions. Zhou et al.'s (2023b) research on risk factors in Gaming Disorder also highlights that prolonged exposure to games can serve as a coping mechanism for stress and anxiety, exacerbating dependency through negative reinforcement and, over time, generating plastic changes that affect behavior long-term.

Functional Connectivity Changes

Another aspect is abnormal functional connectivity in critical regions, such as the frontostriatal circuit, which is directly linked to inhibitory control and motivation. Individuals with Gaming Disorders show reduced functional connectivity in cognitive control networks and increased connectivity in reward networks, resulting in an imbalance between the desire for immediate rewards and the ability to control these impulses (Yuan et al., 2017). This change in functional connectivity is a form of synaptic plasticity that reflects the brain's adaptation to excessive gaming patterns.

Use-Dependent Plasticity Models

The use-dependent plasticity model posits that areas frequently activated in response to specific behaviors, such as gaming, tend to strengthen, while neglected ones may weaken. In the case of Gaming Disorder, reward-related networks strengthen, while executive control and inhibitory networks weaken (Yuan et al., 2013b). This creates a brain architecture adapted to excessive use, making it more challenging to transition to healthier behaviors.

In summary, brain plasticity in individuals with Gaming Disorder is not only a consequence of compulsive gaming patterns but also a factor that contributes to the maintenance of the disorder, increasing susceptibility to compulsive use and making it difficult to reverse the behavior.

Neuropsychological and Behavioral Impact

Individuals with Gaming Disorder show neuropsychological deficits, such as increased impulsivity and reduced inhibitory control. Studies using tasks like the *Cambridge Gambling Task* (CGT)[1] and the *Monetary Incentive Delay Task* (MID)[2] have shown that excessive gamers tend to prefer immediate rewards, even when long-term losses are involved, a phenomenon known as *delay discounting*[3] (Kuss, 2013; Lorenz et al., 2015). These results suggest that risk-taking behavior is exacerbated by an imbalance between the reward system and inhibitory control, complicating behavior regulation.

Psychosocial Impacts

For many individuals, gaming is a recreational activity carried out periodically without causing harm to daily life. However, for some people, gaming can significantly interfere with daily routines. With the widespread use of the Internet and smartphones, excessive use of technological resources and electronic games has become a relevant public health issue (Calado et al., 2017; Clemens et al., 2018). The impacts of excessive gaming are broad, affecting areas from academic and

[1] The *Cambridge Gambling Task* (CGT) is a neuropsychological task used to assess decision-making under risk. It measures impulsivity and risk-taking by presenting subjects with a series of trials where they must place bets on the probability of different outcomes based on limited information (Rogers et al., 1999).

[2] The *Monetary Incentive Delay Task* (MID) is a task designed to evaluate reward anticipation and delay. It involves reacting to visual cues to gain monetary rewards, allowing the measurement of individual differences in sensitivity to reward and impulsivity (Knutson et al., 2001).

[3] *Delay Discounting* is a phenomenon in which the value of a reward decreases as the delay to receive it increases. Individuals with a high rate of delay discounting tend to choose immediate, smaller rewards over larger, delayed ones. This behavioral pattern reflects reduced inhibitory control and is often associated with impulsivity and poor decision-making, characteristics commonly seen in behavioral addictions and substance use disorders. Thus, delay discounting is considered a vulnerability marker for impulsive and addictive behaviors (Green & Myerson, 2004; Madden & Bickel, 2010).

professional performance to social relationships and impairing physical and psychological health (Garcia et al., 2024) (see Table 4.1).

One of the most common risks to physical health associated with excessive gaming is the development of musculoskeletal issues resulting from poor posture and repetitive strain during long gaming sessions. Remaining seated for prolonged periods with poor posture and repetitive movements can lead to muscle pain, tendonitis, and other conditions (Lindberg et al., 2020). Regarding mental health, studies suggest that individuals with Gaming Disorder exhibit elevated levels of anxiety, depression, impulsivity, low self-esteem, and emotional instability, characterized by mood swings (Garcia et al., 2024; Severo et al., 2020).

The consequences of Gaming Disorders extend beyond individual aspects, affecting players' interpersonal relationships. Research with young people indicates that these individuals often exhibit low self-esteem, social anxiety, and feelings of loneliness. The lack of social skills and low emotional support reinforce a repetitive cycle, where gaming becomes a form of experiential avoidance and social connection, albeit virtually (Rojas-Jara et al., 2022). However, some authors argue that while gaming provides social interactions, Gaming Disorder remains associated

Table 4.1 Effects of gaming disorder on individuals' psychosocial life and functioning

Area	Description
Mental health	Individuals with excessive gaming involvement show elevated levels of stress, anxiety, and depression (Alrahili et al., 2023; Aonso-Diego et al., 2024; Idris et al., 2023; Pallavicini et al., 2022; Wang et al., 2022)
Social impairments	Prolonged online engagement can exacerbate difficulties in relationships with family and friends, given the focus on virtual interaction over face-to-face relationships. This can result in feelings of neglect from loved ones and a decline in social skills (Nielsen et al., 2021; Schneider et al., 2017; Szász-Janocha et al., 2023; Throuvala et al., 2019; Zhou et al., 2023a, 2023b)
Academic performance	Prioritizing gaming can reduce interest and dedication to academic or professional tasks, leading to decreased performance due to excessive concentration on gaming at the expense of other activities (Chiang et al., 2022; Ghali et al., 2023; Hawi & Samaha, 2024; Wang et al., 2019)
Physical health issues	Prolonged sitting to play games can cause issues such as sedentary behavior, obesity, poor posture, repetitive strain injuries, and other long-term physical impairments (Fathuldeen et al., 2023; Kohorst et al., 2018; Satish-Kumar et al., 2023; Tholl et al., 2022)
Financial consequences	Games that allow for microtransactions can lead to excessive spending, compromising personal and family financial planning, especially when resources are poorly managed for gaming items or subscriptions (Castrén et al., 2021; King & Delfabbro, 2018; King & Wong-Padoongpatt, 2022; Kleinman & Das, 2020; Saunders et al., 2017)
Cognitive impairments	Studies indicate a correlation between Gaming Disorder and cognitive impairments, such as deficits in executive functioning and decision-making, which can result in impulsivity and risky behaviors (Andrade et al., 2022; Ko et al., 2014; Jang et al., 2021; Lim et al., 2016; Wang et al., 2021; Weinstein & Lejoyeux, 2020)

with social relationship impairments, as screen-mediated interaction does not replace face-to-face relationships (Mills et al., 2016; Rasmussen et al., 2014).

Regarding academic impact, although some studies suggest that moderate use of games for educational purposes can promote cognitive benefits, excessive use has been associated with negative consequences (Fátima & Amin, 2023; Gómez-Gonzalvo et al., 2020; Santos et al., 2021). Excessive gaming time correlates with decreased engagement and academic performance, while excessive online gaming is negatively associated with low educational and professional performance. Difficulty disconnecting from gaming, a characteristic of Gaming Disorder, is linked to reduced study time, concentration difficulties, and lower motivation to learn, resulting in poor grades and challenges in keeping up with academic content (Fátima & Amin, 2023; Footitt et al., 2024; Gómez-Gonzalvo et al., 2020; Mohammad et al., 2023; Paulus et al., 2018; Sun et al., 2023; Wang et al., 2023).

In summary, the impacts of excessive gaming are complex and affect various aspects of life. The difficulty or inability to control gaming time, the prioritization of virtual activities over other life aspects, and the adverse effects on mental health, social relationships, and academic and professional performance underscore the need for prevention and intervention strategies, which will be discussed next.

Prevention

Many individuals with gaming-related disorders are unaware of the negative health impacts associated with their gaming behavior (Ramesh et al., 2023). Understanding these effects enables individuals, especially young people, to actively engage in prevention efforts aimed at fostering autonomy, reducing psychological distress, and promoting health, well-being, and quality of life (Chau et al., 2019; Isralowitz et al., 2022; Kuss, 2018; Lim et al., 2016; Long et al., 2022; Müller et al., 2023; Phan et al., 2019; Torres-Rodríguez et al., 2017).

Involving parents and educators in prevention strategies reinforces the message regarding the importance of balance in gaming usage. These agents play a critical role in monitoring gaming habits and encouraging the adoption of healthy leisure activities as alternatives to excessive use of electronic devices (Ramesh et al., 2023). Table 4.2 lists several alternative activities that can be pursued (Chen et al., 2023; Király et al., 2018; Stevens et al., 2021; Zhang et al., 2024).

Health professionals, teachers, and families can create environments that promote healthy gaming habits and continuously monitor adolescent gaming behaviors. In this context, integrated tools in electronic devices can assist in screen time monitoring (Clemens et al., 2018). These resources allow caregivers to track the duration of gaming sessions in real time, collecting data and other relevant information, which facilitates the development and implementation of alternative interventions tailored to each gaming session (Chen et al., 2023; Krossbakken et al., 2018; Li et al., 2019; She et al., 2022; Werner et al., 2024).

Table 4.2 Activities to stimulate cognitive, emotional, and social development in youth

Activities	Description
Sports and physical activities	Team sports (soccer, basketball) or individual sports (swimming, cycling, martial arts) promote physical health, teamwork, and discipline
Arts and crafts	Creative activities such as painting, drawing, or crafting allow youth to express themselves and develop new skills
Music and performing arts	Playing a musical instrument, participating in a choir, and joining a theater group are alternatives that foster creativity and enhance self-esteem, self-confidence, and self-efficacy
Outdoor adventures	Hiking, camping, or exploring nature helps youth connect with the environment and develop an appreciation for thc outdoors
Volunteering	Involvement in community services or volunteer activities provides adolescents with a sense of purpose and belonging, promoting a positive impact

Source: Based on Chen et al. (2023), Király et al. (2018), Stevens et al. (2021), and Zhang et al. (2024)

Treatment

Cognitive Behavioral Therapy (CBT), developed by Aaron T. Beck in the 1960s, is a psychotherapeutic approach based on the premise that thoughts influence emotions and behaviors. Clinical practice in the cognitive-behavioral approach primarily focuses on identifying and restructuring thoughts and beliefs, aiming at behavioral modification (Bass, 2015; Beck, 2013; Fong, 2005). With a solid empirical foundation, CBT has proven to be effective in treating a wide range of mental disorders, including gaming-related disorders (Beck & Liese, 2024; Ribeiro et al., 2021). CBT is widely recognized in the literature as one of the most effective therapeutic approaches for treating gambling disorder, applicable in both individual and group therapy (Bore et al., 2024; Casey et al., 2017; Dong & Potenza, 2014; Han et al., 2020; Hofstedt et al., 2023; Ji & Wong, 2023; Lindenberg et al., 2022; Stevens et al., 2019).

CBT aims to assist individuals in identifying dysfunctional thoughts, cognitive distortions, and misconceptions about gaming, which perpetuate maladaptive and harmful behaviors (Bass, 2015; Beck, 2013; Beck & Liese, 2024; Fong, 2005; Ribeiro et al., 2021). The efficacy of CBT is supported by a robust body of evidence from randomized clinical trials, positioning it as one of the most effective therapeutic interventions for treating gambling disorders (Carlbring et al., 2009; Casey et al., 2017; Dowling et al., 2007; Petry et al., 2006; Ribeiro et al., 2021; Sylvain et al., 1997). Moreover, CBT has demonstrated effectiveness not only in treating Internet addiction but also in mitigating symptoms of anxiety, impulsivity, and social avoidance (Han et al., 2020).

Group CBT fosters a collaborative learning environment in which group cohesion and mutual support among participants contribute to restoring self-esteem and self-efficacy. Observational learning, in this context, allows individuals to benefit from the shared experiences of others, including both successes and challenges

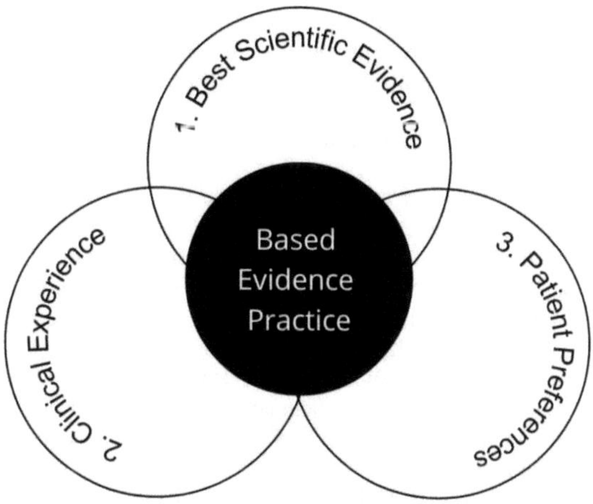

Fig. 4.1 Integrated model of Evidence-Based Practice in treating Gaming Disorder. (Source: Developed based on Leonardi and Meyer (2015))

encountered by group members, thereby enhancing the therapeutic process (Myrseth et al., 2009).

However, despite promising evidence regarding treatments for gambling disorder, it is essential to emphasize that this is a complex disorder with multiple determinants involving biological, psychological, and social factors. Following a clinical approach grounded in Evidence-Based Practice (see Fig. 4.1), in addition to considering the best available evidence and the expertise of mental health professionals, it is essential to ensure the active participation of individuals in decisions related to their health and well-being. For the success of any intervention, it is crucial to consider the particularities of each individual, including their goals, values, beliefs, preferences, sociocultural context, and clinical condition (Leonardi & Meyer, 2015).

References

Alrahili, N., Alreefi, M., Alkhonain, I. M., Aldakhilallah, M., Alothaim, J., Alzahrani, A., Alshargi, A., & Baabbad, N. (2023). The prevalence of video game addiction and its relation to anxiety, depression, and attention deficit hyperactivity disorder (ADHD) in children and adolescents in saudi arabia: a cross-sectional study. *Cureus, 15*(8), e42957. https://doi.org/10.7759/cureus.42957

American Psychiatric Association (APA). (1980). *Diagnostic and statistical manual of mental disorders* (3rd ed.). American Psychiatric Association.

American Psychiatric Association (APA). (1994). *Diagnostic and statistical manual of mental disorders* (4th ed.). American Psychiatric Association.

American Psychiatric Association (APA). (2013). *Diagnostic and statistical manual of mental disorders* (5th ed.). American Psychiatric Association.

American Psychiatric Association (APA). (2022). *Diagnostic and statistical manual of mental disorders* (5th ed., text rev.). American Psychiatric Association.

Andrade, F. R. T., Marin, M. G., & de Almeida, R. M. M. (2022). Use of alcohol and impulsivity during adolescence: A systematic review. *Journal of Drug and Alcohol Research, 11*, 236200. https://doi.org/10.4303/jdar/236200

Aonso-Diego, G., González-Roz, A., Weidberg, S., & Secades-Villa, R. (2024). Depression, anxiety, and stress in young adult gamers and their relationship with addictive behaviors: A latent profile analysis. *Journal of Affective Disorders, 366*, 254–261. https://doi.org/10.1016/j.jad.2024.08.203

Bass, P. F. (2015). Gaming addiction: When going online goes off-kilter. *Contemporary Pediatrics, 32*(11), 16–21.

Beck, S. J. (2013). *Cognitive behavioral therapy* (2nd ed.). Artmed Editora.

Beck, A., & Liese, B. (2024). *Terapia Cognitivo-Comportamental para transtornos por uso de substâncias e dependências comportamentais*. Artmed.

Bonner, J., Allen, A., Katsikitis, M., Love, S., & Kannis-Dymand, L. (2022). Metacognition, desire thinking and craving in problematic video game use. *Journal of Technology in Behavioral Science, 7*(4), 532–546. https://doi.org/10.1007/s41347-022-00272-4

Bore, P., Nilsson, S., Andersson, M., Oehm, K., Attvall, J., Håkansson, A., & Claesdotter-Knutsson, E. (2024). Effectiveness and acceptability of cognitive behavioral therapy and family therapy for gaming disorder: Protocol for a nonrandomized intervention study of a novel psychological treatment. *JMIR Research Protocols, 13*, e56315. https://doi.org/10.2196/56315

Borsato, M., Brasil, M. R., Mattes, V. V., de Oliveira, V. M., & de Souza, J. (2020). Aspectos sobre a esportivização, mercantilização e espetacularização dos jogos eletrônicos. *Pensar a Prática, 23*, 57704. https://doi.org/10.5216/rpp.v23.57704

Bowman, N. D., & Wulf, T. (2023). Nostalgia in video games. *Current Opinion in Psychology, 49*, 101544. https://doi.org/10.1016/j.copsyc.2022.101544

Calado, F., Alexandre, J., & Griffiths, M. D. (2017). Prevalence of adolescent problem gambling: A systematic review of recent research. *Journal of Gambling Studies, 33*(2), 397–424. https://doi.org/10.1007/s10899-016-9627-5

Carlbring, P., Jonsson, J., Josephson, H., & Forsberg, L. (2009). Motivational interviewing versus cognitive behavioral group therapy in the treatment of problem and pathological gambling: A randomized controlled trial. *Cognitive Behaviour Therapy, 39*(2), 92–103. https://doi.org/10.1080/16506070903190245

Casey, L. M., Oei, T. P. S., Raylu, N., Horrigan, K., Day, J., Ireland, M., & Clough, B. A. (2017). Internet-based delivery of cognitive behaviour therapy compared to monitoring, feedback, and support for problem gambling: A randomized controlled trial. *Journal of Gambling Studies, 33*(3), 993–1010. https://doi.org/10.1007/s10899-016-9666-y

Castrén, S., Järvinen-Tassopoulos, J., & Raitasalo, K. (2021). Money used in gaming is associated with problem gambling: Results of the ESPAD 2019 Finland. *Journal of Behavioral Addictions, 10*(4), 932–940. https://doi.org/10.1556/2006.2021.00076

Cepni, A. B., Ledoux, T. A., & Johnston, C. A. (2019). Screen media: A powerful reinforcement. *American Journal of Lifestyle Medicine, 14*(2), 126–129. https://doi.org/10.1177/1559827619892543

Chau, C. L., Tsui, Y. Y., & Cheng, C. (2019). Gamification for internet gaming disorder prevention: Evaluation of a Wise IT-Use (WIT) Program for Hong Kong primary students. *Frontiers in psychology, 10*, 2468. https://doi.org/10.3389/fpsyg.2019.02468

Chen, Y., Lu, J., Wang, L., & Gao, X. (2023). Effective interventions for gaming disorder: A systematic review of randomized control trials. *Frontiers in Psychiatry, 14*, 1098922. https://doi.org/10.3389/fpsyt.2023.1098922

Chiang, C. L. L., Zhang, M. W. B., & Ho, R. C. M. (2022). Prevalence of internet gaming disorder in medical students: A meta-analysis. *Frontiers in Psychiatry, 12*, 760911. https://doi.org/10.3389/fpsyt.2021.760911

Clemens, F., Hanewinkel, R., & Morgenstern, M. (2018). Exposure to gambling advertisements and gambling behavior in young people. *Journal of Gambling Studies, 33*(1), 1–13. https://doi.org/10.1007/s10899-016-9606-x

Dong, G., & Potenza, M. N. (2014). A cognitive-behavioral model of internet gaming disorder: Theoretical underpinnings and clinical implications. *Journal of Psychiatric Research, 58*, 7–11. https://doi.org/10.1016/j.jpsychires.2014.07.005

Dong, G., Lu, Q., Zhou, H., & Zhao, X. (2011). Impulse inhibition in people with internet addiction disorder: Electrophysiological evidence from a Go/NoGo study. *Neuroscience Letters, 485*(2), 138–142.

Dowling, N., Smith, D., & Thomas, T. (2007). A comparison of individual and group cognitive-behavioural treatment for female pathological gambling. *Behaviour Research and Therapy, 45*(9), 2192–2202. https://doi.org/10.1016/j.brat.2006.11.003

Fathuldeen, A., Alshammiri, M. F., & Abdulmohsen, A. (2023). Prevalence and awareness of musculoskeletal injuries associated with competitive video gaming in Saudi Arabia. *Cureus, 15*(4), e37733. https://doi.org/10.7759/cureus.37733

Fátima, A., & Amin, R. (2023). Academic performance and internet gaming disorder: A cross-sectional study. *Journal of Professional & Applied Psychology, 4*(4), 531–544. https://doi.org/10.52053/jpap.v4i4.243

Fong, W. T. (2005). Types of psychotherapy for pathological gamblers. *Psychiatry (Edgmont), 2*(5), 40–46. https://pubmed.ncbi.nlm.nih.gov/21152147/

Footitt, T., Christofi, N., Poulus, D. R., Colder Carras, M., & Stavropoulos, V. (2024). Gaming disorder: The role of a gamers flow profile. *Addictive Behaviors Reports, 19*, 100555. https://doi.org/10.1016/j.abrep.2024.100555

Garcia, B. T. D., Merlotto, A. C., Domingos, F. C., Siqueira, A., & Carolina, A. (2024). The impact of the abuse of electronic games in children and adolescents: Scoping review. *Brazilian Journal of Health Review, 7*(1), 111–133. https://doi.org/10.34119/bjhrv7n1-010

Gentile, D. A., Anderson, C. A., Yukawa, S., Ihori, N., Saleem, M., Ming, L. K., Shibuya, A., Liau, A. K., Khoo, A., Bushman, B. J., Rowell Huesmann, L., & Sakamoto, A. (2009). The effects of prosocial video games on prosocial behaviors: International evidence from correlational, longitudinal, and experimental studies. *Personality & Social Psychology Bulletin, 35*(6), 752–763. https://doi.org/10.1177/0146167209333045

Ghali, S., Afifi, S., Suryadevara, V., Habab, Y., Hutcheson, A., Panjiyar, B. K., Davydov, G. G., Nashat, H., & Nath, T. S. (2023). A systematic review of the association of internet gaming disorder and excessive social media use with psychiatric comorbidities in children and adolescents: Is it a curse or a blessing? *Cureus, 15*(8), e43835. https://doi.org/10.7759/cureus.43835

Gómez-Gonzalvo, F., Devís-Devís, J., & Molina-Alventosa, P. (2020). Video game usage time in adolescents' academic performance. *Comunicar, 28*(65), 89–99. https://doi.org/10.3916/c65-2020-08

Green, L., & Myerson, J. (2004). A discounting framework for choice with delayed and probabilistic rewards. *Psychological Bulletin, 130*(5), 769–792. https://doi.org/10.1037/0033-2909.130.5.769

Han, D. H., Kim, S. M., Lee, Y. S., & Renshaw, P. F. (2012). The effect of family therapy on the changes in the severity of on-line game play and brain activity in adolescents with on-line game addiction. *Psychiatry Research: Neuroimaging, 202*(2), 126–131.

Han, J., Seo, Y., Hwang, H., Kim, M. S., & Han, D. H. (2020). Efficacy of cognitive behavioral therapy for internet gaming disorder. *Clinical Psychology & Psychotherapy, 27*(2), 147–154. https://doi.org/10.1002/cpp.2419

Hawi, N., & Samaha, M. (2024). Relationships of gaming disorder, ADHD, and academic performance in university students: A mediation analysis. *PLoS One, 19*(4), e0300680. https://doi.org/10.1371/journal.pone.0300680

Hofstedt, A., Mide, M., Arvidson, E., Ljung, S., Mattiasson, J., Lindskog, A., & Söderpalm-Gordh, A. (2023). Pilot data findings from the Gothenburg treatment for gaming disorder: A cognitive behavioral treatment manual. *Frontiers in Psychiatry, 14*, 1162492. https://doi.org/10.3389/fpsyt.2023.1162492

Idris, M. F., Saini, S. M., Sharip, S., Idris, N. F., & Ab Aziz, N. F. (2023). Association between the internet gaming disorder and anxiety and depression among university students during COVID-19 pandemic. *Healthcare (Basel, Switzerland), 11*(8), 1103. https://doi.org/10.3390/healthcare11081103

Imakata, T., Izumi, W., & Miyamoto, R. (2024). Gaming disorders: Navigating the fine line between entertainment and addiction—Gaming history, health risks, social consequences, and pathways to prevention. *Journal of Clinical Medicine, 13*(17), 5122. https://doi.org/10.3390/jcm13175122

Isralowitz, R., Romem Porat, S. L., Zolotov, Y., Yehudai, M., Dagan, A., & Reznik, A. (2022). Gaming disorder and psycho-emotional wellbeing among male university students and other young adults in Israel. *International Journal of Environmental Research and Public Health, 19*(23), 15946. https://doi.org/10.3390/ijerph192315946

Jang, J. H., Chung, S. J., Choi, A., Lee, J. Y., Kim, B., Park, M., Park, S., & Choi, J. S. (2021). Association of general cognitive functions with gaming use in young adults: A comparison among excessive gamers, regular gamers and non-gamers. *Journal of Clinical Medicine, 10*(11), 2293. https://doi.org/10.3390/jcm10112293

Ji, Y., & Wong, D. F. K. (2023). Effectiveness of an integrated motivational cognitive-behavioral group intervention for adolescents with gaming disorder: A randomized controlled trial. *Addiction (Abingdon, England), 118*(11), 2093–2104. https://doi.org/10.1111/add.16292

King, D. L., & Delfabbro, P. H. (2018). Predatory monetization schemes in video games (e.g. 'loot boxes') and internet gaming disorder. *Addiction (Abingdon, England), 113*(11), 1967–1969. https://doi.org/10.1111/add.14286

King, A., & Wong-Padoongpatt, G. (2022). Do gamers play for money? A moderated mediation of gaming motives, relative deprivation, and upward mobility. *International Journal of Environmental Research and Public Health, 19*(22), 15384. https://doi.org/10.3390/ijerph192215384

King, D. L., Russell, A., & Hing, N. (2020). Adolescent land-based and internet gambling: Australian and international prevalence rates and measurement issues. *Current Addiction Reports, 7*(2), 137–148. https://doi.org/10.1007/s40429-020-00278-z

Király, O., Griffiths, M. D., King, D. L., Lee, H. K., Lee, S. Y., Bányai, F., Zsila, Á., Takács, Z. K., & Demetrovics, Z. (2018). Policy responses to problematic video game use: A systematic review of current measures and future possibilities. *Journal of Behavioral Addictions, 7*(3), 503–517. https://doi.org/10.1556/2006.7.2018.48

Kleinman, R. A., & Das, S. (2020). Excessive spending in a "free-to-play" smartphone game. *The American Journal on Addictions, 29*(6), 528–530. https://doi.org/10.1111/ajad.13049

Knutson, B., Westdorp, A., Kaiser, E., & Hommer, D. (2001). FMRI visualization of brain activity during a monetary incentive delay task. *NeuroImage, 12*(1), 20–27.

Ko, C.-H., Yen, J.-Y., Chen, S.-H., Wang, P.-W., & Chen, C.-S. (2014). Evaluation of the diagnostic criteria of internet gaming disorder in the DSM-5 among young adults in Taiwan. *Journal of Psychiatric Research, 53*, 103–110. https://doi.org/10.1016/j.jpsychires.2014.02.008

Kohorst, M. A., Warad, D. M., Nageswara Rao, A. A., & Rodriguez, V. (2018). Obesity, sedentary lifestyle, and video games: The new thrombophilia cocktail in adolescents. *Pediatric Blood & Cancer, 65*(7), e27041. https://doi.org/10.1002/pbc.27041

Krossbakken, E., Torsheim, T., Mentzoni, R. A., King, D. L., Bjorvatn, B., Lorvik, I. M., & Pallesen, S. (2018). The effectiveness of a parental guide for prevention of problematic video gaming in children: A public health randomized controlled intervention study. *Journal of Behavioral Addictions, 7*(1), 52–61. https://doi.org/10.1556/2006.6.2017.087

Kühn, S., Romanowski, A., Schilling, C., Lorenz, R., Morsen, C., & Gallinat, J. (2011). The neural basis of video gaming: A systematic review of functional and structural MRI studies. *Translational Psychiatry, 1*(e53), 1–11.

Kuss, D. J. (2013). Internet gaming addiction: Current perspectives. *Psychology Research and Behavior Management, 6*, 125–137.

Kuss, D. J. (2018). Policy, prevention, and regulation for internet gaming disorder. *Journal of Behavioral Addictions, 7*(3), 553–555. https://doi.org/10.1556/2006.7.2018.79

Kuss, D. J., & Griffiths, M. D. (2018). Internet gaming addiction: A systematic review of empirical research. *International Journal of Mental Health and Addiction, 10*(2), 278–296.

Leonardi, J. L., & Meyer, S. B. (2015). Prática baseada em evidências em psicologia e a história da busca pelas provas empíricas da eficácia das psicoterapias. *Psicologia: Ciência E Profissão, 35*(4), 1139–1156. https://doi.org/10.1590/1982-3703001552014

Li, A. Y., Chau, C. L., & Cheng, C. (2019). Development and validation of a parent-based program for preventing gaming disorder: The game over intervention. *International Journal of Environmental Research and Public Health, 16*(11), 1984. https://doi.org/10.3390/ijerph16111984

Li, L., Niu, Z., Song, Y., Griffiths, M. D., Wen, H., Yu, Z., & Mei, S. (2023). Relationships between gaming disorder, risk factors, and protective factors among a sample of Chinese University students utilizing a network perspective. *International Journal of Mental Health and Addiction*, 1–19. https://doi.org/10.1007/s11469-023-01049-3

Liao, Z., Huang, Q., Huang, S., Tan, L., Shao, T., Fang, T., Chen, X., Lin, S., Qi, J., Cai, Y., & Shen, H. (2020). Prevalence of internet gaming disorder and its association with personality traits and gaming characteristics among Chinese adolescent gamers. *Frontiers in Psychiatry, 11*, 598585. https://doi.org/10.3389/fpsyt.2020.598585

Lim, J. A., Lee, J. Y., Jung, H. Y., Sohn, B. K., Choi, S. W., Kim, Y. J., Kim, D. J., & Choi, J. S. (2016). Changes of quality of life and cognitive function in individuals with internet gaming disorder: A 6-month follow-up. *Medicine, 95*(50), e5695. https://doi.org/10.1097/MD.0000000000005695

Limone, P., Ragni, B., & Toto, G. A. (2023). The epidemiology and effects of video game addiction: A systematic review and meta-analysis. *Acta Psychologica, 241*, 104047. https://doi.org/10.1016/j.actpsy.2023.104047

Lindberg, L., Nielsen, S. B., Damgaard, M., Sloth, O. R., Rathleff, M. S., & Straszek, C. L. (2020). Musculoskeletal pain is common in competitive gaming: A cross-sectional study among Danish esports athletes. *BMJ Open Sport & Exercise Medicine, 6*(1), 000799. https://doi.org/10.1136/bmjsem-2020-000799

Lindenberg, K., Kindt, S., & Szász-Janocha, C. (2022). Effectiveness of cognitive behavioral therapy-based intervention in preventing gaming disorder and unspecified internet use disorder in adolescents: A cluster randomized clinical trial. *JAMA Network Open, 5*(2), e2148995. https://doi.org/10.1001/jamanetworkopen.2021.48995

Long, J., Bhad, R., Potenza, M. N., Orsolini, L., Phan, V., Kanabar, M., & Achab, S. (2022). Public health approaches and policy changes after the inclusion of gaming disorder in ICD-11: Global needs. *BJPsych International, 19*(3), 63–66. https://doi.org/10.1192/bji.2021.57

Lorenz, R. C., Gleich, T., Gallinat, J., & Kühn, S. (2015). Video game training and the reward system. *Frontiers in Human Neuroscience, 9*, 40. https://doi.org/10.3389/fnhum.2015.00040

Madden, G. J., & Bickel, W. K. (Eds.). (2010). *Impulsivity: The behavioral and neurological science of discounting*. American Psychological Association. https://doi.org/10.1037/12069-000

Mardon, A. (2021). *The history of board games*. Golden Meteorite Press.

Marin, M. G., Nuñez, X., & de Almeida, R. M. M. (2021). Internet addiction and attention in adolescents: A systematic review. *Cyberpsychology, Behavior, and Social Networking, 24*(4), 237–245. https://doi.org/10.1089/cyber.2020.0665

Mills, D., Mettler, J., Sornberger, M., & Heath, N. (2016). Adolescent problematic gaming and domain-specific perceptions of self. *International Journal of Cyber Behavior, Psychology and Learning, 6*(4), 44–56. https://doi.org/10.4018/ijcbpl.2016100104

Mohammad, S., Jan, R. A., & Alsaedi, S. L. (2023). Symptoms, mechanisms, and treatments of video game addiction. *Cureus, 15*(3), e36957. https://doi.org/10.7759/cureus.36957

Müller, K. W., Dreier, M., Beutel, M. E., Ruckes, C., Batra, A., Mann, K., Musalek, M., & Wölfling, K. (2023). The impact of life satisfaction in the treatment of gaming disorder and other internet use disorders: Results from a randomized controlled trial. *Journal of Behavioral Addictions, 12*(1), 159–167. https://doi.org/10.1556/2006.2022.00091

Myrseth, H., Litlerè, I., Støylen, I., & Pallesen, S. (2009). Um estudo controlado do efeito da terapia cognitivo-comportamental em grupo para jogadores patológicos. *Nordic Journal of Psychiatry, 63*(1), 22–31. https://doi.org/10.1080/08039480802055139

Nielsen, P., Christensen, M., Henderson, C., Liddle, H. A., Croquette-Krokar, M., Favez, N., & Rigter, H. (2021). Multidimensional family therapy reduces problematic gaming in adolescents: A randomised controlled trial. *Journal of Behavioral Addictions, 10*(2), 234–243. https://doi.org/10.1556/2006.2021.00022

Northrup, J. C., & Shumway, S. (2024). Gamer widow: A phenomenological study of spouses of online video game addicts. *American Journal of Family Therapy, 42*(4), 269–281. https://doi.org/10.1080/01926187.2024.1914313

Pallavicini, F., Pepe, A., & Mantovani, F. (2022). The effects of playing video games on stress, anxiety, depression, loneliness, and gaming disorder during the early stages of the COVID-19 pandemic: PRISMA systematic review. *Cyberpsychology, Behavior and Social Networking, 25*(6), 334–354. https://doi.org/10.1089/cyber.2021.0252

Paulus, F. W., Ohmann, S., von Gontard, A., & Popow, C. (2018). Internet gaming disorder in children and adolescents: A systematic review. *Developmental Medicine and Child Neurology, 60*(7), 645–659. https://doi.org/10.1111/dmcn.13754

Petry, N. M., Ammerman, Y., Bohl, J., Doersch, A., Gay, H., Kadden, R., Molina, C., & Steinberg, K. (2006). Cognitive-behavioral therapy for pathological gamblers. *Journal of Consulting and Clinical Psychology, 74*(3), 555–567. https://doi.org/10.1037/0022-006X.74.3.555

Phan, O., Prieur, C., Bonnaire, C., & Obradovic, I. (2019). Internet gaming disorder: Exploring its impact on satisfaction in life in PELLEAS adolescent sample. *International Journal of Environmental Research and Public Health, 17*(1), 3. https://doi.org/10.3390/ijerph17010003

Ramesh, D., Navalagund, S., Peerapur, S. M., & Sunil, M. B. (2023). Effectiveness of an awareness programme to assess the knowledge regarding gaming disorder among adolescents in selected schools of Hubballi. *International Journal of Nursing Education and Research.* https://doi.org/10.52711/2454-2660.2023.00067

Rasmussen, M., Meilstrup, C., Bendtsen, P., Pedersen, T., Nielsen, L., Madsen, K., & Holstein, B. (2014). Perceived problems with computer gaming and internet use are associated with poorer social relations in adolescence. *International Journal of Public Health, 60*(2), 179–188. https://doi.org/10.1007/s00038-014-0633-z

Reichert, R. A., Martins, G. D. G., da Silva, A. M. B., Scatena, A., Barbugli, B. C., De Micheli, D., & Andrade, A. L. M. (2021a). New forms of addiction: Digital media. In A. L. M. Andrade, D. De Micheli, E. Aparecida da Silva, F. M. Lopes, B. O. Pinheiro, & R. A. Reichert (Eds.), *Psychology of substance abuse: Psychotherapy, clinical management and social intervention* (pp. 43–53). Springer. https://doi.org/10.1007/978-3-030-62106-3_3

Reichert, R. A., Calixto, F., da Silva, A. M. B., Martins, G. D. G., Barbugli, B. C., Scatena, A., Lessa, R. T., De Micheli, D., & Andrade, A. L. M. (2021b). Digital games, shopping, sex, and other addictions: Neuropsychological and behavioral correlates. In D. De Micheli, A. L. M. Andrade, R. A. Reichert, E. Aparecida da Silva, B. O. Pinheiro, & F. M. Lopes (Eds.), *Drugs and human behavior: Biopsychosocial aspects of psychotropic substances use* (pp. 443–458). Springer. https://doi.org/10.1007/978-3-030-62855-0_32

Ribeiro, E. O., Afonso, N. H., & Morgado, P. (2021). Non-pharmacological treatment of gambling disorder: A systematic review of randomized controlled trials. *BMC Psychiatry, 21*(1). https://doi.org/10.1186/s12888-021-03097-2

Rogers, R. D., Everitt, B. J., Baldacchino, A., Blackshaw, A. J., Swainson, R., Wynne, K., et al. (1999). Dissociable deficits in the decision-making cognition of chronic amphetamine abusers, opiate abusers, patients with focal damage to prefrontal cortex, and tryptophan-depleted normal volunteers: Evidence for monoaminergic mechanisms. *Neuropsychopharmacology, 20*(4), 322–339.

Rojas-Jara, C., Polanco-Carrasco, R., Navarro-Castillo, R., Faúndez-Castillo, F., & Chamorro-Gallardo, M. (2022). "Game (not) over": A systematic review of video game disorder in adolescents. *Revista Colombiana de Psicología, 31*(2), 45–64. https://doi.org/10.15446/rcp.v31n2.90741

Sandín, B., Chorot, P., & Valiente, R. M. (2012). Transdiagnostic: A new frontier in clinical psychology. *Revista de Psicopatología Y Psicología Clínica, 17*(3), 185. https://doi.org/10.5944/rppc.vol.17.num.3.2012.11839

Santos, I. K. D., Medeiros, R. C. S. C., Medeiros, J. A., Almeida-Neto, P. F., Sena, D. C. S., Cobucci, R. N., Oliveira, R. S., Cabral, B. G. A. T., & Dantas, P. M. S. (2021). Active video games for improving mental health and physical fitness—An alternative for children and adolescents during social isolation: An overview. *International Journal of Environmental Research and Public Health, 18*(4). https://doi.org/10.3390/ijerph18041641

Satish-Kumar, C. R., Sharma, M. K., Amudhan, S., Arya, S., Mahapatra, S., Anand, N., Sahu, A., Kumar, R., & Tripathi, R. (2023). Digital gaming, musculoskeletal, and related health hazards among adolescents and young adults. *Indian Journal of Psychiatry, 65*(6), 698–700. https://doi.org/10.4103/indianjpsychiatry.indianjpsychiatry_818_22

Saunders, J. B., Hao, W., Long, J., King, D. L., Mann, K., Fauth-Bühler, M., Rumpf, H. J., Bowden-Jones, H., Rahimi-Movaghar, A., Chung, T., Chan, E., Bahar, N., Achab, S., Lee, H. K., Potenza, M., Petry, N., Spritzer, D., Ambekar, A., Derevensky, J., … Poznyak, V. (2017). Gaming disorder: Its delineation as an important condition for diagnosis, management, and prevention. *Journal of Behavioral Addictions, 6*(3), 271–279. https://doi.org/10.1556/2006.6.2017.039

Schneider, L. A., King, D. L., & Delfabbro, P. H. (2017). Family factors in adolescent problematic internet gaming: A systematic review. *Journal of Behavioral Addictions, 6*(3), 321–333. https://doi.org/10.1556/2006.6.2017.035

Severo, R. B., Soares, J. M., Affonso, J. P., Giusti, D. A., de Souza Junior, A. A., de Figueiredo, V. L., Pinheiro, K. A., & Pontes, H. M. (2020). Prevalence and risk factors for internet gaming disorder. *Brazilian Journal of Psychiatry, 42*(5), 532–535. https://doi.org/10.1590/1516-4446-2019-0760

She, R., Zhang, Y., & Yang, X. (2022). Parental factors associated with internet gaming disorder among first-year high school students: Longitudinal study. *JMIR Serious Games, 10*(4), e33806. https://doi.org/10.2196/33806

Stevens, M. W. R., King, D. L., Dorstyn, D., & Delfabbro, P. H. (2019). Cognitive-behavioral therapy for internet gaming disorder: A systematic review and meta-analysis. *Clinical Psychology & Psychotherapy, 26*(2), 191–203. https://doi.org/10.1002/cpp.2341

Stevens, M. W., Dorstyn, D., Delfabbro, P. H., & King, D. L. (2021). Global prevalence of gaming disorder: A systematic review and meta-analysis. *The Australian and New Zealand Journal of Psychiatry, 55*(6), 553–568. https://doi.org/10.1177/0004867420962851

Sun, R. Q., Sun, G. F., & Ye, J. H. (2023). The effects of online game addiction on reduced academic achievement motivation among Chinese college students: The mediating role of learning engagement. *Frontiers in Psychology, 14*, 1185353. https://doi.org/10.3389/fpsyg.2023.1185353

Sylvain, C., Ladouceur, R., & Boisvert, J. M. (1997). Cognitive and behavioral treatment of pathological gambling: A controlled study. *Journal of Consulting and Clinical Psychology, 65*(5), 727–732. https://doi.org/10.1037/0022-006X.65.5.727

Szász-Janocha, C., Magann, M., Gold, H., Lindenberg, K., Delfabbro, P., & King, D. L. (2023). Problem gaming-related harm experienced by partners and parents of individuals with gaming problems and their help-seeking experiences. *Journal of Behavioral Addictions, 12*(1), 137–147. https://doi.org/10.1556/2006.2023.00003

Tholl, C., Bickmann, P., Wechsler, K., Froböse, I., & Grieben, C. (2022). Musculoskeletal disorders in video gamers—A systematic review. *BMC Musculoskeletal Disorders, 23*(1), 678. https://doi.org/10.1186/s12891-022-05614-0

Throuvala, M. A., Janikian, M., Griffiths, M. D., Rennoldson, M., & Kuss, D. J. (2019). The role of family and personality traits in internet gaming disorder: A mediation model combining cognitive and attachment perspectives. *Journal of Behavioral Addictions, 8*(1), 48–62. https://doi.org/10.1556/2006.8.2019.05

Torres-Rodríguez, A., Griffiths, M. D., & Carbonell, X. (2017). The treatment of internet gaming disorder: A brief overview of the PIPATIC program. *International Journal of Mental Health and Addiction, 16*(4), 1000–1015. https://doi.org/10.1007/s11469-017-9825-0

Wang, Q., Ren, H., Long, J., Liu, Y., & Liu, T. (2019). Research progress and debates on gaming disorder. *General Psychiatry, 32*(3), e100071. https://doi.org/10.1136/gpsych-2019-100071

Wang, L., Yang, G., Zheng, Y., Li, Z., Wei, P., Li, Q., Hu, K., & Liu, X. (2021). Neural substrates of deficient cognitive control in individuals with severe internet gaming disorder. *NeuroImage. Clinical, 32*, 102828. https://doi.org/10.1016/j.nicl.2021.102828

Wang, Y., Liu, B., Zhang, L., & Zhang, P. (2022). Anxiety, depression, and stress are associated with internet gaming disorder during COVID-19: Fear of missing out as a mediator. *Frontiers in Psychiatry, 13*, 827519. https://doi.org/10.3389/fpsyt.2022.827519

Wang, X., Liu, Y., Chu, H. K., Wong, S. Y., & Yang, X. (2023). Relationships of internet gaming engagement, history, and maladaptive cognitions and adolescent internet gaming disorder: A cross-sectional study. *PLoS One, 18*(9), e0290955. https://doi.org/10.1371/journal.pone.0290955

Wardle, H. (2021). *Games without frontiers?: Socio-historical perspectives at the gaming/gambling intersection.* Palgrave Macmillan.

Weinstein, A. M. (2017). An update overview on brain imaging studies of internet gaming disorder. *Frontiers in Psychiatry, 8*, 185.

Weinstein, A., & Lejoyeux, M. (2020). Neurobiological mechanisms underlying internet gaming disorder. *Dialogues in Clinical Neuroscience, 22*(2), 113–126. https://doi.org/10.31887/DCNS.2020.22.2/aweinstein

Werner, M., Kapetanovic, S., & Claesdotter-Knutsson, E. (2024). Family-centered treatment program for problematic gaming and excessive screen use in a clinical child and youth population (FAME): Protocol for a feasibility pilot mixed method study. *JMIR Research Protocols, 13*, e56387. https://doi.org/10.2196/56387

World Health Organization (WHO). (2018). *International classification of diseases for mortality and morbidity statistics* (11th Revision). World Health Organization. https://icd.who.int/browse11/l-m/en

Yuan, K., Qin, W., Yu, D., Bi, Y., Xing, L., Jin, C., & Tian, J. (2013a). Microstructural abnormalities in adolescents with internet addiction disorder. *PLoS One, 8*(6), e63597.

Yuan, K., Yu, D., Cai, C., Feng, D., Li, Y., Bi, Y., & Tian, J. (2013b). Cortical thickness abnormalities in late adolescence with online gaming addiction. *PLoS One, 8*(1), e53055. https://doi.org/10.1371/journal.pone.0053055

Yuan, K., Cheng, P., Dong, T., Bi, Y., Xing, L., Yu, D., & Tian, J. (2016). Dysfunctional connectivity in the ventral tegmental area-accumbens pathway in internet gaming disorder. *Brain Imaging and Behavior, 10*(3), 719–728. https://doi.org/10.1007/s11682-015-9358-8

Yuan, K., Cheng, P., Dong, T., Bi, Y., Xing, L., Yu, D., & Tian, J. (2017). Frontostriatal circuits, resting state functional connectivity and cognitive control in internet gaming disorder. *Addiction Biology, 22*(3), 813–822. https://doi.org/10.1111/adb.12348

Zhang, Z., Wang, S., Du, X., Qi, Y., Wang, L., & Dong, G. H. (2023). Brain responses to positive and negative events in individuals with internet gaming disorder during real gaming. *Journal of Behavioral Addictions, 12*(3), 758–774. https://doi.org/10.1556/2006.2023.00039

Zhang, L., Han, J., Liu, M., Yang, C., & Liao, Y. (2024). The prevalence and possible risk factors of gaming disorder among adolescents in China. *BMC Psychiatry, 24*(1). https://doi.org/10.1186/s12888-024-05826-9

Zhou, Y., Lin, F. C., Du, Y. S., Qin, L. D., Zhao, Z. M., Xu, J. R., & Lei, H. (2011). Gray matter abnormalities in internet addiction: A voxel-based morphometry study. *European Journal of Radiology, 79*(1), 92–95.

Zhou, H., Dang, L., Wells, A., & Wu, A. M. S. (2023a). Risk factors for internet gaming disorder: Testing the contribution of metacognitions, stress, and coping. *Addictive Behaviors, 147*, 107836. https://doi.org/10.1016/j.addbeh.2023.107836

Zhou, J., Zhao, H., Wang, L., & Zhu, D. (2023b). The vicious cycle of family dysfunction and problematic gaming and the mediating role of self-concept clarity among early adolescents: A within-person analysis using random intercept cross-lagged panel modeling. *Journal of Behavioral Addictions, 12*(4), 920–937. https://doi.org/10.1556/2006.2023.00054

Chapter 5
Exploring the Intersection of Cyberbullying and Digital Addiction

Cláudio Romualdo, Antônio Marcos Neves Esteca, and Wanderlei Abadio de Oliveira

Introduction

Cyberbullying is characterized by the intentional and repetitive use of digital tools such as social networks, emails, and messaging applications to intimidate, humiliate, or cause emotional distress to an individual (Zhang et al., 2022a). According to Kowalski et al. (2014), cyberbullying differs from traditional bullying as it transcends physical boundaries, allowing the perpetrator to reach the victim at any time and place, amplifying the violence's impact.

Among its primary characteristics are intentionality, which reflects the deliberate intent to cause harm; repetition, evidencing a continuous and systematic behavior; power imbalance, which can manifest through the perpetrator's technological or social superiority; anonymity, often encouraging aggressive actions due to the difficulty of identification; and public exposure, which extends the violence's reach to a larger audience, increasing the victim's humiliation (Zhang et al., 2022b). While this phenomenon can occur at any age, it is particularly impactful during childhood and adolescence due to the unique developmental conditions of these age groups.

The types and forms of cyberbullying vary based on the media used and the nature of aggression. Main types include verbal cyberbullying, such as insults, threats, and online humiliation; social cyberbullying, involving exclusion and defamation; psychological cyberbullying, marked by emotional manipulation and harassment; and sexual cyberbullying, encompassing practices like sexting and cyberflashing. These aggressions can occur through text messages and social networks, with frequent offensive comments and negative posts; images and videos, including sharing humiliating or inappropriate content; emails and online chats,

C. Romualdo (✉) · A. M. N. Esteca · W. A. de Oliveira
Pontifical Catholic University of Campinas, Campinas, Brazil
e-mail: romualdo@didaciebe.com.br; tecnologia@faculdademetropolitana.edu.br

A. L. M. Andrade (ed.), *Digital Addictions*,
https://doi.org/10.1007/978-3-031-87986-9_5

involving hate messages or real-time threats; and even blogs and websites created specifically to defame and intimidate (Krešić Ćorić & Kaštelan, 2020).

The impacts of cyberbullying are multifaceted. Studies indicate that victims often experience low self-esteem, feeling devalued, and insecure (Craig et al., 2020; Gohal et al., 2023). Furthermore, anxiety and depression are common consequences. Social isolation is also frequent, with victims avoiding interactions and struggling to establish interpersonal relationships. Physical health issues, such as sleep disturbances like insomnia and nightmares, may lead to self-destructive behaviors, including self-harm and suicidal tendencies.

While scientific literature recognizes the severity of cyberbullying and its consequences, there is still a lack of studies exploring the relationship between this phenomenon and increasingly prevalent online behaviors. The massive use of social networks, instant messaging platforms, and other digital tools has changed the dynamics of social interactions, creating new spaces that may facilitate cyberbullying. Therefore, it is essential to conduct in-depth studies to investigate how the contemporary digital context shapes and intensifies cyberbullying occurrences.

The Present Study

This review aimed to document the relationships between the problematic use of social networks or digital media and the perpetration or victimization of cyberbullying among adolescents aged 10 to 19 years. Other variables of interest, such as mental health issues and social support (familial, school, or peer-based), were also analyzed to elucidate these relationships.

Method

This study employed a rapid review (RR) methodology following the guidelines of the Cochrane Rapid Reviews Methods Group. A RR applies modified systematic review methods to accelerate the review process while maintaining rigor, transparency, and reproducibility (Gartlehner et al., 2024). The steps for conducting a RR include formulating a guiding question, designing a search protocol, streamlining the selection process, extracting data, and ensuring quality (Smela et al., 2023).

The guiding question for this RR was: What is the relationship between cyberbullying and adolescents' (aged 10 to 19 years) experiences in digital media or social networks? Searches were conducted in three databases (Web of Science, Scopus, and SciELO) using the following terms: "cyberbullying AND digital media" and "cyberbullying AND social media." Inclusion criteria were empirical research articles involving adolescents aged 10 to 19 years, published in Portuguese, English, or Spanish between 2020 and 2024. Exclusion criteria included editorials, commentaries, and literature reviews.

After conducting the searches, the identified texts were exported to the Rayyan platform (Ouzzani et al., 2016). Titles and abstracts of the identified articles underwent initial screening. Subsequently, preselected articles were retrieved in full and evaluated against the guiding question and inclusion and exclusion criteria. Finally, the data were analyzed descriptively and qualitatively using the tool "requalify.ai."

Results

Initially, duplicates identified across databases were removed. Subsequently, using Rayyan's tools, studies that could be easily excluded, very easily excluded, or marked as without recommendation were identified. Excluded studies did not meet the established inclusion criteria, particularly regarding participants' profiles, study types (e.g., theoretical, reflective, or review studies), and outcomes that did not address the research question. Most exclusions were due to a lack of clarity or absence of cyberbullying as an analytical variable. Studies focusing on neurodivergent or disabled populations were also excluded. Similarly, studies developed during or about the COVID-19 pandemic, as well as studies on online gaming or the deep web, were excluded.

A total of 20 articles were selected for this RR, and the selection process flow is presented in Fig. 5.1.

The inclusion criteria focused on the clear relationship between social media use and cyberbullying among adolescents, as well as detailed analyses of behavioral or emotional predictors and consequences associated with this phenomenon. Studies

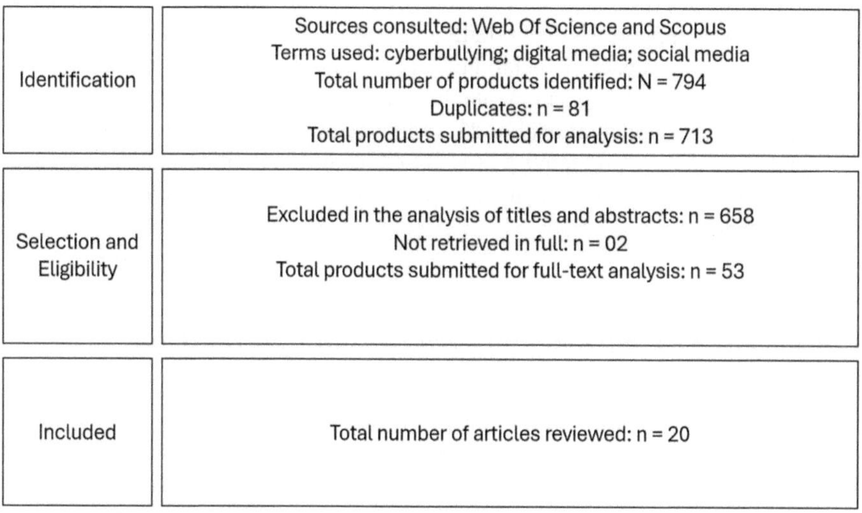

Fig. 5.1 Flowchart of the search and selection process

examining mediating variables like problematic media use, familial factors, and personal characteristics in the cyberbullying context were included.

The reviewed articles were published in English across diverse health and education journals. Nineteen studies were quantitative with cross-sectional designs, and one was qualitative (Felice et al., 2022). China, Spain, and Italy were the most represented countries, each contributing three articles. Table 5.1 presents bibliometric data, objectives, and key findings of the reviewed studies.

It is noted that all the reviewed studies, to some extent, indicate a relationship between behaviors or problematic use of social networks or digital media and involvement in cyberbullying situations. The results show that different mechanisms should be considered when evaluating these issues in adolescence. Furthermore, aspects such as gender and lack of social support emerged as risk factors. At the same time, positive family support and interaction were identified as protective factors. These findings should be discussed in terms of how they can support practices for the prevention and treatment of these problems, and in this regard, Table 5.2 presents the most critical findings.

The results of the reviewed studies were also subjected to qualitative analysis using the "requalify.ai" tool. This analysis identified 24 analytical tags with a high similarity coefficient: 1. predictors of cyberbullying perpetration, 2. impact of parental control, 3. importance of emotional regulation, 4. problematic Internet use and cyberbullying, 5. relationship between bullying experience and online aggression, 6. analysis of the role of the aggressor and the victim, 7. experience with aggression and cyberbullying, 8. relationship between screen time and cyberbullying, 9. psychological risk model on social networks, 10. impact of social support on victimization, 11. prevalence of cyberbullying among adolescents, 12. gender differences in cyberbullying experiences, 13. emotional intelligence and aggressive behavior, 14. impact of family support on mental health, 15. complexity of digital interactions, 16. prevalence of cyberbullying among genders, 17. relationship between family support and cyberbullying victimization, 18. protective effect of social support, 19. impact of social media addiction on victimization, 20. intersection between cyberbullying and mental health, 21. prevalence of cyberbullying, 22. impact of threats on mental health, 23. influence of family support, and 24. emotional intelligence as a protective factor. Based on the similarities and convergences of themes, the 24 tags were organized into three analytical categories that will be presented below.

Category 1: Risk Factors and Predictors of Cyberbullying

The reviewed studies exhibited varying prevalence rates. For instance, a study documenting cyberbullying and cybervictimization within the past 30 days and over a lifetime reported the following rates: 14.4% cyberbullying and 19.8% cybervictimization in the recent past and 24.2% cyberbullying and 42.2% cybervictimization over a lifetime (Kunwar et al., 2024). Problematic Internet, network, or social media

Table 5.1 Bibliometric data, main objectives, and results of the reviewed articles

Reference	Country	Objectives	Main results
Lahti et al. (2024)	Finland	Investigate the prevalence of nine social media threats in adolescence	Adolescents face social media threats, including misinformation, dangerous challenges, and aesthetic pressures. Although cyberbullying is less prevalent than other threats, adolescents reporting problematic social media use and communication with strangers are more exposed to cyberbullying. Mental health issues were also observed
Topan et al. (2024)	Turkey	Investigate the relationship between cyberbullying/victimization and technology addiction among adolescents	72.5% of the sample reported spending a lot of time on social media, with 77.7% not considering the platforms safe. Those exposed to cyberbullying showed higher levels of distress and reactivity to humiliating comments. Acts such as sharing photos without permission or unfriending online increased levels of victimization and digital aggression

(continued)

Table 5.1 (continued)

Reference	Country	Objectives	Main results
Peprah et al. (2024)	Intercultural	Examine the mediating effect of problematic social media use (PSMU) on the association between cyberbullying victimization and psychosomatic complaints among adolescents in high-income countries	Cyberbullying victimization is associated with higher psychosomatic complaints, such as physical pain and stress symptoms. Problematic social media use moderated this relationship, with adolescents involved in cyberbullying and exhibiting PSMU showing higher levels of complaints. Family and peer support partially reduced the negative impact, but cyberbullying remained a significant predictor of physical and psychological distress
Kunwar et al. (2024)	Nepal	Assess the prevalence and factors associated with cyberbullying and cyber-victimization among adolescents	The prevalence of cyberbullying and cyber-victimization among adolescents was 14.4% (30 days prior to data collection) and 24.2% lifetime. Risk factors included being male, living in urban areas, and frequent internet use. Verbal attacks and offensive comments were the most common forms of cyberbullying and victimization, with daily internet users at higher risk. Adolescents using specific social networks (Facebook and Instagram) were less likely to engage in cyberbullying compared to WhatsApp and Twitter users

(continued)

Table 5.1 (continued)

Reference	Country	Objectives	Main results
Göksu et al. (2024)	Turkey	Examine the relationship between social media use, perceived social support, and cyberbullying among adolescent girls with or without major depressive disorder	Adolescents with depression showed higher levels of involvement in cyberbullying situations. Depressed adolescents reported greater social media use to seek social support and express needs but also experienced greater social isolation and less family and peer support. Social media use among depressed adolescents was associated with exposure to depressive content, increasing vulnerability to cyberbullying and its mental health impact
Torrecillas-Lacave et al. (2022)	Spain	Analyze the characteristics of youth digitalization and examine in depth the consequences of problematic internet use	Boys tended to use the internet for gaming and news; girls preferred social networks and communication. Girls also perceived online risks, including cyberbullying and harassment, more intensely and were more likely to report these experiences to family or friends. Cyberbullying affected girls more strongly, especially regarding physical appearance and public exposure
Aljasir and Alsebaei (2022)	Saudi Arabia	Investigate adolescents'perspectives on different parental mediation strategies concerning cyberbullying and cyber-victimization	Restrictive and online safety strategies were associated with lower levels of cyberbullying and cyber-victimization. Age moderated this relationship, with strategies being more effective among older adolescents. The results suggest that active parental mediation can reduce cyberbullying involvement, especially among older adolescents, highlighting the role of parents in positively influencing online behavior

(continued)

Table 5.1 (continued)

Reference	Country	Objectives	Main results
Lareki et al. (2023)	Intercultural	Determine associations between creating fake user accounts and involvement in cyberbullying behaviors	The use of fake accounts was correlated with cyberbullying involvement, being more common on platforms like Facebook and Twitter. Older male adolescents were more frequently involved in cyberbullying behaviors
Badrakh et al. (2023)	Mongolia	Investigate cyberbullying and cyber-victimization experiences and the relationship between psychosocial well-being and social media use	Adolescents with lower psychosocial well-being showed higher levels of cyberbullying and victimization. Problematic social media use partially mediated the relationship between well-being and cyberbullying involvement, suggesting that problematic social media use can exacerbate aggressive online behaviors. Male adolescents were more likely to be perpetrators, while both genders reported similar victimization rates
Borraccino et al. (2022)	Italy	Explore the role of family, peer, and teacher support in the association between cyberbullying and problematic media use	Cyber-victimization was more frequent among girls, especially at ages 11 and 13. Problematic media use was more common among younger adolescents and strongly associated with cyber-victimization risk. Social support (school, peer, and family) showed a significant protective effect against victimization and perpetration of cyberbullying

(continued)

Table 5.1 (continued)

Reference	Country	Objectives	Main results
Geng et al. (2022)	China	Investigate associations between social comparison orientation, cyberbullying perpetration, and victimization, considering envy on social media as a mediator and body satisfaction as a moderator	Adolescents with high social comparison orientation and low body satisfaction were more involved in cyberbullying, both as victims and perpetrators. Social media envy mediated this relationship, indicating that envious adolescents were more likely to engage in cyberbullying. High body satisfaction reduced the impact of social comparison orientation on envy, which in turn reduced cyberbullying involvement
Wong et al. (2022)	China	Examine the moderating role of inclusive norms in cyberbullying behaviors	Controlled and impulsive cyber aggression was positively associated with social media addiction and cyberbullying perpetration. Controlled and impulsive aggression mediated the effect of social media addiction on cyberbullying. Inclusive norms moderated the relationship between cyberbullying and social media addiction, with adolescents valuing inclusive norms showing a stronger association between these factors, suggesting they might engage in cyberbullying to reinforce group belonging
Nagata et al. (2022)	United States	Determine the prevalence and sociodemographic correlates of cyberbullying victimization and perpetration	Cyberbullying prevalence was higher among girls and adolescents from sexual and economic minorities. Adolescents with higher screen time, particularly on social media and the internet, showed increased rates of cyberbullying as both victims and perpetrators. Digital media platforms, especially social media, were associated with increased exposure to cyberbullying

(continued)

Table 5.1 (continued)

Reference	Country	Objectives	Main results
Zhang et al. (2022a)	China	Examine how sensation seeking (personality trait), boredom, and exposure to antisocial media content are associated with cyberbullying	Sensation seeking predisposes adolescents to cyberbullying, mediated by experiences of boredom and exposure to antisocial content on social media. Eighth-grade students reported higher levels of boredom and antisocial media exposure, increasing their likelihood of involvement in cyberbullying. Seeking intense emotions through social media as an escape from boredom exposed adolescents to negative content and aggressive behaviors
Felice et al. (2022)	Italy	Investigate the uses and dangers of social networks among adolescents and build a model of how they become hazardous	Social networks influence adolescents'self-image and can lead to dangerous behaviors, including cyberbullying and negative self-assessments. Using social networks for approval put adolescents at risk, especially those seeking external validation, exposing them to offenses and bullying situations
Marengo et al. (2021)	Italy	Investigate the prevalence and association between cyberbullying and problematic social media behaviors	Girls reported more cyber-victimization and greater problematic social media use compared to boys, especially at age 13. School, family, and peer support were protective against cyber-victimization, with the effect being more significant for girls
Duin et al. (2021)	Luxembourg	Investigate predictors of problematic social media use	Cyberbullying perpetration was one of the main predictors of problematic social media use, particularly among adolescents reporting high stress levels and psychosomatic complaints. Adolescents involved in cyberbullying tended to use social media more problematically

(continued)

Table 5.1 (continued)

Reference	Country	Objectives	Main results
Sivabalan et al. (2020)	Malaysia	Determine the prevalence of cyberbullying among adolescents and its association with gender, internet use patterns, and offline bullying	Girls reported greater cyber-victimization, especially at age 13, while boys reported higher incidence of cyberbullying perpetration across all age groups. Intense and problematic social media use was associated with both victimization and perpetration, particularly among girls. Frequent contact with strangers was also a risk factor for victimization
Yudes et al. (2020)	Spain	Examine the predictive value of personal resources (emotional intelligence, gratitude, and self-assessment) and risk factors (cyber-victimization, problematic internet use) and parental control over adolescents'involvement in cyberbullying perpetration	31.6% reported being victims of cyberbullying and 20.9% perpetrators. Daily internet use increased the likelihood of involvement in cyberbullying. Adolescents with a history of offline bullying were at greater risk of being victims or perpetrators of cyberbullying. Owning electronic devices and frequent use of social media and messaging apps increased the chances of involvement in cyberbullying situations
Martínez-Ferrer et al. (2021)	Spain	Examine the mediating role of problematic social media use in the relationship between cyber-victimization, offline victimization, and cyberbullying	Problematic social media use intensified the impact of online and offline victimization on cyberbullying. Boys tended to show a stronger link between victimization and cyberbullying, while girls were more likely to engage in problematic social media use in response to victimization

use was the most strongly associated with cyberbullying, both as a perpetrator and a victim. This finding is further supported by the review's focus on search and selection processes. Additionally, involvement in traditional school bullying was also associated with engaging in cyberbullying. Gender differences emerged as risk factors for cyberbullying, but these were often mediated by other variables such as mental health issues.

Table 5.2 Critical findings of the reviewed studies

Discovery	Definition
Direct relationship between problematic use of media or social networks and cyberbullying	Adolescents who present problematic use of media or social networks have an increased risk of victimization or engaging in cyberbullying
Relationship between mental health and cyberbullying	Adolescents with greater involvement in cyberbullying present major problems in mental health; experiences on social media or digital platforms intensify mental health problems
Social support or backing	Social support, such as family, school, or peer support, acts as a significant protective factor against cyberbullying victimization; this protective effect is more noticeable among girls and adolescents who communicate their experiences; the perception of lack of support increases the probability of problematic use of social media and involvement in cyberbullying situations
Gender differences	Girls report more cases of online victimization and perceive cyberbullying risks more, especially regarding physical appearance and exposure; boys tend to show more aggressive behaviors and frequent contact with strangers, and the intense use of social networks is also associated with higher levels of victimization among girls
Search for approval and validation	Adolescents who use social media or digital platforms in search of external validation and approval from peers are more vulnerable to cyberbullying and negative self-evaluations

Category 2: Individual and Mental Health Factors

The analyzed results indicate that adolescent personality traits and mood can significantly influence digital behaviors, particularly regarding cyberbullying. Adolescents seeking intense stimuli and novel experiences were more likely to engage in risky online activities, such as aggression and antisocial interactions. This behavior is intensified by high levels of boredom, leading adolescents to impulsively use the Internet and interact with harmful content. In terms of mental health, social media use among adolescents with depression exposed them to depressive content, increasing their exposure to cyberbullying (Göksu et al., 2024). Moreover, problematic use of social media and cyberbullying appeared to elevate stress levels and psychosomatic symptoms.

Category 3: Protective Factors Against Cyberbullying

Protective factors for cyberbullying and problematic social media use among adolescents primarily include elements of emotional regulation and restrictions on unrestricted Internet access. In this sense, adolescents with higher emotional intelligence and emotional regulation skills have lower involvement in cyberbullying situations, both as victims and perpetrators, demonstrating that the ability to manage emotions serves as a significant protective factor. Another important aspect is the active mediation of online use by adults (mainly parents or guardians), with strategies such as screen time limits and monitoring of online interactions, which have proven effective in reducing aggressive and impulsive online behaviors. A reviewed study further evidenced that parents have the power to positively influence adolescents' online behavior, especially when they are older (Aljasir & Alsebaei, 2022).

Discussion

This chapter examined the interconnected and complex phenomena of cyberbullying and problematic use of social media, highlighting their significant impact on adolescent health. The existing literature indicates that there is "hidden" information within digital interactions that can help identify risk factors, predictors, and protective influences associated with cyberbullying and inappropriate social media use. However, as with traditional school bullying, studies on cyberbullying still face methodological challenges, such as variability in approaches and lack of standardization, often hindering the reproducibility and generalizability of results.

Specifically, this chapter explored risk factors, individual mental health issues, and protective influences that can mitigate the impacts of cyberbullying and problematic use of social media. One of the main findings is the identification of risk factors and predictors, such as impulsivity, low emotional regulation, and prolonged exposure to harmful content. These factors frequently increase the likelihood of engaging in cyberbullying behaviors or exacerbate the negative effects of continuous exposure to social media. Additionally, mental health issues such as depression, anxiety, and low self-esteem have been consistently associated with both victims and aggressors, highlighting the need for interventions that address these underlying vulnerabilities (Craig et al., 2020; Gohal et al., 2023). Another critical point is the role of protective influences, such as social support, digital literacy, and parental regulation.

Although studies show that building support networks can reduce the impacts of cyberbullying and problematic use of social media, the evidence is still limited and dispersed, reinforcing the need for more research to identify effective interventions (Zhang et al., 2022a). Additionally, there is a significant gap in studies investigating how rapid changes in digital platforms affect these protective influences. As with other areas, the emerging and constantly evolving nature of technologies and the Internet requires interdisciplinary and collaborative approaches to advance knowledge on the subject (Krešić Ćorić & Kaštelan, 2020). In the near future, it will be necessary to discuss the issue of artificial intelligence use and how it may exacerbate the problem of cyberbullying.

Practical Implications in Terms of Prevention and Treatment

The implications of the reviewed studies encompass strategies that span both awareness and education as well as psychological and social support. In terms of prevention, family dialogue plays a crucial role. Studies show that regular conversations between parents and children about the risks of cyberbullying and ways to protect themselves can reduce exposure to risky situations and strengthen the emotional resilience of children and adolescents (Livingstone & Helsper, 2008; Oliveira et al., 2023). Additionally, media education, promoted through school activities, is a powerful tool for fostering conscious and responsible use of digital media. Educational programs can also teach skills such as critical thinking, digital empathy, and safe Internet practices, preventing harmful behaviors. Complementing these measures, the implementation of prevention programs in schools and communities has proven effective in creating environments that promote collective awareness and encourage proactive interventions against cyberbullying (Kowalski et al., 2014; Oliveira et al., 2023).

In the field of treatment, psychological support is essential to address the emotional and behavioral impacts of cyberbullying. Individual psychotherapy or cognitive-behavioral therapy can help victims rebuild self-esteem, overcome trauma, and develop strategies to cope with future situations, for example (Bansal et al., 2024). Moreover, support groups and family-based therapy can be a valuable approach to address the consequences of cyberbullying, strengthen bonds, and create more effective collective support, as well as promote more prosocial and less aggressive behaviors in schools.

Conclusion

This chapter documented the relationships established between problematic use of social media and perpetration or victimization by cyberbullying among adolescents aged 10 to 19. Various aspects were highlighted, contributing to the advancement of current and relevant topics considering the advancement and increased access of adolescents to the Internet or technologies. While it was already evident that cyberbullying is closely linked to technology or the Internet, this review revealed risk factors, predictors, individual and mental health issues, as well as protective factors and influences.

Even recognizing the strengths of this rapid review, its limitations must be observed. One important limitation identified is the predominance of retrospective studies and the lack of prospective investigations that longitudinally follow the effects of cyberbullying and problematic use of social media or digital media. This makes it difficult to identify causalities and formulate effective prevention and intervention strategies. In addition, methodological heterogeneity made it challenging to compare studies. To advance in this area, it is crucial to conduct high-quality prospective research that explores, for example, how specific interventions can modify problematic online behaviors or reduce the occurrence of cyberbullying cases. Interventions with adolescents should also contribute to a healthier and more responsible use of technology and the Internet.

References

Aljasir, S. A., & Alsebaei, M. O. (2022). Cyberbullying and cybervictimization on digital media platforms: The role of demographic variables and parental mediation strategies. *Humanities and Social Sciences Communications, 9*, 320. https://doi.org/10.1057/s41599-022-01318-x

Badrakh, A., Larkin, R. F., Betts, L. R., & Buglass, S. L. (2023). Psychosocial well-being, problematic social media use, and cyberbullying involvement among Mongolian adolescents. *International Journal of Bullying Prevention*. https://doi.org/10.1007/s42380-023-00202-9

Bansal, S., Garg, N., Singh, J., & Van Der Walt, F. (2024). Cyberbullying and mental health: Past, present and future. *Frontiers in Psychology, 14*, 1279234. https://doi.org/10.3389/fpsyg.2023.1279234

Borraccino, A., Marengo, N., Dalmasso, P., Marino, C., Ciardullo, S., Nardone, P., Lemma, P., & The Hbsc-Italia Group. (2022). Problematic social media use and cyber aggression in Italian adolescents: The remarkable role of social support. *International Journal of Environmental Research and Public Health, 19*(15), 9763. https://doi.org/10.3390/ijerph19159763

Craig, W., Boniel-Nissim, M., King, N., Walsh, S. D., Boer, M., Donnelly, P. D., Harel-Fisch, Y., Malinowska-Cieślik, M., Gaspar de Matos, M., Cosma, A., Van den Eijnden, R., Vieno, A., Elgar, F. J., Molcho, M., Bjereld, Y., & Pickett, W. (2020). Social media use and cyber-bullying: A cross-national analysis of young people in 42 countries. *The Journal of Adolescent Health, 66*(6S), S100–S108. https://doi.org/10.1016/j.jadohealth.2020.03.006

Duin, C., Heinz, A., & Willems, H. (2021). Predictors of problematic social media use in a nationally representative sample of adolescents in Luxembourg. *International Journal of Environmental Research and Public Health, 18*(22), 11878. https://doi.org/10.3390/ijerph182211878

Felice, G., Burrai, J., Mari, E., Paloni, F., Lausi, G., Giannini, A. M., & Quaglieri, A. (2022). How do adolescents use social networks and what are their potential dangers? A qualitative study of gender differences. *International Journal of Environmental Research and Public Health, 19*(9), 5691. https://doi.org/10.3390/ijerph19095691

Gartlehner, G., Nussbaumer-Streit, B., Devane, D., Kahwati, L., Viswanathan, M., King, V. J., Qaseem, A., Akl, E., Schuenemann, H. J., & Cochrane Rapid Reviews Methods Group. (2024). Rapid reviews methods series: Guidance on assessing the certainty of evidence. *BMJ Evidence Based Medicine, 29*(1), 50–54. https://doi.org/10.1136/bmjebm-2022-112111

Geng, J., Wang, Y., Wang, H., Wang, P., & Lei, L. (2022). Social comparison orientation and cyberbullying perpetration and victimization: Roles of envy on social networking sites and body satisfaction. *Journal of Interpersonal Violence, 37*(17–18), NP16060–NP16083. https://doi.org/10.1177/08862605211023486

Gohal, G., Alqassim, A., Eltyeb, E., Rayyani, A., Hakami, B., Al Faqih, A., Hakami, A., Qadri, A., & Mahfouz, M. (2023). Prevalence and related risks of cyberbullying and its effects on adolescent. *BMC Psychiatry, 23*(1), 39. https://doi.org/10.1186/s12888-023-04542-0

Göksu, M., Rodopman Arman, A., Gündoğdu, Ü., & Gümüştaş, F. (2024). Social media use in adolescent girls with depression: The relationship between social media use purposes, lack of social support, and cyber victimization. *Marmara Medical Journal, 37*(1), 29–36. https://doi.org/10.5472/marumj.1379988

Kowalski, R. M., Giumetti, G. W., Schroeder, A. N., & Lattanner, M. R. (2014). Bullying in the digital age: A critical review and meta-analysis of cyberbullying research among youth. *Psychological Bulletin, 140*(4), 1073–1137. https://doi.org/10.1037/a0035618

Krešić Ćorić, M., & Kaštelan, A. (2020). Bullying through the internet—Cyberbullying. *Psychiatria Danubina, 32*(2), 269–272. Retrieved from https://pubmed.ncbi.nlm.nih.gov/32970646/

Kunwar, S., Sharma, S., Marasini, S., Joshi, A., Adhikari, A., Ranjit, A., Byanju Shrestha, I., Shrestha, A., Shrestha, A. K., & Karmacharya, B. M. (2024). Cyberbullying and cyber-victimisation among higher secondary school adolescents in an urban city of Nepal: A cross-sectional study. *BMJ Open, 14*(3), e081016. https://doi.org/10.1136/bmjopen-2023-081016

Lahti, H., Kokkonen, M., Hietajärvi, L., Lyyra, N., & Paakkari, L. (2024). Social media threats and health among adolescents: Evidence from the health behaviour in school-aged children study. *Child and Adolescent Psychiatry and Mental Health, 18*(1), 62. https://doi.org/10.1186/s13034-024-00754-8

Lareki, A., Altuna, J., & Martínez-de-Morentin, J.-I. (2023). Fake digital identity and cyberbullying. *Media, Culture and Society, 45*(2), 338–353. http://hdl.handle.net/10810/64316

Livingstone, S., & Helsper, E. J. (2008). Parental mediation of children's internet use. *Journal of Broadcasting & Electronic Media, 52*(4), 581–599. https://doi.org/10.1080/08838150802437396

Marengo, N., Borraccino, A., Charrier, L., Berchialla, P., Dalmasso, P., Caputo, M., & Lemma, P. (2021). Cyberbullying and problematic social media use: An insight into the positive role of social support in adolescents-data from the health behaviour in school-aged children study in Italy. *Public Health, 199*, 46–50. https://doi.org/10.1016/j.puhe.2021.08.010

Martínez-Ferrer, B., León-Moreno, C., Suárez-Relinque, C., Del Moral-Arroyo, G., & Musitu-Ochoa, G. (2021). Cybervictimization, offline victimization, and cyberbullying: The mediating role of the problematic use of social networking sites in boys and girls. *Psychosocial Intervention, 30*(3), 155–162. https://doi.org/10.5093/pi2021a5

Nagata, J. M., Trompeter, N., Singh, G., Ganson, K. T., Testa, A., Jackson, D. B., Assari, S., Murray, S. B., Bibbins-Domingo, K., & Baker, F. C. (2022). Social epidemiology of early adolescent cyberbullying in the United States. *Academic Pediatrics, 22*(8), 1287–1293. https://doi.org/10.1016/j.acap.2022.07.003

Oliveira, W. A., Esteca, A. M. N., Romualdo, C., Andrade, A. L. M., & Santos, M. A. (2023). Programas de intervenção contra o cyberbullying na adolescência: mapping review. In A. V. Craveiro & E. P. Priotto (Eds.), *Violências na atualidade. Olhares e Perspectivas* (pp. 495–522). Nova Práxis.

Ouzzani, M., Hammady, H., Fedorowicz, Z., & Elmagarmid, A. (2016). Rayyan—A web and mobile app for systematic reviews. *Systematic Reviews, 5*(1), 210. https://doi.org/10.1186/s13643-016-0384-4

Peprah, P., Oduro, M. S., Atta-Osei, G., Addo, I. Y., Morgan, A. K., & Gyasi, R. M. (2024). Problematic social media use mediates the effect of cyberbullying victimisation on psychosomatic complaints in adolescents. *Scientific Reports, 14*(1), 9773. https://doi.org/10.1038/s41598-024-59509-2

Sivabalan, T. V., Zaki, R. A., & Yuen, C. W. (2020). The prevalence of cyberbullying and its associated factors among young adolescents in Penang, Malaysia. *Journal of Health and Translational Medicine, 23*(1), 202–211. Retrieved from https://mjs.um.edu.my/index.php/jummec/article/view/25856

Smela, B., Toumi, M., Świerk, K., Francois, C., Biernikiewicz, M., Clay, E., & Boyer, L. (2023). Rapid literature review: Definition and methodology. *Journal of Market Access & Health Policy, 11*(1), 2241234. https://doi.org/10.1080/20016689.2023.2241234

Topan, A., Anol, S., Taşdelen, Y., & Kurt, A. (2024). Exploring the relationship between cyberbullying and technology addiction in adolescents. *Public Health Nursing, 42*, 33. https://doi.org/10.1111/phn.13433

Torrecillas-Lacave, T., Vázquez-Barrio, T., & Suárez-Álvarez, R. (2022). Cyberbullying among adolescents and its effect on their internet use. *Revista de Comunicación y Tecnologías Emergentes, 20*(1), e1624. https://doi.org/10.7195/ri14.v20i1.1624

Wong, N., Yanagida, T., Spiel, C., & Graf, D. (2022). The association between appetitive aggression and social media addiction mediated by cyberbullying: The moderating role of inclusive norms. *International Journal of Environmental Research and Public Health, 19*(16), 9956. https://doi.org/10.3390/ijerph19169956

Yudes, C., Rey, L., & Extremera, N. (2020). Predictive factors of cyberbullying perpetration amongst Spanish adolescents. *International Journal of Environmental Research and Public Health, 17*(11), 3967. https://doi.org/10.3390/ijerph17113967

Zhang, X., Chu, X., Fan, C., Andrasik, F., Shi, H., & Hu, X. (2022a). Sensation seeking and cyberbullying among Chinese adolescents: Examining the mediating roles of boredom experience and antisocial media exposure. *Computers in Human Behavior, 130*, 107185. https://doi.org/10.1016/j.chb.2022.107185

Zhang, W., Huang, S., Lam, L., Evans, R., & Zhu, C. (2022b). Cyberbullying definitions and measurements in children and adolescents: Summarizing 20 years of global efforts. *Frontiers in Public Health, 10*, 1000504. https://doi.org/10.3389/fpubh.2022.1000504

Chapter 6
Hazardous Gambling and Online Sports Betting: A New Frontier of Behavioral Addiction—Overview, Clinical Correlates, and Interventions

Richard Alecsander Reichert, Filipe Reis Teodoro Andrade, Manoela Fontelles, Nicoly Camile Mendes Reichert, Rosa Maria Martins de Almeida, and Denise De Micheli

Introduction

The twenty-first century has revolutionized the ways of betting and the situations in which people place their bets (Vieira et al., 2023). In this context, sports betting, broadly defined as the act of wagering money on the prediction of outcomes of sporting events (Otis et al., 2022), has gained prominence in recent decades, driven by legislative changes (Anderson et al., 2012; Bengel & McCarriston, 2022; Humphreys, 2021; Ukhova et al., 2024), the introduction of new modalities (Granero et al., 2020; Grubbs & Kraus, 2023), and the increase in the availability of betting options (Espadafor & Martínez, 2021). In addition to sports betting, gambling generally encompasses activities involving placing money or valuables at risk based on the uncertain outcome of competitions, draws, or other events. The advancement of digital platforms and the ease of access through mobile devices have contributed to the growing popularity of these practices, enabling global audiences to engage in different types of betting and gambling (Hing et al., 2023, 2024a; Otis et al., 2022).

R. A. Reichert · D. De Micheli (✉)
Universidade Federal de São Paulo, São Paulo, SP, Brazil
e-mail: reichert@unifesp.br

F. R. T. Andrade
Zentralinstitut für seelische Gesundheit, Mannheim, Germany

M. Fontelles
Universidade do Vale do Itajaí, Itajaí, SC, Brazil

N. C. M. Reichert
Fundação Universidade Regional de Blumenau, Blumenau, SC, Brazil

R. M. M. de Almeida
Universidade Federal do Rio Grande do Sul, Porto Alegre, RS, Brazil

A. L. M. Andrade (ed.), *Digital Addictions*,
https://doi.org/10.1007/978-3-031-87986-9_6

Indications suggest that betting on games predates historical records, being present at various moments in ancient history (Matheson, 2021). In Greek mythology, the gods Hades, Poseidon, and Zeus used games to divide control over the heavens, seas, and underworld among themselves. Throughout history, organized sports have also been closely linked to betting. From the Olympic Games of Ancient Greece to the Circus Maximus in Rome—the most prominent entertainment stadium in the city, where chariot races, horse races, and gladiatorial competitions attracted numerous spectators—betting was an integral part of the sporting landscape (Dmochowski, 2023; Matheson, 2021). In the seventeenth century, betting on events such as street races, horse racing, and boxing matches gained significance, being viewed not only as entertainment but also as drivers of developing and disseminating sports rules (Brohm, 1982; Dunning, 2014). However, in the twenty-first century, sports betting solidified as a globally booming industry, propelled by the advent of the Internet, which allowed for unprecedented expansion. The ease of betting from mobile devices, such as smartphones,[1] completely transformed access to and the popularity of sports betting, making it widely accessible and profitable (Cavalcante, 2024; Divos et al., 2018; Etuk et al., 2022; Killick & Griffiths, 2021; Lopez-Gonzalez et al., 2021; Nelson et al., 2021).

The expansion of modern technologies and ongoing legalization efforts have facilitated a significant increase in engagement with sports betting (Bengel & McCarriston, 2022; Vieira et al., 2023), especially in North America, where a 2021 report revealed an 80% increase in the proportion of US citizens who regularly bet on sports (Silverman, 2022; Vieira et al., 2023). In Australia, one of the most liberalized gambling environments in the world, online sports betting has also proliferated, with an increase in expenditures and profit margins for bookmakers, despite a concurrent rise in the number of individuals seeking help for gambling-related issues (Bengel & McCarriston, 2022; Davidson et al., 2016; Deans et al., 2017; Hing et al., 2022; Statista, 2018). In the United Kingdom, there was an approximately 46% increase in gamblers, with about 30% of online gamblers using mobile devices for their bets, reflecting a 10% rise in mobile device usage between 2016 and 2017 (Gambling Commission, 2018). Furthermore, a comparison between samples of individuals seeking treatment for gambling-related issues in 2015 and 2002 revealed that, in 2015, there was a significant increase in the number of people reporting having gambled online compared to the 2002 samples (Nelson et al., 2021; Sharman et al., 2019). In Brazil, Law 13.756, enacted in 2018 (Brasil, 2018), enabled exponential growth in the sports betting market, which generates approximately 150 billion reais (roughly \$30 billion or €28 billion as of September 27, 2024) and leads the global ranking in access to betting websites, with 3.2 billion accesses in 2022,

[1] The study by Hing et al. (2024a), for example, investigated the impact of smartphone use on sports betting among young adults, comparing it with the use of computers and physical betting facilities. The results revealed that the features offered by smartphones, such as online gambling and betting applications, enable instant access to betting anywhere and anytime, which may facilitate harmful behaviors such as increased participation, frequency, and spending on bets. Furthermore, there was an observed increase in the variety and impulsivity of bets, a higher likelihood of riskier betting, the recurrence of losses, and the influence of social incentives to gamble.

surpassing countries such as the United Kingdom and the United States (Cavalcante, 2024; Parrela, 2023; Magri, 2021).

The commercial growth of gambling options, along with the diversification of their modalities, has increased exposure to the risks associated with gambling behaviors, especially among populations already predisposed to gambling problems, such as younger individuals, people with higher levels of impulsivity, and those who use substances (Hing et al., 2015; Russell et al., 2019a, 2019b). This phenomenon has received increasing attention in the field of public health (Goyder et al., 2020; Nyemcsok et al., 2022; The Lancet, 2017), highlighting its unequal consequences, which disproportionately impact individuals and populations in situations of greater psychological, social, and economic vulnerability (Espadafor & Martínez, 2021).

Advertising has significantly contributed to this scenario, promoting the popularization of sports betting, which, combined with other factors of biopsychosocial vulnerability, may elevate the risk of developing disorders related to these behaviors. This condition is characterized by persistent and recurrent behavioral patterns of betting that result in significant distress and functional impairment (American Psychiatric Association (APA), 2013, 2022; World Health Organization (WHO), 2018). Studies show that individuals who report a higher frequency of betting and/or involvement in other forms of gambling tend to exhibit more intense symptoms of stress, anxiety, and depression, as well as more frequent problematic use of alcohol and other substances (Gainsbury et al., 2020; Lopez-Gonzalez et al., 2018). Furthermore, the harms can affect not only the gamblers but also their social networks and the community as a whole (Gainsbury et al., 2014; Johnstone & Regan, 2020; Seal et al., 2022), potentially generating or exacerbating financial problems, affecting family functioning dynamics, causing interpersonal conflicts, contributing to severe mental disorders, and, in extreme cases, leading to suicidal situations (Langham et al., 2016; McGee, 2020; Valleur et al., 2016).

These data emphasize the urgent need to implement public health policies that prioritize both prevention and harm reduction, especially for the groups most vulnerable to gambling-related problems. Although a growing body of evidence suggests that betting during games is linked to a specific profile of individual characteristics and associated harms, the current literature on the topic still needs to be expanded in its scope (Russell et al., 2019a, 2019b; Vieira et al., 2023). In light of this, this chapter aims to provide an overview of aspects related to behavioral addictions—disorders not related to substances—focusing on sports betting and its impacts, addressing topics such as the definition of these disorders in the ICD-11 (WHO, 2018) and the DSM-5-TR (APA, 2022), the differentiation between substance-related disorders and other behavioral addictions, and the state of the art of research on these conditions. Epidemiological data will also be discussed, including the prevalence of sports betting and other forms of gambling in different groups and age ranges and the impact of online betting on growth and accessibility. Furthermore, the chapter will examine neurobiological and psychosocial aspects, comorbidities with other psychiatric disorders, clinical interventions, and future directions for research.

Definition and Diagnostic Criteria

In the category of *Substance-Related and Addictive Disorders* of the Diagnostic and Statistical Manual of Mental Disorders (Chapter II, Section II of the DSM-5-TR; APA, 2022), the classification of *Gambling Disorder*[2,3] is used, referring to a persistent and recurrent pattern of involvement with gambling that results in clinically significant distress. For diagnosis, individuals must meet at least four of the established criteria within 12 months, including the need to gamble with increasing amounts of money to achieve excitement, frequent thoughts about gambling, and seeking ways to obtain money to gamble, among others. The severity of the disorder is assessed based on the number of criteria met, classifying it as mild (4–5 criteria), moderate (6–7 criteria), or severe (8–9 criteria) (APA, 2022).

According to the definition of the DSM-5-TR, gambling involves risking something of value with the expectation of obtaining a greater return. Although many individuals participate in gaming and gambling without developing problems, some experience significant impairments related to these behaviors. The central characteristic of gambling disorder is the persistent and recurrent pattern of harmful behaviors that interfere with personal, familial, and professional activities (Criterion A). The disorder is diagnosed when an individual exhibits four or more symptoms listed in Criterion A within 12 months. A common aspect is the "pursuit of one's losses," where the gambler feels an urgency to continue gambling, often increasing the stakes or taking more significant risks to recover previous losses. While many may experience this "chasing" temporarily, the frequency and duration of this behavior are distinguishing features of the disorder (Criterion A6). Additionally, many lie to family members, therapists, or others about the extent of their involvement in gambling, which may involve fraudulent behaviors, such as forgery or theft, to obtain money to continue gambling (Criterion A7). It is also common for

[2]Gambling disorder was recognized as a psychiatric diagnosis for the first time in 1980 when it was included in the category of *Impulse Control Disorders*. In the last decade, international studies have evidenced several similarities between gambling disorder and substance use disorders, pointing to significant neurobiological overlaps. Although some investigations have explored the comparability with obsessive-compulsive disorders, support for the inclusion of gambling disorder in a "compulsive spectrum" has been inconsistent. As a result, the DSM-5 reclassified gambling disorder under the category of addictions, highlighting the importance of this inclusion for advancing research on behavioral addictions in general (Clark et al., 2013; Hollander & Wong, 1995; Leeman & Potenza, 2012; Petry, 2006; Petry et al., 2014).

[3]The DSM-5-TR presents diagnostic criteria for *Internet Gaming Disorder*, which encompasses only online games that do not involve gambling; therefore, it is not the focus of this chapter. However, to contextualize within the scope of this book on digital addictions, it is relevant to share that Internet gaming disorder is characterized by persistent and recurrent use of the Internet for gaming, often in interaction with other players, resulting in clinically significant impairment or distress. The diagnosis requires the endorsement of at least five of the following criteria within a 12-month period: excessive concern about gaming, withdrawal symptoms when not gaming, the need for increased time to achieve satisfaction, unsuccessful attempts to control the behavior, loss of interest in other activities, continued use despite social problems, deception of family members and professionals about the amount of time spent gaming, use of gaming as an escape or avoidance of emotional issues, and impairment in interpersonal relationships and responsibilities (APA, 2022).

individuals to turn to family members or other sources for help in dealing with financial crises generated by gambling (Criterion A9).

Chart 6.1 Diagnostic Criteria for Gambling Disorder in the DSM-5-TR

A. Problematic gambling behavior that is persistent and recurrent, leading to clinically significant impairment or distress, as indicated by the individual exhibiting four (or more) of the following criteria within a 12-month period:

1. Needs to gamble with increasing amounts of money to achieve the desired excitement.
2. Is restless or irritable when attempting to cut down or stop gambling.
3. Has made repeated unsuccessful efforts to control, reduce, or stop gambling.
4. Is often preoccupied with gambling (e.g., having persistent thoughts of reliving past gambling experiences, making up losses, or planning the next venture, thinking about ways to get money to gamble).
5. Often gambles when feeling distressed (e.g., feelings of helplessness, guilt, anxiety, depression).
6. After losing money gambling, often returns another day to get even ("chasing" losses).
7. Lies to conceal the extent of involvement with gambling.
8. Has jeopardized or lost a significant relationship, job, or educational or career opportunity because of gambling.
9. Relies on others to provide money to relieve desperate financial situations caused by gambling.

B. The gambling behavior is not better explained by a manic episode.
Specify if:

- **Episodic**: Meeting diagnostic criteria at more than one time, with symptoms dissipating between periods of gambling disorder for at least several months.
- **Persistent**: Experiencing continuous symptoms, meeting diagnostic criteria for several years.

Specify if:

- **Early remission**: After having previously met all criteria for gambling disorder, none of the criteria for gambling disorder have been met for at least 3 months but for less than 12 months.
- **Sustained remission**: After having previously met all criteria for gambling disorder, none of the criteria for gambling disorder have been met for a period of 12 months or more.

Specify current severity:

- **Mild**: 4–5 criteria met.
- **Moderate**: 6–7 criteria met.
- **Severe**: 8–9 criteria met.

In the International Classification of Diseases and Related Health Problems (ICD-11; WHO, 2018), code QE21 refers to *hazardous gambling and/or betting*. This classification, included in the category of problems associated with health behaviors, encompasses a pattern of gambling or betting that results in a significant increase in the risk of harmful consequences to the physical and/or psychological health of individuals or others in their social circle. The risks may be related to the frequency of gambling or betting activities, the amount of time spent, the context in which they occur, the neglect of other priorities, and the occurrence of associated risk behaviors. The pattern persists even when individuals are aware of the increased risk of harm. This classification can justify the need for attention and counseling from health professionals. However, it does not meet the diagnostic criteria for gambling disorder (WHO, 2018), as defined in the DSM-5-TR (APA, 2022).

Epidemiological Data

The prevalence of problematic involvement with gambling shows significant variations depending on the population and cultural context. In the United States, estimates suggest that gambling disorder may affect between 0.2% and 0.3% of the general population, while international studies indicate a variation of 0.1% to 0.7%. It is estimated that between 0.4% and 1.0% of Americans exhibit this behavior throughout their lifetime. Demographic factors such as gender and ethnicity also influence these rates. Among men, the lifetime prevalence has been estimated at around 0.6%, while for women, it is approximately 0.2%. Differences have also been observed among ethnoracial groups, with previous studies suggesting gambling disorder prevalences of 0.52% among African Americans, 0.25% among Latinos, and 0.23% among non-Latino whites (APA, 2022).

In Seville, Spain, Legarda et al. (1992) identified that 1.7% of the population exhibited behaviors that could be associated with gambling-related difficulties, while 5.2% were in at-risk situations. In New Zealand, a national study conducted by Volberg and Abbott (1994) revealed a prevalence of 2.7% for gambling-related difficulties and 4.2% for at-risk situations among 4053 interviewed adults, with significant risk factors associated with ethnicity, age, and gender. In Nigeria, Bankole (2019) estimated that over 60 million Nigerians participated in sports betting, with four in ten individuals involved in this type of activity. In Madrid, a study conducted by Labrador and Vallejo-Achón (2020) indicated that 42.6% of students had wagered on sports, with a higher prevalence among men (81%). In Europe, Grall-Bronnec et al. (2016) found a prevalence of 8.2% for gambling-related problems among professional athletes. A more recent Nigerian study conducted by Afe et al. (2022) recorded a prevalence of 30.5% for gambling disorders associated with lower educational levels and job market instability. In Brazil, Carvalho (2024) reported that beneficiaries of social programs allocated R$ 3 billion (approximately US$ 540 million and € 480 million, considering the conversion of September 27, 2024) to sports betting just in August 2024, with an average of R$ 100 (around

US$ 18 and € 16) per bet, suggesting a rising risk behavior, especially among the younger population.

Vulnerability Factors

The vulnerability factors associated with harmful behaviors involving gambling and/or betting, as described in the DSM-5-TR, encompass genetic, physiological, and temperamental dimensions. Evidence suggests that these behaviors may manifest in familial contexts, with a higher prevalence among monozygotic twins than dizygotic twins. Additionally, the occurrence of gambling behaviors is more common among first-degree relatives of individuals with moderate to severe alcohol use disorders when compared to the general population. Early onset of gambling, particularly in childhood or adolescence, is associated with high rates of challenging behaviors. Furthermore, these behaviors often coexist with antisocial personality disorders, depressive disorders, bipolar disorders, and other substance use disorders. Lastly, although many individuals, including adolescents and young adults, may overcome their problematic behaviors over time, previous experiences of problematic gambling serve as significant predictors of future difficulties. The presence of psychopathology, such as attention-deficit/hyperactivity disorder and anxiety disorders, has also been linked to an increased risk of developing and maintaining harmful gambling-related behaviors (APA, 2022) (Table 6.1).

The study conducted by Wang et al. (2021) explored the factors influencing the behavioral intention and behavior of university students regarding sports betting, with the participation of 334 students from four universities in the United States. The results highlighted that the attitude toward sports betting was the most relevant factor for predicting the intention to bet, followed by subjective norms. Intention and perceived behavioral control were significant predictors of betting behavior. The authors suggest that prevention and education programs should focus on shaping appropriate attitudes toward sports betting, emphasizing that this activity should be viewed as entertainment, not as a means of generating income. The influence of media and social norms was also identified as critical elements to be considered in intervention strategies.

The study by Wirkus et al. (2024) investigated the individual risk factors associated with the development and maintenance of gambling disorders in online sports bettors, with a sample of 607 German participants, predominantly male (92%), and an average age of 34 years. The researchers conducted an initial online survey and a 1-year follow-up with 325 participants. The results showed that impulsivity, difficulties in identifying emotions, emotional suppression, the presence of comorbid psychological disorders, and stress were associated with gambling disorder, with impulsivity and the perception of helplessness standing out as significant predictors over time. The authors emphasize integrating these risk factors and coping mechanisms into prevention and intervention strategies to identify at-risk individuals early and adapt treatment accordingly.

Table 6.1 Vulnerabilities associated with harmful involvement in betting and/or gambling

Authors (year)	Participants	Main results
Hing et al. (2017)	4594 Australian gamblers, focusing on harmful gambling modes	Risk factors for sports betting included being male, younger, having a lower income, and experiencing greater psychological distress. Substance use during gambling was also a significant risk factor
Bodor et al. (2018)	140 members of alcohol dependency clubs in the city of Zagreb (Croatia)	Pathological gambling was more prevalent among individuals with alcohol dependence than in general populations. Problematic gambling behaviors were associated with games that have a higher potential for addiction, such as sports betting and slot machines, although the intensity of gambling problems did not significantly correlate with alcohol dependence
Gainsbury et al. (2019)	998 Australians who gambled online in the past 30 days	Problematic gambling was positively associated with the frequency of online gambling, particularly in sports betting and electronic gaming machines. Psychological distress was exclusively associated with a higher frequency of gambling in venues, including electronic gaming machines, sports betting, and card/table casino games
Granero et al. (2020)	4516 patients seeking treatment for pathological gambling at the Bellvitge University Hospital (Barcelona)	The prevalence of sports betting as a gambling disorder was 7.2%. Two clusters were identified: the first, with more affected individuals, showed higher comorbidity with other addictions, lower socioeconomic status, and less adaptive personality characteristics. The second group was less affected, with higher social levels and more adaptive personality traits
Jiménez-Murcia et al. (2021)	352 Spanish sports bettors in treatment for gambling disorder	Older age, more significant psychological distress, lower educational level, higher dependence scores, lower self-direction, and greater novelty-seeking were predictors of the severity and higher frequency of gambling involvement
Cooper et al. (2022)	1280 participants, 596 sports bettors, in Ontario, Canada	Sports bettors exhibited a higher risk of problematic gambling due to differences in attitudes, personality traits, and cognitive biases, including higher levels of impulsivity, sensation-seeking, and positive urgency (the predisposition to seek immediate rewards) and negative urgency (the need to avoid undesirable consequences). The association between predictors and problematic gambling was stronger for sports bettors, indicating that preventive methods should be targeted based on the type of gambler

Neurobiology and Cognitive Basis

The neurobiological aspects of problematic involvement with gambling are closely related to alterations in decision-making, as demonstrated in studies that analyzed lesions in specific regions of the brain. Lesions in the basolateral amygdala distorted subjects' preferences, leading them to choose high-risk, high-reward options. This observation reflects the association between damage in this region and disadvantageous choices, as evidenced in the Iowa gambling task. When lesions occur before task acquisition, subjects struggle to develop effective strategies and correctly discriminate between available options. Similarly, lesions in the orbitofrontal cortex impair task acquisition, suggesting that disruptions in decision-making may stem from difficulties in learning strategies rather than an increased preference for risky outcomes. The interaction between the prefrontal cortex and the striatum also plays a significant role in choice behavior, with contemporary hypotheses highlighting the relevance of this connectivity in both action selection and reinforcement learning, factors that are important in the context of behavioral addictions and problematic gambling (Bechara et al., 1994, 1999, 2000; Clark et al., 2013; Fellows & Farah, 2005; Seo et al., 2012; Zeeb & Winstanley, 2011).

Functional neuroimaging studies have significantly expanded the understanding of reward-related circuits in individuals engaged in gambling behaviors. Research utilizing fMRI has revealed blunted neural responses to monetary gains and appetitive cues, particularly in the ventral striatum and the orbital/lateral prefrontal cortex, indicating a possible alteration in reward sensitivity. Furthermore, investigations into sensitivity to non-monetary rewards have revealed that individuals engaged in gambling behaviors exhibit diminished responses to erotic cues, correlating with the severity of gambling-related symptoms. These findings suggest that the response to monetary rewards, in contrast to other appetitive cues, may be a central variable in understanding gambling behaviors. Finally, experiments focused on cognitive distortions related to gambling highlight the involvement of reward circuits, evidencing the interaction between emotional and cognitive decision-making mechanisms (Clark et al., 2013; Goldstein et al., 2007; Schott et al., 2008; Sescousse et al., 2013; Shiv et al., 2005).

Brevers et al. (2018) investigated the neural responses of football fans to stimuli representing sporting events with and without the betting opportunity, utilizing a cue exposure task and functional magnetic resonance imaging. The study included 42 participants who viewed cues from football matches that would take place after the brain imaging session. In the "betting" condition, each individual indicated which games and teams they wished to bet on, while in the "watching" condition, they selected the games they preferred to follow. The results revealed that events with the possibility of betting generated greater activation in frontostriatal regions and the insular cortex and more excellent functional connectivity compared to events without the betting option. Games, where participants expressed more confidence regarding the winning team, resulted in intensified activations in regions associated with affective decision-making, inhibitory control, and reward processing, such as the ventromedial prefrontal cortex and the striatum. These findings suggest that the widespread availability of sports betting directly influences reward systems and cognitive control.

In the field of behavioral economics, one of the central concepts is *loss aversion,* which demonstrates that individuals tend to react more intensely to losses than to equivalent gains (Kahneman & Tversky, 1979; Schonberg et al., 2011; Trepel et al., 2005). This aversion is evident when people avoid bets with equal chances of winning or losing. Research suggests that loss aversion is linked to valuation mechanisms in the ventral striatum and the amygdala, with modulation influenced by norepinephrine (De Martino et al., 2010; Takahashi et al., 2013; Tom et al., 2007). Additionally, the theory proposes that the value functions for gains and losses exhibit different shapes, with the gain function being concave (indicating that perceived value increases at a decreasing rate with additional gains) and the loss function being convex (suggesting that the impact of losses increases as the magnitude of the loss grows), which contributes to risk aversion in gain situations and risk-seeking behavior in loss situations (Campbell-Meiklejohn et al., 2008). The theory also suggests a nonlinear calibration of probabilities, where small and medium to high chances are often overestimated (Tobler et al., 2008). This dynamic is associated with alterations in value representations in the brain, particularly in the ventral striatum, and is frequently observed in individuals with problematic gambling involvement (Campbell-Meiklejohn et al., 2008; Clark et al., 2013; Miedl et al., 2012; Peters et al., 2012; Trepel et al., 2005).

The cognitive mechanisms associated with gambling reveal a significant role of distortions in how individuals perceive and interpret randomness, chance, and the skills involved. These distortions, which include incorrect beliefs about the probability of winning, generate unduly optimistic expectations during gambling practice (Clark, 2010; Fortune & Goodie, 2012; Ladouceur & Walker, 1996). A notorious example is the *gambler's fallacy*, in which the expectation of a specific outcome, such as heads in a coin toss, becomes less likely after a prolonged sequence of the same result, such as three consecutive tails. This belief is often attributed to the representativeness heuristic, which suggests that small samples should reflect the overall distribution (Ayton & Fischer, 2004; Rabin, 2002; Sundali & Croson, 2006). Another common distortion is the illusion of control, where participants mistakenly believe that their skills influence the outcomes of chance-based games, such as selecting a lottery ticket or engaging in actions involving dice rolls (Langer, 1975). Additionally, *near-miss* experiences—situations where the outcomes are close to a win—can further motivate gamblers to continue, even if these outcomes do not represent actual wins (Clark et al., 2009, 2013). Despite evidence that individuals who frequently participate in gambling show a greater inclination toward these distortions, there is still a scarcity of studies that empirically demonstrate hypersensitivity to specific biases in this group (Clark et al., 2013).

Sociocultural Aspects

The DSM-5-TR explores cultural and diagnostic differences related to gambling and betting behavior, highlighting that the prevalence and type of gambling activity vary across different cultural contexts and ethnic-racial groups. For instance, activities such as pai gow (a traditional Chinese game played with dominoes), cockfighting, blackjack (a card game commonly known as 21), and horse racing are more pronounced in certain cultures, often influenced by specific social and economic factors. In Indigenous communities in Canada, New Zealand, and the United States, high rates of gambling problems may be associated with limited economic opportunities,[4] the belief that gambling can contribute to social goals and the presence of casinos on American tribal lands. Gambling problem rates also differ between individuals born in the United States and first-generation immigrants, being higher among the former. Additionally, there are variations in the manifestation of diagnostic criteria among ethnic groups: while Asian Americans with gambling issues may be less likely to report excessive concern about their behavior (Criterion A4), African Americans and Latinos tend to face more significant difficulties in controlling their gambling (Criterion A3), demonstrating that cultural issues and the adaptation process to the North American cultural context are important factors in the development and maintenance of these behaviors (APA, 2022).

Psychiatric Comorbidities: Associated Clinical Conditions

The presence of harmful behaviors related to gambling and betting is often associated with a range of comorbidities, negatively impacting the overall health of affected individuals. Research conducted in the United States has revealed a high rate of comorbidity with various mental disorders, including depressive disorders, anxiety disorders, personality disorders, and substance use disorders. In many cases, these other mental disorders may precede or coexist with problematic gambling behaviors, particularly highlighting the occurrence of bipolar disorders, anxiety disorders, and substance use disorders. A national analysis found that in about 75% of situations where individuals exhibited harmful gambling behaviors alongside another mental disorder, the associated psychopathology had emerged before the involvement with gambling (APA, 2022).

The systematic review conducted by Valenciano-Mendoza et al. aimed primarily to investigate the clinical correlates associated with sports betting. The results indicated a strong relationship between psychological distress and the frequency of

[4] This phenomenon can be understood in relation to the limited economic opportunities faced by these beneficiaries, who are mostly from contexts marked by socioeconomic inequalities. The absence of access to safer financial alternatives, combined with the increase in the number of betting modalities and intense media promotion, has led to an increase in engagement in gambling activities, with many individuals perceiving betting as a form of economic ascension. However, this behavior often results in negative consequences, such as exacerbation of problems related to gambling behavior (financial difficulties, family conflicts, and psychological distress). The relationship between socioeconomic vulnerability and problematic gambling involvement is illustrated by the study conducted by Latvala et al. (2021) in Finland, which analyzed representative population data ($N = 7186$) and found a higher prevalence of risky gambling behavior among unemployed individuals or those receiving social security benefits. The study revealed that the likelihood of problematic involvement was significantly greater among these groups, with an odds ratio of 5.6 for those receiving social assistance. This suggests that, even in contexts of public policies aimed at resource redistribution, the harms associated with gambling disproportionately affect the most disadvantaged populations, deepening existing social inequalities.

sports betting, with evidence that problematic online betting is correlated with higher levels of emotional distress. Additionally, the use of alcohol and other substances was significantly reported among individuals involved in sports betting, ranging from 22.1% to 71.2%. The study also highlighted impulsivity, especially negative urgency (the tendency to act impulsively in response to negative emotions), as one of the main predictors for participation in sports betting, with sensation-seeking proving to be a relevant characteristic. Overall, problematic sports betting was associated with personality profiles that include traits such as impulsivity and sensitivity to rewards, suggesting a biological predisposition that may increase vulnerability to behavioral addictions. This combination of factors may not only facilitate involvement in problematic sports betting but also perpetuate such behaviors over time.

Psychosocial Impacts.

According to the DSM-5-TR, involvement in gambling and/or betting can lead to a disorder[5] characterized by impairments in various areas of life, including compromised social and family relationships, as well as academic and professional losses (APA, 2022). Behaviors such as repeatedly lying to conceal the extent of time and money invested or asking for financial resources to pay off incurred debts are common and significantly affect personal relationships. Persistent thoughts about gambling or betting, along with the negative consequences arising from these activities, often hinder academic and professional performance. In addition to social and professional impacts, there is an observed increase in the use of health services and a deterioration in overall physical condition (APA, 2022).

[5] Psychological disorders are described by Banaco et al. (2015), Barlow and Durand (2015), and Dalgalarrondo (2019) as behavioral patterns that, due to their frequency, intensity, or context in which they occur, result in significant impairments at the individual and/or interpersonal level. The DSM-5-TR distinguishes these disorders from culturally expected responses to stressors or losses, suggesting that the clinical utility of the diagnosis does not, in itself, imply the need for treatment (APA, 2022). Furthermore, the manual emphasizes the consideration of sociocultural contexts in the assessment of symptoms, promoting a culturally sensitive approach in interpretation and treatment. In alignment, Banaco et al. (2015) expand the discussion and argue that the definition of pathological behaviors includes a cultural component, based on the norms established by the scientific community, highlighting the influence of language and culture in the classification of behaviors considered pathological. It is recommended to read the chapter *Psicopatologia* (Banaco et al., 2015), present in the book *Temas Clássicos da Psicologia sob a Ótica da Análise do Comportamento* (pp. 154–166), for a detailed analysis of how the definition of behaviors considered pathological is influenced by the verbal determination of the scientific community, emphasizing its relevance as a significant cultural component.

Assessment

Case Formulation[6]

Evidence-based practice (EBP) in mental health involves the integration of scientific evidence with clinical expertise to provide effective treatments tailored to individuals' needs. Implementing EBP consists of several stages, as Leonardi et al. (2023) described: a survey of the most relevant clinical issues must be conducted. Next, seeking the best available evidence, such as clinical guidelines and systematic reviews of randomized controlled trials (RCTs), is essential. A critical analysis of this evidence allows professionals to assess the applicability of the information found. After the analysis, the intervention is carried out by qualified professionals, and finally, the measurement of the obtained results takes place. However, the implementation of EBP faces significant challenges, such as the difficulty of applying interventions in diverse contexts and the inflexibility of therapeutic manuals, as pointed out by Gonçalves (2023). Additionally, the suboptimal administration of available treatments, highlighted by Shafran et al. (2009), limits the reach and effectiveness of evidence-based practices, underscoring the need for more flexible and contextually adapted approaches.

Case formulation (CF) constitutes a structured clinical tool essential for understanding and addressing the complexity of cases presented in mental health contexts. Its goal is to integrate nomothetic approaches, which deal with general principles, and idiographic approaches, which focus on the specificities of individuals (Eells, 2022; Gonçalves, 2023). Through CF, the clinical reasoning of professionals is translated into specific intervention strategies tailored to individual needs. Among the main benefits of CF is its assistance in adapting the components of therapeutic protocols to individual demands and integrating theory, research, and practices from different psychotherapeutic models. CF also enables a comprehensive understanding of the predisposing, precipitating, and perpetuating factors[7] of distress, facilitating the development of more precise and effective interventions.

---

[6] This topic was developed based on Mattos and Pinho (2024), from the chapter *Prática Baseada em Evidências em Psicologia Clínica*, in the book *Neuropsicologia e Dependência de Drogas: Neurobiologia, Cognição e Comportamento*, edited by Reichert and De Micheli.

[7] In the field of mental health, the terms "predisposing," "precipitating," and "perpetuating" are used to categorize different influences on the development, manifestation, and continuity of mental disorder symptoms. *Predisposing* factors refer to individual or contextual characteristics that increase the likelihood of a person developing a mental disorder, including genetic aspects, a family history of disorders, and traumatic experiences. *Precipitating* factors pertain to specific situations or events that trigger the immediate expression of symptoms, such as psychosocial stressors, recent traumas, or significant changes in living conditions. *Perpetuating* factors, in turn, are conditions or behaviors that contribute to the maintenance and recurrence of symptoms over time, such as dysfunctional thought patterns, avoidance behaviors, or negative environmental contexts (Barlow, 2022; Barlow & Durand, 2015; Dalgalarrondo, 2019).

The development of the CF follows specific steps that ensure a systematic and structured approach. The first step consists of obtaining a comprehensive list of problems and describing them across various domains, such as physiological, cognitive, emotional, and behavioral. Next, it is necessary to assign an anchoring diagnosis, which corresponds to the diagnosis that most impacts the individual's overall functioning. In the third step, a nomothetic evidence-based case formulation is selected, utilizing clinical manuals or adapting existing models to the case at hand. Finally, the individualization of the idiographic CF occurs, which involves the detailed collection of information about the problems and related factors, the generation of explanatory hypotheses, and the development of a treatment plan tailored to the specific needs of the patient (Eells, 2013, 2022; Gonçalves, 2023).

Cognitive Conceptualization

Cognitive conceptualization is a fundamental tool in Cognitive-Behavioral Therapy, especially when treating the diversity of profiles of individuals with behavioral dependencies, such as sports betting and gambling. There is no uniformity among these profiles, reflecting significant variability in the severity of problems, mental health indicators and quality of life, willingness to seek treatment and level of readiness for behavioral change, socioeconomic conditions, personal resources, and social support networks. Cultural practices and individual characteristics, such as thought patterns and emotions, also play a relevant role. Thus, the differences in each individual's needs require an adapted approach to their treatment plans. In this sense, case conceptualization underpins the understanding of these particularities and guides the formulation of interventions that consider the complexity of the individual and contextual factors involved in maintaining addiction behaviors (Beck & Liese, 2024).

In the case conceptualization process in Cognitive-Behavioral Therapy, various questions can be addressed to understand the dynamics of addiction behaviors better. Among them, investigating how and why individuals developed these behaviors and how they evolved to their current level stands out. It is essential to examine the psychosocial functioning of individuals before the onset of dependencies and to identify which environmental stimuli act as triggers for addictive behaviors or relapses. Equally relevant is the analysis of schemas (cognitive structures that organize information and influence how people perceive the world), thoughts (the momentary cognitions people have in response to situations), or beliefs (deep convictions that shape the interpretation of reality) that sustain these behaviors, as well as the role of the environment in their maintenance. Additionally, it is crucial to consider which aspects of the environment may reduce the frequency of behaviors, contributing to their cessation. It is also necessary to investigate whether other mental health problems are associated with these dependencies, such as anxiety and/or depression disorders, which may complicate the situation and require more comprehensive interventions (Beck & Liese, 2024).

Figure 6.1 describes the process of developing addictive behaviors, which is essential for cognitive assessment and conceptualization. Understanding this process allows for the identification of the stages through which individuals evolve into addictive behaviors, such as sports betting and gambling. The first stage involves early life experiences characterized by distal antecedents, which include genetic, neurobiological, psychosocial, and environmental risk factors. These factors contribute to the development of cognitive vulnerabilities, such as dysfunctional schemas and beliefs, behavioral vulnerabilities related to ineffective coping strategies, and emotional vulnerabilities, which often involve states of anxiety, anger, or depression. Subsequent exposure to risk behaviors, such as initial engagement in gambling or betting, usually leads to experimentation and, later, ongoing involvement. Over time, the reinforcement of distorted beliefs, such as the illusion of control or unrealistic optimism about outcomes, and the increased emotional response promote a cycle that perpetuates the occurrence of these behaviors.

Based on these issues, Beck and Liese (2024, pp. 41–42) propose ten essential elements for case conceptualization: (1) *basic problems*, including behavioral dependencies and related mental and physical health conditions; (2) *social context*, which encompasses life history, current situation, interpersonal relationships, sociocultural practices, and membership in vulnerable groups, along with socioeconomic circumstances and legal issues, referring to the social determinants of health as defined by the Office of Disease Prevention and Health Promotion (ODPHP) of the United States; (3) *distal antecedents*, which consider genetic, neurobiological, and psychosocial vulnerabilities; (4) *proximal antecedents*, involving internal and external stimuli, triggers, and high-risk circumstances; (5) *cognitive processes*, which include schemas, beliefs, and cognitive distortions, with reference to the thinking

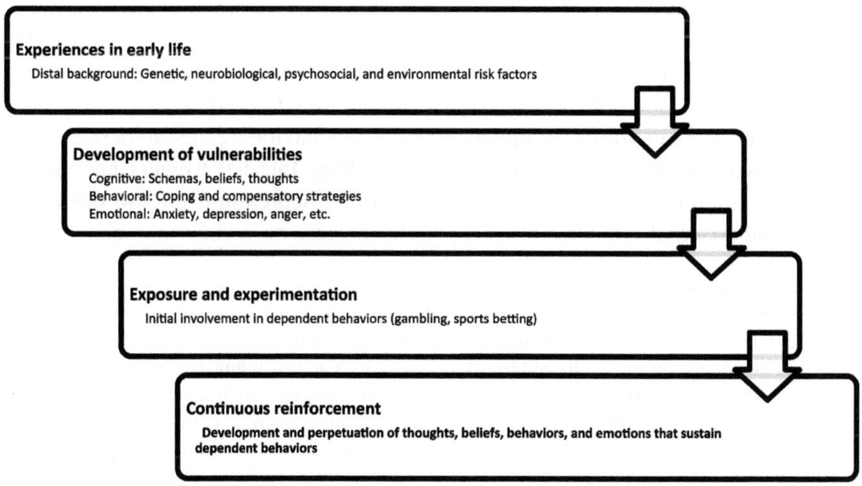

Fig. 6.1 Flowchart of the process of developing addictive behaviors in betting and gambling. (Source: Elaborated by the authors based on Beck and Liese (2024))

systems proposed by Kahneman (2012)[8]; (6) *affective processes*, addressing emotions and mood states; (7) *behavior patterns*, which consider adaptive behaviors and coping skills; (8) *readiness for change and goals*, encompassing the stages of change (Table 6.2) and associated goals; (9) *data integration*, which seeks to identify patterns and causal relationships among context, thoughts, emotions, and behaviors; and (10) *treatment implications*, which aim to identify the most appropriate strategies and techniques based on the information collected.

At the core of Cognitive-Behavioral Therapy lies a theoretical model that facilitates understanding behavioral dependencies, allowing for the analysis of individuals involved in these behaviors. The cognitive processes that underpin this understanding can be organized into three main categories: core beliefs, thoughts, and beliefs associated with addictive behaviors, as well as automatic thoughts and other specific cognitive processes, such as self-efficacy, outcome expectations, permissive beliefs, and instrumental thoughts (Table 6.3). Automatic thoughts are characterized by being brief, spontaneous, and not resulting from deliberate reasoning. In contrast, beliefs are more stable cognitive processes that form over time and generate thoughts. Core beliefs, also known as nuclear beliefs, refer to principles, ideas, or values central to an individual's identity, encompassing areas such as self-image, worldview, future expectations, relationships, and perceptions of others. These core beliefs are fundamental in emotions and recurring behaviors, including behavioral dependencies. Individuals who hold generalized negative beliefs about themselves, their future expectations, others, and interpersonal relationships tend to be at greater risk of developing anxiety and depression, resulting in significant emotional suffering. This suffering may lead to the pursuit of relief through substance use or addictive behaviors, a behavior often identified as "self-medication" (Beck & Liese, 2024; Lee et al., 2017; Smith et al., 2017; Turner et al., 2018) (Fig. 6.2).

Since the emergence of Cognitive-Behavioral Therapy, the "ABC" model (Fig. 6.3) has been widely utilized, considering stimuli (internal and external) that precede behaviors, such as signals, situations, and circumstances, which activate beliefs and thoughts, directly influencing emotions, behaviors, and physiological responses. These stimuli, known as triggers, elicit thoughts and beliefs, being identified as high-risk situations for the occurrence of behaviors related to dependence, such as involvement in sports betting or gambling. Internal triggers encompass physical or emotional sensations, such as anxiety, depression, intense desire, or pain, while external triggers involve people, places, or objects associated with

[8] The thinking systems proposed by Kahneman (2012) include *System 1*, which operates automatically and quickly, often without the perception of voluntary control. This system is responsible for instinctive reactions and rapid decisions, which can contribute to impulsive behaviors, such as recurrent involvement in sports betting and gambling. In contrast, *System 2* allocates attention to cognitive activities that require more effort and concentration, such as complex calculations or detailed analyses. The operations of this system are often associated with the subjective experience of activity, choice, and deliberate concentration. The activation of System 2 allows for a more careful assessment of the consequences of behaviors (such as betting), promoting reflection that may lead to a reduction in risk behaviors. However, the predominance of System 1 can hinder this analysis, perpetuating dependencies (Beck & Liese, 2024).

Table 6.2 Stages of motivation in changing behaviors related to sports betting and gambling

Stage	Description	Examples	Motivational tasks for professionals
Pre-contemplation	The period before considering change may be when there is little or no recognition of addictive behaviors and potential associated harms. At this stage, information and feedback are needed	A gambler who continues to gamble regularly without recognizing the risks associated with their behavior	Reflect and raise doubts to stimulate awareness of the risks and issues related to gambling patterns
Contemplation	This is when individuals begin to consider the possibility of change. Ambivalence is prevalent, and individuals may oscillate between changing or not	A gambler starts to think about reducing their bets but is still determining if they should do so	"Tip the balance" to evoke reasons for change, highlight the risks of not changing, and strengthen self-efficacy
Preparation	It occurs between contemplation and action when individuals begin to plan how to stop engaging in addictive behaviors	A gambler decides to set a weekly spending limit and seeks strategies to avoid situations that may lead to gambling behavior	Collaboratively assist in determining the best course of action to follow for change
Action	The period in which individuals implement planned changes, facing vulnerabilities to lapses or relapses	A gambler starts to restrict their bets and participate in support groups to maintain control over their behavior	Monitor and assist in the steps toward change, reinforcing the importance of ongoing support
Maintenance	This is the stage in which individuals integrate changes into their daily lives, consolidating new behaviors and avoiding relapse	A former gambler who now invests their time in alternative activities, such as sports or hobbies, and avoids risky situations	Assist and guide in identifying and utilizing relapse prevention strategies

Source: Elaborated by the authors based on Miller and Rollnick (2001, 2023) and Beck and Liese (2024)

addictive behaviors. Behaviors are actions performed to achieve a goal or outcome, and over time, many become automatic and repetitive, mediated by automatic thoughts. This automatic nature is particularly prominent in dependence-related behaviors, making them frequent and habitual. Emotions, in turn, are subjective experiences closely associated with these behaviors, and it is widely accepted that individuals seek to maximize positive emotions and minimize negative emotions. Those who struggle to regulate their emotions exhibit greater vulnerability to addictive behaviors, often using them as a means to alleviate emotional discomfort (Beck & Liese, 2024).

Chain analysis is a technique used to identify and connect thoughts, beliefs, and feelings related to dependent behaviors, such as sports betting and gambling

Table 6.3 Specific cognitive processes in behavioral addictions related to sports betting and gambling

Process	Definition	Examples
Self-efficacy	Assessments by individuals regarding their abilities to perform specific tasks or achieve particular goals	Gamblers believe they can control their ability to limit the time spent on betting
Outcome expectations	Thoughts and beliefs about the consequences associated with specific addictive behaviors	Individuals may believe they will win large prizes if they bet more frequently on sporting events
Permissive beliefs	Beliefs arise during times of greater vulnerability, where people tend to justify or minimize addictive behaviors	A gambler may think that "today is a special day" and therefore "deserves" to make an extra bet, ignoring the consequences
Instrumental thoughts	Guide the logistics or mechanics of addictive behaviors, addressing the "how" of performing these behaviors	Considering the odds and statistics, a gambler may plan the best strategy for betting on a sporting event

Source: Elaborated by the authors based on Beck and Liese (2024)

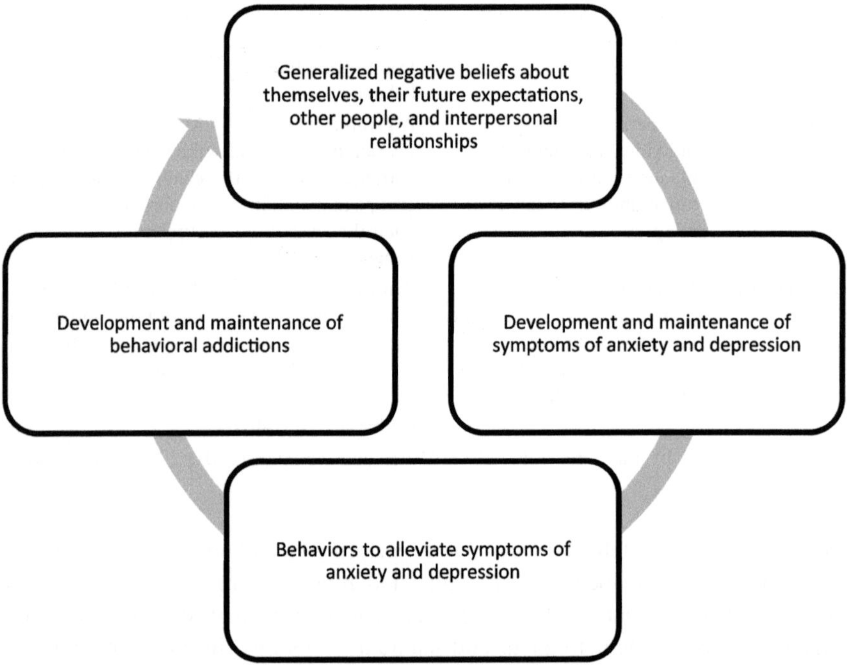

Fig. 6.2 Repetitive cycle involving behavioral addictions and co-occurrence of anxiety and depression symptoms. (Source: Adapted from Beck and Liese (2024))

(Table 6.4). This process aids in examining the triggers, thoughts, emotions, and behaviors associated with the functioning of risk behaviors. The first step involves identifying the most relevant processes, such as circumstances, thoughts, beliefs,

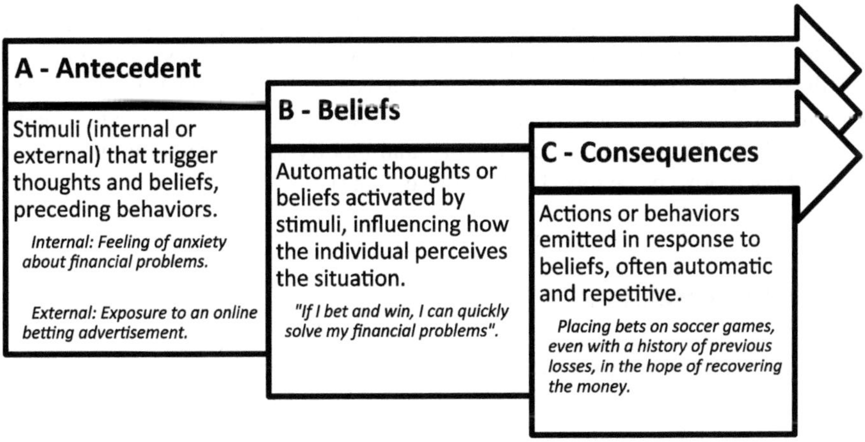

Fig. 6.3 ABC model applied to sports betting and gambling involvement. (Source: Prepared by the authors based on Beck and Liese (2024))

Table 6.4 Chain analysis: flowchart of triggers, thoughts, and behaviors in sports betting and gambling

Triggers →	Thoughts →	Behaviors →	Thoughts →	Behaviors
Feeling of boredom →	*"If I place a bet, it will entertain me"* →	Places a bet on a sporting event →	*"If I keep going, I might recover what I lost"* →	Makes another bet to try to recover the money
Previous loss on a bet →	*"I need to recover the money I lost"* →	Bets more money on a game →	*"I can't stop now; I just need one win"* →	Increases the bet amount
Feeling of anxiety →	*"Betting will help me relax and forget my problems"* →	Bets impulsively to relieve anxiety →	*"Betting really helped me; I should continue"* →	Repeats the bet to prolong emotional relief
Pressure from friends at a sporting event →	*"Everyone is betting; I'll look weak if I don't do the same"* →	Places a bet to follow the group →	*"If I win, I'll impress everyone"* →	Makes another bet to maintain social image
Bonus offer on a betting site →	*"I can't waste this opportunity to win more"* →	Bets using the available bonus →	*"Luck will turn in my favor; I just need to try one more time"* →	Bets again to maximize potential gains

Source: Elaborated by the authors based on Beck and Liese (2024)

feelings, and behaviors contributing to the dependence cycle. In the second step, a flowchart illustrates the causal relationships between these elements, facilitating the understanding of how this pattern operates. When individuals experience emotions and physiological triggers (such as anger, anxiety, boredom, or craving), the cycle begins with automatic thoughts that influence subsequent emotions. These emotions, in turn, provoke a behavioral response, which may include the action of betting again. Following the action, new thoughts and justifications arise, reinforcing the behavior. During interventions, the goal is to assist individuals in identifying the circumstances and thought patterns that maintain the behaviors in question to evaluate these thoughts, test their validity, and modify them, promoting the enactment of alternative behaviors (Beck & Liese, 2024).

Clinical Interventions

Cognitive-Behavioral Therapy Techniques

Table 6.5, developed by the authors based on Beck and Liese (2024), synthesizes the main standardized techniques of Cognitive Behavioral Therapy applicable to managing sports betting and gambling behaviors. Each technique is described in terms of its definition and is accompanied by practical examples of application, demonstrating how these strategies can be used to intervene in patterns of dependent behavior.

An Understanding of Gambling from Behavior Analysis: Contributions to Interventions[9]

Behavior Analysis is a natural science dedicated to studying human behavior as an independent discipline, as proposed by Skinner (1953). This approach to psychology is structured into three interconnected subdivisions: (1) *Radical Behaviorism*, which represents the underlying philosophy; (2) *Experimental Analysis of Behavior*, which focuses on basic research; and (3) *Applied Behavior Analysis*, which involves the practical application of concepts derived from these investigations (Carvalho-Neto, 2002; Tourinho, 1999).

This science redefines the concept of behavior, understanding it not only as individual manifestations but as a dynamic interaction between these manifestations and the environmental stimuli that influence them (De Rose, 1999; Matos, 1999; Todorov, 2020). Thus, behaviors classified as "psychopathological" (psychological or mental disorders; APA, 2022) are analyzed within this perspective, considering them as learned responses that occur and are maintained in relation to the environment. Behavior Analysis, therefore, investigates the environmental variables that

[9] This topic was developed based on Aranha and Oshiro (2024), from the chapter '*Uma Possibilidade de Compreensão dos Transtornos por Uso de Substâncias a partir da Análise do Comportamento: Subsídios para Intervenções Clínicas e Psicossociais*', in the book '*Neuropsicologia e Dependência de Drogas: Neurobiologia, Cognição e Comportamento*', edited by Reichert and De Micheli.

establish and perpetuate behaviors, even when these generate aversive consequences for the individuals or the social community to which they belong (Banaco et al., 2015).

Radical Behaviorism proposes that human behavior should be the focus of its own discipline, in contrast to approaches that regard it as a result of underlying events. This perspective critiques the tendency to attribute the causes of behavior to internal events, arguing that by asserting an internal event is responsible for a behavior, it remains necessary to explain what provokes that internal event (Skinner,

Table 6.5 Standardized Cognitive-Behavioral Therapy techniques for behaviors related to sports betting and gambling

Techniques	Definition	Example of application to gambling and/or betting behaviors
Stimulus control	Involves identifying and managing stimuli that trigger desires, impulses, and opportunities to engage in dependent behaviors. This technique is organized into four steps: (1) list and describe problematic triggers (high-risk circumstances); (2) discuss past strategies to manage these triggers; (3) identify triggers that generate the most concern; and (4) debate strategies to manage these triggers	When working with an individual struggling with gambling, a professional may help them identify that seeing advertisements for sporting events (external trigger) and feeling anxious (internal trigger) are factors that trigger the urge to gamble. The professional can then discuss strategies such as avoiding certain media channels or developing relaxation techniques to cope with anxiety
Delay gratification and distraction	Refers to creating time and distance between a desire/impulse and the actual behavior. Techniques for delaying gratification and distraction help control impulses by redirecting attention to alternative stimuli. This technique can include creating a list of alternative activities that can be performed. It is used to avoid, cancel, interrupt, or neutralize the progression of dependency rituals, allowing individuals time to implement self-help skills and seek social support	An individual feeling an urge to gamble after a loss may use this technique to distract themselves by calling a friend, going to the park, or engaging in a hobby. They may create a list of alternative activities, such as reading a book or watching a movie, to divert their attention from the urge to gamble
Cost-benefit analysis	This technique highlights the tendency of people with behavioral addictions to amplify the benefits and minimize the drawbacks of their behaviors. The cost-benefit analysis identifies the potential benefits of engaging in dependent behaviors compared to the harms of not engaging. A practical method is to use a quadrant matrix, starting with the "benefits of engaging" quadrant, which provides insights into underlying motivations	A professional can help an individual create a matrix listing the benefits of gambling, such as excitement and the possibility of financial gain, alongside the drawbacks, such as debt and negative impacts on relationships. This can help the individual reflect on their choices and consider the consequences of their behavior

(continued)

Table 6.5 (continued)

Techniques	Definition	Example of application to gambling and/or betting behaviors
Value hierarchy	Values are deeply rooted core beliefs, such as moral and ethical standards principles, that guide desired behaviors. When asked about their values, many people cite relationships with family, friends, and the community, as well as virtues like reliability, honesty, and compassion. The value hierarchy technique involves listing important values and narrowing them down to the top five. After this step, professionals review the results with individuals, identifying conflicts and establishing strategies aligned with their personal values* * It is important to emphasize that this approach focuses on the values individuals consider valuable in their lives, avoiding a moralizing perspective that could deter them from treatment. Additionally, psychological reactance[a] should be considered, as it may arise when individuals feel that their values are being challenged or disregarded	A professional can help individuals identify that honesty and commitment to family are core values for them. By exploring the conflicts between these values and gambling behavior, the professional can help them develop strategies more aligned with their personal beliefs, such as prioritizing time with family instead of gambling on sporting events
Activity monitoring and scheduling	This technique is used to uncover and address deficits in self-care, outline patterns of dependent behavior, and identify opportunities for alternative activities. By collecting data on activities, professionals and individuals can assess the impact of these behaviors and identify strengths and resources in their lives. A daily activity schedule can be utilized, covering all days of the week and divided into time blocks, instructing individuals to monitor their activities. This allows for a better understanding of time use and serves as a guide for planning future activities that may replace dependent behaviors	A professional may instruct an individual to create a daily schedule that includes time slots for activities such as exercise, hobbies, social interactions, and relaxation time. By analyzing this schedule, the individual may realize they spend many hours watching betting games and may start to fill that time with healthier alternative activities

(continued)

Table 6.5 (continued)

Techniques	Definition	Example of application to gambling and/or betting behaviors
Behavioral activation[b]	This approach aims to improve the quality of life for individuals by increasing positive behaviors that align with their values. Behavioral activation emerges from monitoring and scheduling activities, where the initiated behaviors result from the monitoring process and the completion of the value hierarchy, ensuring that the chosen actions are consistent with the individual's deeper values. Key elements include (1) daily monitoring; (2) identification of important areas of life (relationships, education, career, recreation); (3) review of values; and (4) planning of activities	A professional can work with an individual to identify areas of life that need attention, such as relationships and leisure. After reviewing their values, the client may plan activities like spending more time with family or enrolling in a course, promoting a more fulfilling life, and reducing gambling behaviors
Automatic thought recording	Fundamental for helping individuals understand the relationships between situations, automatic thoughts, beliefs, emotions, and behaviors. Well-constructed alternative responses in these records reinforce positive and healthy processes and identify areas for potential change. The recording helps identify and optimize thoughts, feelings, and behaviors that are important to individuals	An individual may use automatic thought recording to note recurring thoughts like "I'm going to win this time" or "Just one more bet." By analyzing these thoughts with a professional, they can formulate more rational and balanced alternative responses, such as *the odds of winning are low, and I've already lost a lot of money*
Relaxation training	Provides individuals with methods to reduce the arousal and tension associated with impulses and desires, allowing for a time lag after the initial urge, during which it may decrease. Techniques include controlled breathing and progressive muscle relaxation. Individuals are informed that they are more likely to make mistakes and harm themselves when making significant decisions or performing important tasks while hyper-aroused	An individual may practice controlled breathing when feeling an intense urge to gamble, helping to calm the body and reduce agitation before making an impulsive decision. This can include breathing exercises or a routine of progressive muscle relaxation to decrease anxiety associated with the urge
Mindfulness and meditation training	Aims to encourage individuals to be aware of their present experiences and each moment in a conscious and receptive manner. The techniques help observe sensations (such as tension, anxiety, sadness, impulses) and accept them with the understanding that they are temporary states	The individual may use mindfulness practices to observe their impulses and desires without acting immediately. For example, when feeling a strong urge to gamble, they may observe their physical and emotional sensations, recognizing that the urge will pass with time

(continued)

Table 6.5 (continued)

Techniques	Definition	Example of application to gambling and/or betting behaviors
Contingency management[c]	Involves rewarding positive changes. Individuals can create their own contingency management strategies, rewarding themselves with resources that would otherwise be spent on dependent behaviors	The individual may create a reward system, such as setting aside an amount that would be used for betting and using it for enjoyable and healthy activities, such as a trip or a gift, after a period without gambling
Role-play	Interaction between individuals, in which one or both act as a character different from themselves to facilitate the learning process. It can be used to teach a variety of skills, including active listening, assertiveness, empathy, and emotional regulation	The professional and the individual in treatment may simulate a situation where the individual declines an invitation to gamble with friends, practicing assertiveness skills and developing confidence to handle real social pressure situations

Source: Elaborated by the authors based on Beck and Liese (2024)

[a]Psychological reactance is a phenomenon that refers to the predictable pattern of emotion and behavior that arises when individuals perceive that their personal freedom is being restricted or threatened, often leading to behaviors that are contrary to what is being imposed (Brehm, 1966; Miller & Rollnick, 2001, 2009, 2023)

[b]For a deeper reading on behavioral activation, its theoretical foundations, current research, and applications, it is recommended to read *Transtornos Psicológicos: Terapias Baseadas em Evidências'* by Abreu and Abreu (2022a)

[c]Dorey et al. (2022a) identified that contingency management can facilitate prolonged engagement in the treatment of individuals with disorders related to gambling and gaming, increasing motivation and helping to initiate the therapeutic process earlier. However, some participants pointed out the possibility of manipulation for obtaining money intended for gambling, as well as the risk that this approach could trigger relapses. In another study, Dorey et al. (2022b) observed that healthcare professionals reported concerns about the compatibility of contingency management with their therapeutic philosophies, highlighting similarities with gambling, which could compromise trust in the therapeutic relationship. Petry et al. (2006) demonstrated that contingency management, by providing rewards to individuals, is effective in maintaining treatment and reducing drug use, without increasing gambling behaviors. Christensen et al. (2018) also suggested that this approach may be effective for the treatment of gambling-related disorders. In Brazil, contingency management has proven effective in promoting abstinence from crack cocaine (Miguel et al., 2016) and in retaining cocaine users in treatment (Miguel et al., 2022)

1953). In opposition to internalist explanations, Radical Behaviorism advocates a model in which all behaviors—the behavioral repertoire (Da Silva et al., 2018)—are products of the individual's interaction with the environment. Thus, behaviors are understood as natural events, possessing physical dimensions and being determined by specific conditions rather than being considered random or the result of agents' free will.

Based on the model of natural selection, Skinner (1981) introduced the idea that the environment shapes behavior through three interconnected levels of selection: phylogeny, ontogeny, and culture. Phylogenetic history refers to how human ancestors interacted with essential environmental factors for organism regulation and survival, resulting in the selection of behaviors that became "automatic" and did not require prior learning. This evolutionary basis also influenced individuals' sensitivity to learning processes. From conception to adulthood, each human encounters a diverse range of environmental stimuli that contribute to the formation of individual behavioral repertoires (Skinner, 1974). Respondent conditioning allows stimuli that initially do not provoke reactions to generate responses similar to those caused by unconditioned stimuli.

On the other hand, operant selection, which resembles phylogenetic selection, pertains to the emission, variability, and selection of responses whose consequences influence their repetition. These consequences are divided into four categories: positive reinforcement, negative reinforcement, positive punishment, and negative punishment, which can increase or decrease the likelihood of behavior recurrence. Additionally, cultural history represents a level of selection that involves the transmission of practices with adaptive value among group members, enhancing collective survival chances (Skinner, 1981).

In summary, according to Behavior Analysis, all behaviors—unconditioned respondents, conditioned respondents, and operants—are functionally connected to specific aspects of the environment (Skinner, 1981). In the context of psychopathology, the criterion of suffering generated by behavior is applied, both for the individuals exhibiting the behavior and for others around them, as an indication that this behavior is susceptible to intervention (Banaco et al., 2015). Suffering can be operationalized as a set of behaviors that manifest in situations where the behavioral repertoire of individuals, within a given context, results in a scarcity of positive reinforcers and/or fails to eliminate aversive stimuli, both in the short and/or long term (Guilhardi, 2004).

The behavior of gambling or betting is interpreted as an operant behavior maintained by reinforcing positive and negative consequences (Delfabbro et al., 2023). In a respondent relationship, the gambling environment can be understood as an unconditioned stimulus that provokes unconditioned responses (euphoria and hyperarousal, for example). From an operant perspective, betting can be seen as an unconditioned positive reinforcer. When initiating the activity of betting, for instance, motivated by the observation of other bettors, the sequence of behaviors culminating in the bet (such as planning, going to the betting location, placing the bet) is positively reinforced by financial gains or the excitement generated, increasing the likelihood that the behavior will be repeated. For example, an individual may win a sum of money in a game, and this gain positively reinforces the behavior of betting, raising the chance that they will bet again in the future (Cardwell et al., 2022; Clark, 2010; James et al., 2016; Mathieu et al., 2020; Mravčík et al., 2020). Furthermore, antecedent events referred to as discriminative stimuli (Catania, 1998/1999) present at the moment of the bet (such as the casino environment company of friends) become marked in such a way that, in future interactions, contact with these stimuli also increases the likelihood of repeating the betting behavior.

Social reinforcers can sustain the behavior of betting, such as attention and approval from peers (Deans et al., 2016; Gordon et al., 2015; Hing et al., 2024b; Mazar et al., 2018; Nyemcsok et al., 2018; Seal et al., 2022; Sirola et al., 2021;

Sztainert et al., 2014). For example, in a context where betting is admired, an individual may be seen betting and receiving praise from friends (such as *"she's amazing"* or *"he always wins!"*). These social reinforcers encourage betting behavior and increase its probability of recurrence, especially in the presence of people who provide this validation.

Betting behavior may also be sustained by negative reinforcement. Aversive stimuli, both unconditioned and conditioned, can induce the practice of betting. By betting, individuals may temporarily attenuate or eliminate the influence of the aversive condition (in this case, the behavior is not driven by the addition of a positive reinforcer but by the removal of the aversive stimulus) (Ferro et al., 2024). For example, a bettor may feel anxiety in situations of financial difficulty and gamble to relieve this condition, with the act of betting acquiring a reinforcing function of alleviating tension.

Behavioral Interventions: Applications of Behavior Analysis

The applied Behavior Analysis is grounded in the philosophy of Radical Behaviorism and the principles derived from the experimental analysis of behavior, which aims to assess and intervene in human problems (Baer et al., 1968). In the context of the services provided, professionals seek to (1) identify behaviors related to gambling or betting that result in a decrease of positive reinforcers and/or an increase in aversive stimuli, both in the short and long term, as well as understand the environmental variables that establish and sustain such behaviors and (2) promote the adoption of behaviors that facilitate access to positive reinforcers and reduce exposure to aversive stimuli (Ferster, 1972).

According to Skinner's (1981) model of selection by consequences, each individual's behavioral repertoire is unique and influenced by a specific set of environmental variables that sustain gambling-related behaviors. Analyzing reinforcement contingencies is essential for identifying the antecedent and consequent factors that maintain these behaviors (Britto et al., 2020). From this understanding, it is possible to modify the environmental variables and assist individuals in developing alternative and more effective behavioral repertoires.

The clinical evaluation process can begin with identifying the conditions that maintain gambling behavior, considering that the stimuli that provoke this behavior and its consequences vary among individuals. Professionals may investigate the behavioral deficits and excesses that hinder the adoption of alternatives in situations that evoke gambling. Additionally, the analysis of positive and negative punishments related to gambling behavior is vital for understanding the mechanisms that control engagement in gambling. When an individual is not fully aware of the adverse consequences associated with gambling, they may resist treatment, remaining in contact with reinforcers that encourage them to gamble. Effective interventions may include describing the punitive consequences of gambling, questioning the effects of betting, and guiding family members to avoid reinforcing gambling behavior.

The development of self-awareness regarding the antecedent factors and consequences that control gambling behavior is fundamental, as is the identification of specific situations that trigger gambling practices. Finally, different behavioral approaches may be utilized to help individuals adopt alternative or incompatible behaviors to gambling, generating new reinforcers that break the gambling cycle. If these new behaviors are properly reinforced, it is more likely that the antecedents associated with them will be evoked, leading to the extinction of the compensatory responses linked to gambling behavior (for some behavioral intervention techniques, see Table 6.5).

Acceptance and Commitment Therapy

In the models of cognitive and behavioral therapies, since their early formulations for the treatment of depression (Beck et al., 1979) and later for addictions (Beck et al., 1993), it is assumed that it is crucial to distinguish what can cognitively and cannot be changed, promoting personal behavioral changes to maintain health and quality of life. Following these principles, Acceptance and Commitment Therapy has been widely and effectively applied to the treatment of behavioral addictions, based on four processes that contribute to its development: (1) *cognitive fusion*, which refers to excessive identification with negative thoughts; (2) *experiential avoidance*, which involves avoiding uncomfortable feelings or experiences; (3) *poorly defined values*, which implies a lack of clarity about what is truly important in life; and (4) *lack of commitment* to behaviors that support well-defined values. In this sense, the main objectives of therapy are to help individuals flexibly accept what they cannot change and commit to changing what they can, aligning their actions with their personal values (Beck & Liese, 2024).

When applied to individuals involved in sports betting and gambling, these concepts can be exemplified through strategies that encourage acceptance of feelings of anxiety and impulsivity rather than avoiding them. This may include identifying values such as financial stability and healthy relationships, which are often compromised by gambling behavior. By promoting an active commitment to activities that reflect these values, individuals can be guided to set limits on their betting practices, reducing the frequency and intensity of impulsive behavior. Furthermore, by reevaluating their beliefs and automatic thoughts that justify gambling, they can develop greater psychological flexibility, facilitating decision-making that is more aligned with their life goals and well-being.

In analytical-behavioral terms, *cognitive fusion* occurs when individuals relate so literally to verbal constructs that they cannot perceive them as what they indeed are—words, rules, instructions, thoughts, among other verbal behaviors. As a result, individuals are highly likely to follow what these verbal constructs prescribe, becoming less sensitive to environmental contingencies (Abreu & Abreu, 2022b; Hayes et al., 2021). In the context of sports betting and gambling, this manifests when gamblers firmly believe in self-imposed rules or superstitions that assert that a win is guaranteed if they follow certain rituals, thus disregarding the realities of gambling.

On the other hand, *experiential avoidance* refers to behaviors aimed at controlling or avoiding private events, such as efforts to feel good and avoid emotional discomfort at any cost. This unavailability to experience emotions can lead individuals to engage in betting behaviors to escape feelings such as sadness or anxiety (e.g., in search of a state of euphoria or hyper-excitation). Although these attempts may provide immediate relief, in the long term, the result is a repetitive cycle of behaviors that entail events that individuals try to avoid (Abreu & Abreu, 2022b). For example, a gambler may initially feel relief by participating in a bet, believing that this will provide the necessary distraction to escape sadness or stress. However, as losses accumulate, this behavior becomes an additional source of anxiety and discontent.

These cognitive fusion and experiential avoidance processes are closely related to inflexible attention and attachment to the conceptualized self. *Inflexible attention* refers to controlling verbal stimuli related to the past, such as rumination, and to the future, such as anticipation. This represents a cognitive fusion that diminishes contact with present stimuli during behavior emission. Generally, this inflexible attention results in a low ability to describe the public or private experiences occurring in the here and now. When individuals have difficulty expressing such experiences, they become less capable of recognizing private events as what they really are—verbal or physical events that are occurring and are transitory. In turn, the *conceptualized self* is based on a rigid narrative about who one is, leading to an inflexible relationship with the concepts that define identity. When individuals are fused with their thoughts, oscillating between ruminations about the past and fears of the future, and engaging in strategies to avoid these emotions and thoughts, it is to be expected that they lack clarity about what makes their lives meaningful (Abreu & Abreu, 2022b; Hayes et al., 2021). This scenario is often observed in individuals involved with sports betting and gambling, who may find themselves in a cycle of impulsive behavior, guided by a need to meet the expectations of their conceptualized self rather than engaging in actions that truly resonate with their values and life goals.

In this sense, through six central processes, Acceptance and Commitment Therapy aims to increase individuals' psychological flexibility. The first process is *acceptance*, which involves the willingness to experience private events without judgment. The second is *cognitive defusion*, where the person learns to recognize that obsessions are just obsessions, thoughts are just thoughts, and feelings are just feelings, all transitory and not entirely under control. *Contact with the present moment*, the third process, pertains to the ability to respond to what is present in the here and now, with full awareness of the stimuli occurring both within and outside oneself. The fourth process, the *self-as-context*, involves observing one's own experience more broadly, recognizing the symbolic and transitory nature of thoughts and feelings. The fifth process consists of identifying *values* and qualities of actions to be cultivated throughout life, making life more meaningful. Finally, *committed actions* represent how values can be implemented in practice (Abreu & Abreu, 2022b; Hayes et al., 2021).

These processes become fundamental when applied to sports betting and gambling. For example, by accepting the feelings of anxiety associated with loss, individuals can develop a healthier and more conscious approach to gambling, shedding cognitive fusion with self-critical thoughts and promoting actions that align with values such as financial stability and healthy relationships. This approach not only encourages greater psychological flexibility but also empowers individuals to make decisions that more authentically reflect what they consider meaningful in their lives. In this way, individuals can avoid the repetition of impulsive behaviors that distance them from their goals and aspirations, allowing for a more balanced and sustainable relationship with betting activities (Beck & Liese, 2024).

Studies and Evidence

Higueruela-Ahijado et al. (2023) conducted a systematic review to synthesize and analyze the evidence regarding the effectiveness of cognitive-behavioral interventions in improving the quality of life of individuals with pathological gambling. The results indicated that such interventions not only enhanced the participants' quality of life but also reduced associated symptoms, such as anxiety and depression, the amount of money spent on gambling, as well as decreased alcohol consumption and scores on gambling behavior assessment instruments. It was observed that combining Cognitive-Behavioral Therapy with manuals or techniques such as mindfulness and support sessions like Gamblers Anonymous yielded better long-term outcomes. The authors concluded that cognitive-behavioral interventions have the potential to promote significant improvements in quality of life and related psychological variables, suggesting that future research should explore the effectiveness of these interventions in different formats and contexts.

Technological innovations have proven promising in the treatment of problematic gambling behaviors, particularly through accessible digital interventions. The positive outcomes of online gambling intervention programs are substantial, as is the emerging evidence indicating that interventions implemented via mobile devices, such as smartphones, have the potential to reach a wide audience. A significant example is the mobile game developed by Humphrey et al. (2020), described in a protocol that presents the design of a randomized clinical trial to evaluate the efficacy and acceptability of Cognitive-Behavioral Therapy delivered through a mobile application for individuals reporting gambling-related issues.

Final Considerations

This chapter addressed the evolution of sports betting as a new frontier of behavioral addictions, outlining a historical panorama from ancient civilizations to the current digital era, marked by technological innovations and a wide range of betting modalities. It presented data on the global prevalence of involvement in gambling, highlighting statistics and epidemiological data that described the impacts associated with gambling-related disorders. The diagnostic criteria from ICD-11 and DSM-5-TR were reviewed, providing an updated description of the characteristics of these disorders. The text explored vulnerability factors, including genetic, physiological, and temperamental dimensions, and discussed the neurobiology and cognitive aspects that influence choice behavior, emphasizing the interaction between the prefrontal cortex and brain regions associated with processing emotions and rewards. The sociocultural and economic contexts that influence involvement in gambling were also examined, along with the psychiatric comorbidities that are often observed. The chapter further addressed assessment and case formulation, presenting principles and applications of cognitive and behavioral approaches, with a description of theoretical models, techniques, and practical examples for planning and conducting effective assessments and interventions. Thus, this chapter aimed to broaden the understanding of the complexities involved in gambling behaviors, highlighting the importance of multidimensional strategies for treating gambling-related disorders and other emerging behavioral addictions in contemporary society.

References

Abreu, P. R., & Abreu, J. H. S. (2022a). *Transtornos psicológicos: terapias baseadas em evidências*. Manole.

Abreu, P. R., & Abreu, J. H. S. (2022b). *Psicopatologia: Tratamento Comportamental Contextual*. Manole.

Afe, T., Ogunsemi, O., Daniel, O., Ale, A., & Adeleye, O. (2022). Prevalence of and factors associated with disordered gambling disorder, and use of DSM-5 based sports betting questionnaire, in a southwest Nigerian community. *Indian Journal of Psychological Medicine, 44*(3), 265–271. https://doi.org/10.1177/02537176211023809

American Psychiatric Association (APA). (2013). *Diagnostic and statistical manual of mental disorders* (5th ed.). American Psychiatric Association.

American Psychiatric Association (APA). (2022). *Diagnostic and statistical manual of mental disorders* (5th ed.). American Psychiatric Association.

Anderson, P. M., Blackshaw, I. S., Siekmann, R. C. R., & Soek, J. (2012). *Sports betting: Law and policy*. https://doi.org/10.1007/978-90-6704-799-9

Ayton, P., & Fischer, I. (2004). The hot hand fallacy and the gambler's fallacy: Two faces of subjective randomness? *Memory & Cognition, 32*(8), 1369–1378. https://doi.org/10.3758/bf03206327

Baer, D. M., Wolf, M. M., & Risley, T. R. (1968). Some current dimensions of applied behavior analysis. *Journal of Applied Behavior Analysis, 1*(1), 91–97. https://doi.org/10.1901/jaba.1968.1-91

Banaco, R. A., Zamignani, D. R., Martone, R. C., Vermes, J. S., & Kovac, R. (2015). Psicopatologia. In M. M. C. Hübner & M. B. Moreira (Eds.), *Temas Clássicos da Psicologia sob a Ótica da Análise do Comportamento* (pp. 154–166). Guanabara Koogan.

Bankole, E. T. (2019). Patterns and prevalence of gambling behavior among youth in Southwest Nigeria: A case study of youth in Oyo and Ekiti states. *British Journal of Psychological Research, 7*(2), 22–46.

Barlow, D. H. (2022). *Manual clínico dos transtornos psicológicos*. Artmed.

Barlow, D. H., & Durand, V. M. (2015). *Psicopatologia: uma abordagem integrada* (2nd ed.). Cengage Learning.

Bechara, A., Damasio, A. R., Damasio, H., & Anderson, S. W. (1994). Insensitivity to future consequences following damage to human prefrontal cortex. *Cognition, 50*(1–3), 7–15. https://doi.org/10.1016/0010-0277(94)90018-3

Bechara, A., Damasio, H., Damasio, A. R., & Lee, G. P. (1999). Different contributions of the human amygdala and ventromedial prefrontal cortex to decision-making. *The Journal of Neuroscience, 19*(13), 5473–5481. https://doi.org/10.1523/JNEUROSCI.19-13-05473.1999

Bechara, A., Tranel, D., & Damasio, H. (2000). Characterization of the decision-making deficit of patients with ventromedial prefrontal cortex lesions. *Brain, 123*(Pt 11), 2189–2202. https://doi.org/10.1093/brain/123.11.2189

Beck, A., & Liese, B. (2024). *Terapia cognitivo-comportamental para transtornos por uso de substâncias e dependências comportamentais*. Artmed.

Beck, A. T., Rush, A. J., Shaw, B. F., & Emery, G. (1979). *Cognitive therapy of depression*. Guilford Press.

Beck, A. T., Wright, F. D., Newman, C. F., & Liese, B. S. (1993). Cognitive therapy of substance abuse.

Bengel, C., & McCarriston, S. (2022). U.S. sports betting: Here's where all 50 states stand on legalizing sports gambling, new mobile bets. *CBS Sports*. Retrieved from https://www.cbssports.com/other/news/u-s-sports-betting-heres-where-all-50-states-stand-on-legalizing-sports-gambling-new-mobile-bets/

Bodor, D., Ricijaš, N., Zoričić, Z., Dodig Hundrić, D., & Filipčić, I. (2018). Prevalence of pathological gambling among alcohol addicts in outpatient treatment in the City of Zagreb: A cross-sectional study. *Psychiatria Danubina, 30*(3), 348–355. https://doi.org/10.24869/psyd.2018.348

Brasil. (2018). *Lei n° 13.756, de 12 de dezembro de 2018*. Retrieved from https://www.planalto.gov.br/ccivil_03/_ato2015-2018/2018/lei/L13756.htm

Brehm, J. W. (1966). *A theory of psychological reactance*. Academic Press.

Brevers, D., Herremans, S. C., He, Q., Vanderhasselt, M. A., Petieau, M., Verdonck, D., Poppa, T., De Witte, S., Kornreich, C., Bechara, A., & Baeken, C. (2018). Facing temptation: The neural correlates of gambling availability during sports picture exposure. *Cognitive, Affective, & Behavioral Neuroscience, 18*(4), 718–729. https://doi.org/10.3758/s13415-018-0599-z

Britto, I. A. G. S., Marcon, R. M., & Oliveira, I. J. S. (2020). Avaliação funcional e a sua prática em contextos aplicados. *Revista Brasileira de Terapia Comportamental e Cognitiva, 22*. https://doi.org/10.31505/rbtcc.v22i1.1045

Brohm, J.-M. (1982). *Sociología política del deporte*. Fondo de Cultura Económica.

Campbell-Meiklejohn, D. K., Woolrich, M. W., Passingham, R. E., & Rogers, R. D. (2008). Knowing when to stop: The brain mechanisms of chasing losses. *Biological Psychiatry, 63*(3), 293–300. https://doi.org/10.1016/j.biopsych.2007.05.014

Cardwell, E., Hoff, R. A., Garakani, A., Krishnan-Sarin, S., Potenza, M. N., & Zhai, Z. W. (2022). An exploratory study of anxiety-motivated gambling in adolescents: Associations with minority status and gambling, health and functioning measures. *Journal of Psychiatric Research, 151*, 445–453. https://doi.org/10.1016/j.jpsychires.2022.03.052

Carvalho, P. (2024, September 26). *Brazil faces an epidemic of addiction to betting: 'I wanted R$ 20,000 a day and left with nothing'*... Retrieved September 28, 2024, from https://noticias.uol.com.br/ultimas-noticias/deutschewelle/2024/09/26/brasil-tem-epidemia-de-vicio-em-bets-queria-r-20-mil-por-dia-e-saia-sem-nada.htm

Carvalho-Neto, M. B. (2002). Análise do comportamento: Behaviorismo radical, análise experimental do comportamento e análise aplicada do comportamento. *Interação em Psicologia, 6*(1), 13–18. https://doi.org/10.5380/psi.v6i1.3188

Catania, A. C. (1999). *Aprendizagem: Comportamento, linguagem e cognição* (4th ed.). Artmed. (Original work published 1998).

Cavalcante, F. R. (2024). In search of more excitement: Reflections on sports bets. *Movimento, 30*, e30010. https://doi.org/10.22456/1982-8918.132978

Christensen, D. R., Witcher, C. S. G., Leighton, T., Hudson-Breen, R., & Ofori-Dei, S. (2018). Piloting the addition of contingency management to best practice counselling as an adjunct treatment for rural and remote disordered gamblers: Study protocol. *BMJ Open, 8*(4), e018804. https://doi.org/10.1136/bmjopen-2017-018804

Clark, L. (2010). Decision-making during gambling: An integration of cognitive and psychobiological approaches. *Philosophical Transactions of the Royal Society of London. Series B, Biological Sciences, 365*(1538), 319–330. https://doi.org/10.1098/rstb.2009.0147

Clark, L., Lawrence, A. J., Astley-Jones, F., & Gray, N. (2009). Gambling near-misses enhance motivation to gamble and recruit win-related brain circuitry. *Neuron, 61*(3), 481–490. https://doi.org/10.1016/j.neuron.2008.12.031

Clark, L., Averbeck, B., Payer, D., Sescousse, G., Winstanley, C. A., & Xue, G. (2013). Pathological choice: The neuroscience of gambling and gambling addiction. *The Journal of Neuroscience, 33*(45), 17617–17623. https://doi.org/10.1523/JNEUROSCI.3231-13.2013

Cooper, A., Olfert, K., & Marmurek, H. H. C. (2022). Predictors of problem gambling for sports and non-sports gamblers: A stochastic search variable selection analysis. *Journal of Gambling Studies, 38*(3), 767–783. https://doi.org/10.1007/s10899-021-10025-2

Da Silva, K. P., Dantas, L. Z., Nascimento, A. R., Melo, C. M., Haydu, V. B., & Pimentel, N. S. (2018). Repertório comportamental: Uma reflexão sobre o conceito. In D. L. O. Vilas Boas, F. Cassas, H. L. Gusso, & P. C. M. Mayer (Eds.), *Comportamento em foco: Processos clínicos e de saúde* (Vol. 6, pp. 155–164). ABPMC.

Dalgalarrondo, P. (2019). *Psicopatologia e semiologia dos transtornos mentais* (3rd ed.). Artmed.

Davidson, T., Rodgers, B., Markham, F., & Taylor-Rodgers, E. (2016). *Gambling expenditure in the ACT (2014): By level of problem gambling, type of activity, and socioeconomic demographic characteristics*. Australian National University.

De Martino, B., Camerer, C. F., & Adolphs, R. (2010). Amygdala damage eliminates monetary loss aversion. *Proceedings of the National Academy of Sciences of the United States of America, 107*(8), 3788–3792. https://doi.org/10.1073/pnas.0910230107

De Rose, J. C. C. (1999). O que é comportamento? In R. A. Banaco (Ed.), *Sobre comportamento e cognição: Aspectos teóricos, metodológicos e de formação em análise do comportamento e terapia cognitivista* (2nd ed., pp. 79–81). ESETec.

Deans, E. G., Thomas, S. L., Daube, M., & Derevensky, J. (2016). The role of peer influences on the normalisation of sports wagering: A qualitative study of Australian men. *Addiction Research & Theory, 25*(2), 103–113. https://doi.org/10.1080/16066359.2016.1205042

Deans, E. G., Thomas, S. L., Derevensky, J., & Daube, M. (2017). The influence of marketing on the sports betting attitudes and consumption behaviours of young men: Implications for harm reduction and prevention strategies. *Harm Reduction Journal, 14*(1), 5. https://doi.org/10.1186/s12954-017-0131-8

Delfabbro, P., King, D., & Parke, J. (2023). The complex nature of human operant gambling behaviour involving slot games: Structural characteristics, verbal rules and motivation. *Addictive Behaviors, 137*, 107540. https://doi.org/10.1016/j.addbeh.2022.107540

Divos, P., Bihari, Z., & Aste, T. (2018). Risk-neutral pricing and hedging of in-play football bets. *Applied Mathematical Finance, 25*(4), 315–335. https://doi.org/10.1080/1350486X.2018.1535275

Dmochowski, J. P. (2023). A statistical theory of optimal decision-making in sports betting. *PLoS One, 18*(6), e0287601. https://doi.org/10.1371/journal.pone.0287601

Dorey, L., McGarrigle, J., May, R., Hoon, A. E., & Dymond, S. (2022a). Client views of contingency management in gambling treatment: A thematic analysis. *International Journal of Environmental Research and Public Health, 19*(24), 17101. https://doi.org/10.3390/ijerph192417101

Dorey, L., Christensen, D. R., May, R., Hoon, A. E., & Dymond, S. (2022b). Gambling treatment service providers' views about contingency management: A thematic analysis. *Harm Reduction Journal, 19*(1), 19. https://doi.org/10.1186/s12954-022-00600-0
Dunning, E. (2014). *Sociologia do esporte e os processos civilizatórios*. Annablume.
Eells, T. D. (2013). The case formulation approach to psychotherapy research revisited. *Pragmatic Case Studies in Psychotherapy, 9*(4), 426–447. https://doi.org/10.14713/pcsp.v9i4.1834
Eells, T. (2022). *Handbook of psychotherapy case formulation* (3rd ed.). The Guilford Press.
Espadafor, M., & Martínez, S. (2021). The negative consequences of sports betting opportunities on human capital formation: Evidence from Spain. *PLoS One, 16*(10), e0258857. https://doi.org/10.1371/journal.pone.0258857
Etuk, R., Xu, T., Abarbanel, B., Potenza, M. N., & Kraus, S. W. (2022). Sports betting around the world: A systematic review. *Journal of Behavioral Addictions, 11*(3), 689–715. https://doi.org/10.1556/2006.2022.00064
Fellows, L. K., & Farah, M. J. (2005). Different underlying impairments in decision-making following ventromedial and dorsolateral frontal lobe damage in humans. *Cerebral Cortex, 15*(1), 58–63. https://doi.org/10.1093/cercor/bhh108
Ferro, L., Monaci, M. G., & Scacchi, L. (2024). Emotions and motivations of gambling: A comparison between scratch card, slot-machines, and casino gamblers. *Brain and Behavior, 14*(3), e3416. https://doi.org/10.1002/brb3.3416
Ferster, C. B. (1972). An experimental analysis of clinical phenomena. *The Psychological Record, 22*, 1–16. https://doi.org/10.1007/BF03394059
Fortune, E. E., & Goodie, A. S. (2012). Cognitive distortions as a component and treatment focus of pathological gambling: A review. *Psychology of Addictive Behaviors, 26*(2), 298–310. https://doi.org/10.1037/a0026422
Gainsbury, S. M., Hing, N., Delfabbro, P., Dewar, G., & King, D. (2014). An exploratory study of interrelationships between social casino gaming, gambling, and problem gambling. *International Journal of Mental Health and Addiction, 13*(1), 136–153. https://doi.org/10.1007/s11469-014-9526-x
Gainsbury, S. M., Angus, D. J., & Blaszczynski, A. (2019). Isolating the impact of specific gambling activities and modes on problem gambling and psychological distress in internet gamblers. *BMC Public Health, 19*(1), 1372. https://doi.org/10.1186/s12889-019-7738-5
Gainsbury, S. M., Abarbanel, B., & Blaszczynski, A. (2020). The relationship between in-play betting and gambling problems in an Australian context of prohibited online in-play betting. *Frontiers in Psychiatry, 11*, 574884. https://doi.org/10.3389/fpsyt.2020.574884
Gambling Commission. (2018). *Gambling participation in 2017: Behaviour, awareness and attitudes (annual report)*. Gambling Commission. Retrieved from https://www.gamblingcommission.gov.uk/pdf/survey-data/gambling-participation-in-2017-behaviour-awareness-and-attitudes.pdf
Goldstein, R. Z., Alia-Klein, N., Tomasi, D., Zhang, L., Cottone, L. A., Maloney, T., Telang, F., Caparelli, E. C., Chang, L., Ernst, T., Samaras, D., Squires, N. K., & Volkow, N. D. (2007). Is decreased prefrontal cortical sensitivity to monetary reward associated with impaired motivation and self-control in cocaine addiction? *The American Journal of Psychiatry, 164*(1), 43–51. https://doi.org/10.1176/ajp.2007.164.1.43
Gonçalves, J. (2023). Proposta de Formulação de Caso Nomotética em Terapia Cognitivo-Comportamental. *Revista Científica Sophia, 15*(1), 5. https://doi.org/10.5281/zenodo.10223550
Gordon, R., Gurrieri, L., & Chapman, M. (2015). Broadening an understanding of problem gambling: The lifestyle consumption community of sports betting. *Journal of Business Research, 68*(10), 2164–2172. https://doi.org/10.1016/j.jbusres.2015.03.016
Goyder, E., Blank, L., Baxter, S., & van Schalkwyk, M. C. (2020). Tackling gambling related harms as a public health issue. *The Lancet. Public Health, 5*(1), e14–e15. https://doi.org/10.1016/S2468-2667(19)30243-9
Grall-Bronnec, M., Caillon, J., Humeau, E., Perrot, B., Remaud, M., Guilleux, A., Rocher, B., Sauvaget, A., & Bouju, G. (2016). Gambling among European professional athletes. Prevalence

and associated factors. *Journal of Addictive Diseases, 35*(4), 278–290. https://doi.org/10.1080/10550887.2016.1177807

Granero, R., Jiménez-Murcia, S., Del Pino-Gutiérrez, A., Mora, B., Mendoza-Valenciano, E., Baenas-Soto, I., et al. (2020). Gambling phenotypes in online sports betting. *Frontiers in Psychiatry, 11*, 482. https://doi.org/10.3389/fpsyt.2020.00482

Grubbs, J. B., & Kraus, S. W. (2023). The relative risks of different forms of sports betting in a U.S. sample: A brief report. *Comprehensive Psychiatry, 127*, 152420. https://doi.org/10.1016/j.comppsych.2023.152420

Guilhardi, H. J. (2004). Terapia por contingências de reforçamento. In C. N. Abreu & H. J. Guilhardi (Eds.), *Terapia comportamental e cognitivo-comportamental: Práticas clínicas* (pp. 3–40). Roca.

Hayes, S. C., Strosahl, K. D., & Wilson, K. G. (2021). *Terapia de aceitação e compromisso: o processo e a prática da mudança consciente*. Artmed.

Higueruela-Ahijado, M., López-Espuela, F., Caro-Alonso, P. Á., Novo, A., & Rodríguez-Martín, B. (2023). Efficacy of cognitive-behavioral therapy in improving the quality of life of people with compulsive gambling, a systematic review. *Archives of Psychiatric Nursing, 43*, 127–142. https://doi.org/10.1016/j.apnu.2022.12.014

Hing, N., Lamont, M., Vitartas, P., & Fink, E. (2015). Sports-embedded gambling promotions: A study of exposure, sports betting intention and problem gambling among adults. *International Journal of Mental Health and Addiction, 13*(1), 115–135. https://doi.org/10.1007/s11469-014-9519-9

Hing, N., Russell, A. M., & Browne, M. (2017). Risk factors for gambling problems on online electronic gaming machines, race betting and sports betting. *Frontiers in Psychology, 8*, 779. https://doi.org/10.3389/fpsyg.2017.00779

Hing, N., Russell, A. M. T., Browne, M., Rockloff, M., Lole, L., Tulloch, C., & Greer, N. (2022). *Smartphone betting on sports, esports and daily fantasy sports amongst young adults*. NSW Responsible Gambling Fund.

Hing, N., Browne, M., Rockloff, M., Russell, A. M. T., Tulloch, C., Lole, L., Thorne, H., & Newall, P. (2023). Situational features of smartphone betting are linked to sports betting harm: An ecological momentary assessment study. *Journal of Behavioral Addictions, 12*(4), 1006–1018. https://doi.org/10.1556/2006.2023.00065

Hing, N., Russell, A. M. T., Tulloch, C., Lole, L., Rockloff, M., Browne, M., Thorne, H., & Newall, P. (2024a). Feature preferences of sports betting platforms: A discrete choice experiment shows why young bettors prefer smartphones. *Journal of Behavioral Addictions, 13*(1), 134–145. https://doi.org/10.1556/2006.2023.00073

Hing, N., Thorne, H., Russell, A. M. T., et al. (2024b). 'Immediate access … everywhere you go': A grounded theory study of how smartphone betting can facilitate harmful sports betting behaviours amongst young adults. *International Journal of Mental Health and Addiction, 22*(5), 1413–1432. https://doi.org/10.1007/s11469-022-00933-8

Hollander, E., & Wong, C. M. (1995). Obsessive-compulsive spectrum disorders. *The Journal of Clinical Psychiatry, 56*(Suppl 4), 3–55.

Humphrey, G., Chu, J., Dowling, N., Rodda, S., Merkouris, S., Parag, V., Newcombe, D., Ho, E., Nosa, V., Ruwhui-Collins, R., Whittaker, R., & Bullen, C. (2020). Manaaki—a cognitive behavioral therapy mobile health app to support people experiencing gambling problems: A randomized control trial protocol. *BMC Public Health, 20*(1), 191. https://doi.org/10.1186/s12889-020-8304-x

Humphreys, B. R. (2021). Legalized sports betting, VLT gambling, and state gambling revenues: Evidence from West Virginia. *Eastern Economic Journal, 47*(1), 9–28. https://doi.org/10.1057/s41302-020-00178-0

James, R. J., O'Malley, C., & Tunney, R. J. (2016). Why are some games more addictive than others: The effects of timing and payoff on perseverance in a slot machine game. *Frontiers in Psychology, 7*, 46. https://doi.org/10.3389/fpsyg.2016.00046

Jiménez-Murcia, S., Giménez, M., Granero, R., López-González, H., Gómez-Peña, M., Moragas, L., Baenas, I., Del Pino-Gutiérrez, A., Codina, E., Mena-Moreno, T., Valenciano-Mendoza, E., Mora-Maltas, B., Valero-Solís, S., Rivas-Pérez, S., Guillén-Guzmán, E., Menchón, J. M., & Fernández-Aranda, F. (2021). Psychopathogical status and personality correlates of problem gambling severity in sports bettors undergoing treatment for gambling disorder. *Journal of Behavioral Addictions, 10*(3), 422–434. Advance online publication. https://doi.org/10.1556/2006.2020.00101

Johnstone, P., & Regan, M. (2020). Gambling harm is everybody's business: A public health approach and call to action. *Public Health, 184*, 63–66. https://doi.org/10.1016/j.puhe.2020.06.010

Kahneman, D. (2012). *Rápido e devagar: duas formas de pensar*. Objetiva.

Kahneman, D., & Tversky, A. (1979). Prospect theory: An analysis of decision under risk. *Econometrica, 47*, 263–291. https://doi.org/10.2307/1914164

Killick, E. A., & Griffiths, M. D. (2021). Why do individuals engage in in-play sports betting? A qualitative interview study. *Journal of Gambling Studies, 37*(1), 221–240. https://doi.org/10.1007/s10899-020-09968-9

Labrador, F. J., & Vallejo-Achón, M. (2020). Prevalence and characteristics of sports betting in a population of young students in Madrid. *Journal of Gambling Studies, 36*(1), 297–318. https://doi.org/10.1007/s10899-019-09863-y

Ladouceur, R., & Walker, M. (1996). A cognitive perspective on gambling. In P. M. Salkovskis (Ed.), *Trends in cognitive and behavioural therapies* (pp. 89–120). Wiley.

Langer, E. J. (1975). The illusion of control. *Journal of Personality and Social Psychology, 32*(2), 311–328. https://doi.org/10.1037/0022-3514.32.2.311

Langham, E., Thorne, H., Browne, M., Donaldson, P., Rose, J., & Rockloff, M. (2016). Understanding gambling related harm: A proposed definition, conceptual framework, and taxonomy of harms. *BMC Public Health, 16*, 80. https://doi.org/10.1186/s12889-016-2747-0

Latvala, T. A., Lintonen, T. P., Browne, M., Rockloff, M., & Salonen, A. H. (2021). Social disadvantage and gambling severity: A population-based study with register-linkage. *European Journal of Public Health, 31*(6), 1217–1223. https://doi.org/10.1093/eurpub/ckab162

Lee, C. H., Chang, F. C., Hsu, S. D., Chi, H. Y., Huang, L. J., & Yeh, M. K. (2017). Inappropriate self-medication among adolescents and its association with lower medication literacy and substance use. *PLoS One, 12*(12), e0189199. https://doi.org/10.1371/journal.pone.0189199

Leeman, R. F., & Potenza, M. N. (2012). Similarities and differences between pathological gambling and substance use disorders: A focus on impulsivity and compulsivity. *Psychopharmacology, 219*(2), 469–490. https://doi.org/10.1007/s00213-011-2550-7

Legarda, J. J., Babio, R., & Abreu, J. M. (1992). Prevalence estimates of pathological gambling in Seville (Spain). *British Journal of Addiction, 87*(5), 767–770. https://doi.org/10.1111/j.1360-0443.1992.tb02722.x

Leonardi, J. L., Mácimo, T., Bacchi, A. D., & Josua, D. (2023). Ciência, análise do comportamento e a prática baseada em evidências em psicologia. *Revista Perspectivas em Análise do Comportamento, 14*(1), 97–119. https://doi.org/10.18761/PACCha0a1

Lopez-Gonzalez, H., Griffiths, M. D., & Estévez, A. (2018). In-play betting, sport broadcasts, and gambling severity: A survey study of Spanish sports bettors on the risks of betting on sport while watching it. *Communication & Sport, 8*(1), 50–71. https://doi.org/10.1177/2167479518816338

Lopez-Gonzalez, H., Griffiths, M., & Jimenez-Murcia, S. (2021). The symbolic construction of sports betting products. *International Gambling Studies, 21*(3), 498–515. https://doi.org/10.1080/14459795.2021.1937274

Magri, D. (2021, September 25). *Casas de aposta esportiva tomam o Brasil, mas movimentam seus bilhões de reais fora do país*. El País. Retrieved from https://brasil.elpais.com/esportes/2021-09-25/casas-de-aposta-esportiva-tomam-o-brasil-mas-movimentam-seus-bilhoes-de-reais-fora-do-pais.html

Matheson, V. (2021). An overview of the economics of sports gambling and an introduction to the symposium. *Eastern Economic Journal, 47*(1), 1–8. https://doi.org/10.1057/s41302-020-00182-4
Mathieu, S., Barrault, S., Brunault, P., & Varescon, I. (2020). The role of gambling type on gambling motives, cognitive distortions, and gambling severity in gamblers recruited online. *PLoS One, 15*(10), e0238978. https://doi.org/10.1371/journal.pone.0238978
Matos, M. A. (1999). Com o que o behaviorismo radical trabalha? In R. A. Banaco (Ed.), *Sobre comportamento e cognição: Aspectos teóricos, metodológicos e de formação em análise do comportamento e terapia cognitivista* (Vol. 1, 2nd ed., pp. 45–53). ARBytes.
Mattos, B. P., & Pinho, J. G. (2024). Prática Baseada em Evidências em Psicologia Clínica. In R. A. Reichert & D. De Micheli (Eds.), *Neuropsicologia e Dependência de Drogas: Neurobiologia, Cognição e Comportamento* (pp. 480–509). UNIFESP.
Mazar, A., Williams, R. J., Stanek, E. J., 3rd, Zorn, M., & Volberg, R. A. (2018). The importance of friends and family to recreational gambling, at-risk gambling, and problem gambling. *BMC Public Health, 18*(1), 1080. https://doi.org/10.1186/s12889-018-5988-2
McGee, D. (2020). On the normalisation of online sports gambling among young adult men in the UK: A public health perspective. *Public Health, 184*, 89–94. https://doi.org/10.1016/j.puhe.2020.04.018
Miedl, S. F., Peters, J., & Büchel, C. (2012). Altered neural reward representations in pathological gamblers revealed by delay and probability discounting. *Archives of General Psychiatry, 69*(2), 177–186. https://doi.org/10.1001/archgenpsychiatry.2011.1552
Miguel, A. Q., Madruga, C. S., Cogo-Moreira, H., Yamauchi, R., Simões, V., da Silva, C. J., McPherson, S., Roll, J. M., & Laranjeira, R. R. (2016). Contingency management is effective in promoting abstinence and retention in treatment among crack cocaine users in Brazil: A randomized controlled trial. *Psychology of Addictive Behaviors, 30*(5), 536–543. https://doi.org/10.1037/adb0000192
Miguel, A. Q. C., McPherson, S. M., Simões, V., Yamauchi, R., Madruga, C. S., Smith, C. L., da Silva, C. J., Laranjeira, R. R., McDonell, M. G., Roll, J. M., & Mari, J. J. (2022). Effectiveness of incorporating contingency management into a public treatment program for people who use crack cocaine in Brazil. A single-blind randomized controlled trial. *The International Journal on Drug Policy, 99*, 103464. https://doi.org/10.1016/j.drugpo.2021.103464
Miller, W., & Rollnick, S. (2001). *Entrevista motivacional: preparando as pessoas para a mudança de comportamentos adictivos*. Artmed.
Miller, W. R., & Rollnick, S. (2023). *Motivational interviewing—Helping people change and grow* (4th ed.). The Guilford Press.
Mravčík, V., Chomynová, P., Grohmannová, K., & Rous, Z. (2020). Gambling products and their risk potential for gambling disorder. Hazardní hry a jejich rizikovost z hlediska rozvoje problémového hráčství. *Casopís Lékařů Ceských, 159*(5), 196–202.
Nelson, S. E., Edson, T. C., Louderback, E. R., Tom, M. A., Grossman, A., & LaPlante, D. A. (2021). Changes to the playing field: A contemporary study of actual European online sports betting. *Journal of Behavioral Addictions, 10*(3), 396–411. Advance online publication. https://doi.org/10.1556/2006.2021.00029
Nyemcsok, C., Thomas, S. L., Bestman, A., Pitt, H., Daube, M., & Cassidy, R. (2018). Young people's recall and perceptions of gambling advertising and intentions to gamble on sport. *Journal of Behavioral Addictions, 7*(4), 1068–1078. https://doi.org/10.1556/2006.7.2018.128
Nyemcsok, C., Pitt, H., Kremer, P., & Thomas, S. L. (2022). Young men's perceptions about the risks associated with sports betting: A critical qualitative inquiry. *BMC Public Health, 22*(1), 867. https://doi.org/10.1186/s12889-022-13164-2
Otis, E., Kim, A. J., Stewart, S. H., Sherry, S. B., & Yakovenko, I. (2022). Changes in sports gambling behavior during the COVID-19 pandemic in Canada. *Frontiers in Psychiatry, 13*, 1018234. https://doi.org/10.3389/fpsyt.2022.1018234

Parrela, L. (2023, May 24). *Sites de apostas: Brasil tem quase 25% dos acessos em todo o mundo*. Itatiaia. Retrieved from https://www.itatiaia.com.br/editorias/esportes/2023/05/24/sites-de-apostas-brasil-tem-quase-25-dos-acessos-em-todo-o-mundo

Peters, J., Miedl, S. F., & Büchel, C. (2012). Formal comparison of dual-parameter temporal discounting models in controls and pathological gamblers. *PLoS One, 7*(11), e47225. https://doi.org/10.1371/journal.pone.0047225

Petry, N. M. (2006). Should the scope of addictive behaviors be broadened to include pathological gambling? *Addiction (Abingdon, England), 101*(Suppl 1), 152–160. https://doi.org/10.1111/j.1360-0443.2006.01593.x

Petry, N. M., Kolodner, K. B., Li, R., Peirce, J. M., Roll, J. M., Stitzer, M. L., & Hamilton, J. A. (2006). Prize-based contingency management does not increase gambling. *Drug and Alcohol Dependence, 83*(3), 269–273. https://doi.org/10.1016/j.drugalcdep.2005.11.023

Petry, N. M., Blanco, C., Auriacombe, M., Borges, G., Bucholz, K., Crowley, T. J., Grant, B. F., Hasin, D. S., & O'Brien, C. (2014). An overview of and rationale for changes proposed for pathological gambling in DSM-5. *Journal of Gambling Studies, 30*(2), 493–502. https://doi.org/10.1007/s10899-013-9370-0

Rabin, M. (2002). Inference by believers in the law of small numbers. *Quarterly Journal of Economics, 117*(3), 775–816. https://doi.org/10.1162/003355302760193896

Russell, A. M. T., Hing, N., Browne, M., Li, E., & Vitartas, P. (2019a). Who bets on micro events (microbets) in sports? *Journal of Gambling Studies, 35*(1), 205–223. https://doi.org/10.1007/s10899-018-9810-y

Russell, A. M. T., Hing, N., & Browne, M. (2019b). Risk factors for gambling problems specifically associated with sports betting. *Journal of Gambling Studies, 35*(4), 1211–1228. https://doi.org/10.1007/s10899-019-09848-x

Schonberg, T., Fox, C. R., & Poldrack, R. A. (2011). Mind the gap: Bridging economic and naturalistic risk-taking with cognitive neuroscience. *Trends in Cognitive Sciences, 15*(1), 11–19. https://doi.org/10.1016/j.tics.2010.10.002

Schott, B. H., Minuzzi, L., Krebs, R. M., Elmenhorst, D., Lang, M., Winz, O. H., Seidenbecher, C. I., Coenen, H. H., Heinze, H. J., Zilles, K., Düzel, E., & Bauer, A. (2008). Mesolimbic functional magnetic resonance imaging activations during reward anticipation correlate with reward-related ventral striatal dopamine release. *The Journal of Neuroscience, 28*(52), 14311–14319. https://doi.org/10.1523/JNEUROSCI.2058-08.2008

Seal, E., Cardak, B. A., Nicholson, M., Donaldson, A., O'Halloran, P., Randle, E., & Staley, K. (2022). The gambling behaviour and attitudes to sports betting of sports fans. *Journal of Gambling Studies, 38*(4), 1371–1403. https://doi.org/10.1007/s10899-021-10101-7

Seo, M., Lee, E., & Averbeck, B. B. (2012). Action selection and action value in frontal-striatal circuits. *Neuron, 74*(5), 947–960. https://doi.org/10.1016/j.neuron.2012.03.037

Sescousse, G., Barbalat, G., Domenech, P., & Dreher, J. C. (2013). Imbalance in the sensitivity to different types of rewards in pathological gambling. *Brain, 136*(Pt 8), 2527–2538. https://doi.org/10.1093/brain/awt126

Shafran, R., Clark, D. M., Fairburn, C. G., Arntz, A., Barlow, D. H., Ehlers, A., Frees-ton, M., Garety, P. A., Hollon, S. D., Ost, L. G., Salkovskis, P. M., Williams, J. M., & Wilson, G. T. (2009). Mind the gap: Improving the dissemination of CBT. *Behaviour Research and Therapy, 47*(11), 902–909. https://doi.org/10.1016/j.brat.2009.07.003

Sharman, S., Murphy, R., Turner, J. J. D., & Roberts, A. (2019). Trends and patterns in UK treatment seeking gamblers: 2000-2015. *Addictive Behaviors, 89*, 51–56. https://doi.org/10.1016/j.addbeh.2018.09.009

Shiv, B., Loewenstein, G., Bechara, A., Damasio, H., & Damasio, A. R. (2005). Investment behavior and the negative side of emotion. *Psychological Science, 16*(6), 435–439. https://doi.org/10.1111/j.0956-7976.2005.01553.x

Silverman, A. (2022, January 18) *2021 Was a banner year for sports betting participation*. Morning Consult. Retrieved from https://morningconsult.com/2022/01/18/sports-betting-trends/

Sirola, A., Savela, N., Savolainen, I., Kaakinen, M., & Oksanen, A. (2021). The role of virtual communities in gambling and gaming behaviors: A systematic review. *Journal of Gambling Studies, 37*(1), 165–187. https://doi.org/10.1007/s10899-020-09946-1

Skinner, B. F. (1953). *Science and human behavior*. Mcmillan.

Skinner, B. F. (1974). *About behaviorism*. Alfred A. Knopf.

Skinner, B. F. (1981). Selection by consequences. *Science, 213*(4507), 501–504. https://doi.org/10.1126/science.7244649

Smith, L. L., Yan, F., Charles, M., Mohiuddin, K., Tyus, D., Adekeye, O., & Holden, K. B. (2017). Exploring the link between substance use and mental health status: What can we learn from the self-medication theory? *Journal of Health Care for the Poor and Underserved, 28*(2S), 113–131. https://doi.org/10.1353/hpu.2017.0056

Statista. (2018). *Statistics and market data on sports and recreation*. https://www.statista.com/markets/409/sports-recreation/

Sundali, J., & Croson, R. (2006). Biases in casino betting: The hot hand and the gambler's fallacy. *Judgment and Decision making, 1*(1), 1–12.

Sztainert, T., Wohl, M. J., McManus, J. F., & Stead, J. D. (2014). On being attracted to the possibility of a win: Reward sensitivity (via gambling motives) undermines treatment seeking among pathological gamblers. *Journal of Gambling Studies, 30*(4), 901–911. https://doi.org/10.1007/s10899-013-9394-5

Takahashi, H., Fujie, S., Camerer, C., Arakawa, R., Takano, H., Kodaka, F., Matsui, H., Ideno, T., Okubo, S., Takemura, K., Yamada, M., Eguchi, Y., Murai, T., Okubo, Y., Kato, M., Ito, H., & Suhara, T. (2013). Norepinephrine in the brain is associated with aversion to financial loss. *Molecular Psychiatry, 18*(1), 3–4. https://doi.org/10.1038/mp.2012.7

The Lancet. (2017). Problem gambling is a public health concern. *Lancet (London, England), 390*(10098), 913. https://doi.org/10.1016/S0140-6736(17)32333-4

Tobler, P. N., Christopoulos, G. I., O'Doherty, J. P., Dolan, R. J., & Schultz, W. (2008). Neuronal distortions of reward probability without choice. *The Journal of Neuroscience, 28*(45), 11703–11711. https://doi.org/10.1523/JNEUROSCI.2870-08.2008

Todorov, J. C. (2020). *Comportamento e cultura: análise de interações*. Technopolitik.

Tom, S. M., Fox, C. R., Trepel, C., & Poldrack, R. A. (2007). The neural basis of loss aversion in decision-making under risk. *Science, 315*(5811), 515–518. https://doi.org/10.1126/science.1134239

Tourinho, E. Z. (1999). Estudos conceituais na análise do comportamento. *Temas em Psicologia, 7*(3), 213–222.

Trepel, C., Fox, C. R., & Poldrack, R. A. (2005). Prospect theory on the brain? Toward a cognitive neuroscience of decision under risk. *Brain Research. Cognitive Brain Research, 23*(1), 34–50. https://doi.org/10.1016/j.cogbrainres.2005.01.016

Turner, S., Mota, N., Bolton, J., & Sareen, J. (2018). Self-medication with alcohol or drugs for mood and anxiety disorders: A narrative review of the epidemiological literature. *Depression and Anxiety, 35*(9), 851–860. https://doi.org/10.1002/da.22771

Ukhova, D., Marionneau, V., Nikkinen, J., & Wardle, H. (2024). Public health approaches to gambling: A global review of legislative trends. *The Lancet. Public Health, 9*(1), e57–e67. https://doi.org/10.1016/S2468-2667(23)00221-9

Valleur, M., Codina, I., Vénisse, J. L., Romo, L., Magalon, D., Fatséas, M., Chéreau-Boudet, I., Gorsane, M. A., Guilleux, A., JEU, G., Grall-Bronnec, M., & Challet-Bouju, G. (2016). Towards a validation of the three pathways model of pathological gambling. *Journal of Gambling Studies, 32*(2), 757–771. https://doi.org/10.1007/s10899-015-9545-y

Vieira, J. L., Coelho, S. G., Snaychuk, L. A., Parmar, P. K., Keough, M. T., & Kim, H. S. (2023). Who makes in-play bets? Investigating the demographics, psychological characteristics, and gambling-related harms of in-play sports bettors. *Journal of Behavioral Addictions, 12*(2), 547–556. https://doi.org/10.1556/2006.2023.00030

Volberg, R. A., & Abbott, M. W. (1994). Lifetime prevalence estimates of pathological gambling in New Zealand. *International Journal of Epidemiology, 23*(5), 976–983. https://doi.org/10.1093/ije/23.5.976

Wang, X., Won, D., & Jeon, H. S. (2021). Predictors of sports gambling among college students: The role of the theory of planned behavior and problem gambling severity. *International Journal of Environmental Research and Public Health, 18*(4), 1803. https://doi.org/10.3390/ijerph18041803

Wirkus, T., Czernecka, R., Bühringer, G., & Kräplin, A. (2024). Individual risk factors and prediction of gambling disorder in online sports bettors—The Longitudinal RIGAB study. *Frontiers in Psychiatry, 15*, 1320592. https://doi.org/10.3389/fpsyt.2024.1320592

World Health Organization (WHO). (2018). *International classification of diseases for mortality and morbidity statistics (11th revision)*. World Health Organization. https://icd.who.int/browse11/l-m/en.

Zeeb, F. D., & Winstanley, C. A. (2011). Lesions of the basolateral amygdala and orbitofrontal cortex differentially affect acquisition and performance of a rodent gambling task. *The Journal of Neuroscience, 31*(6), 2197–2204. https://doi.org/10.1523/JNEUROSCI.5597-10.2011

Chapter 7
Parental Mediation in the Use of Digital Media by Children and Adolescents

Isabela Brasil Correia, Manoela Fontelles, Victor Hugo Silva Turnes, Natália Minatti de Souza, Weliton da Silva, João Vitor Girardi Turqueti da Rocha, Nicoly Camile Mendes Reichert, Eloísa Medeiros Avancini, Richard Alecsander Reichert, and Denise De Micheli

Parental Mediation in the Digital Landscape

When addressing the question of who should take responsibility for monitoring children and adolescents' Internet use and protecting them from potential associated risks, the most immediate answer often points to parents. Traditionally, the role of raising children by instilling values, norms, and socially accepted behaviors has been attributed to parents or other family or community members engaged in caregiving. This responsibility encompasses a wide range of tasks, from assisting with schoolwork to ensuring physical safety. Historically, such responsibilities were primarily guided by personal experience and knowledge accumulated and passed down through generations (Ariès, 1981; Grossman, 1998; Mollborn & Lawrence, 2018; Phillips & Lowenstein, 2011; Schoen-Ferreira et al., 2010).

The digital era has posed significant challenges to parenting, transforming how parents and caregivers address the demands of child development. The growing ubiquity of electronic devices in children's daily lives and the complexity of digital technologies require continuous and demanding adaptations. The rapid pace of technological advancement, coupled with the overwhelming volume of available information, has led to uncertainties and concerns among caregivers. Issues related

I. B. Correia · M. Fontelles · V. H. S. Turnes · N. M. de Souza · W. da Silva · J. V. G. T. da Rocha
Universidade do Vale do Itajaí, Itajaí, SC, Brazil

N. C. M. Reichert · E. M. Avancini
Fundação Universidade Regional de Blumenau, Blumenau, SC, Brazil
e-mail: emavancini@furb.br

R. A. Reichert · D. De Micheli (✉)
Universidade Federal de São Paulo, São Paulo, SP, Brazil
e-mail: reichert@unifesp.br

A. L. M. Andrade (ed.), *Digital Addictions*,
https://doi.org/10.1007/978-3-031-87986-9_7

to excessive screen time, exposure to inappropriate content, and the risk of negative experiences such as cyberbullying have become recurring concerns in family dynamics. In this context, parental mediation emerges as a central strategy to address the challenges posed by the digital contemporary era (Koning et al., 2018; Saputri & Wulandari, 2024).

Parental mediation refers to the set of strategies and practices employed by parents and caregivers to guide, monitor, and discuss children and adolescents' engagement with digital media and online activities. This concept encompasses various approaches, notably active regulation and restrictive regulation, both aiming to mitigate the risks associated with digital exposure. Active regulation involves parental participation in their children's digital lives through the collaborative establishment of rules and limits in a democratic format. This approach includes dialogue about Internet content and its potential implications, aiming to foster children's autonomy within a safe and supervised environment (Koning et al., 2018; Livingstone & Helsper, 2008).

Active regulation is characterized as a bidirectional process, wherein continuous dialogue between parents and children about issues related to the online environment plays a central role in the development of critical thinking among children and adolescents regarding digital content. This approach includes direct parental involvement in their children's online activities, such as jointly exploring games, social media platforms, and other applications. This interaction not only strengthens family bonds but also provides a deeper understanding of the digital universe experienced by children. In addition to protecting against risks associated with digital exposure, active regulation prepares children and adolescents by fostering critical and responsible behaviors in the virtual environment (Coyne et al., 2011; Livingstone et al., 2017).

Restrictive mediation is an approach characterized by the imposition of strict rules regarding the use of digital media, including limits on screen time, the types of content accessed, and permitted activities, such as participation in social networks or gaming platforms. Studies indicate that this approach is often adopted by parents concerned about excessive use of digital technologies and its potential impacts, such as difficulties in academic performance and changes in the dynamics of their children's interpersonal relationships (Koning et al., 2018; Lee, 2012).

Research indicates that adopting restrictive mediation strategies can effectively reduce the time children and adolescents spend online, mitigating risks such as exposure to inappropriate content, privacy violations, and cyberbullying (Chang et al., 2015; Chou et al., 2019; Navarro et al., 2013). However, parental practices rarely adhere exclusively to either an active or restrictive approach. Studies, such as that of Barkin et al. (2006), involving 1831 parents, revealed that 59% employed different mediation strategies simultaneously. This combination of approaches suggests that a balanced and integrated application of active and restrictive practices can foster a more collaborative environment. In this context, children are more likely to accept parental guidance while gradually and appropriately developing autonomy according to their developmental stage (Shin & Ismail, 2014; Steinfeld, 2021).

Parental mediation has proven to be an evolving practice throughout history, accompanying changes in media consumption habits and available technologies. With the advancement of digital technologies and the growing integration of the virtual world into the daily lives of children and adolescents, mediation strategies have had to adapt to new demands. Between the 1960s and 1980s, the focus of parental mediation predominantly revolved around supervising television use, emphasizing screen time limitations and the selection of accessible content. During this period, research concentrated on exploring the impacts of television on various aspects, including academic performance, reduced time spent on activities such as reading and sports, and changes in interpersonal relationships (Comstock, 1978; Desmond et al., 1985; Modecki et al., 2022; Nikken & Schols, 2015).

After the 2000s, with the expansion of access to social networks, platforms such as YouTube and Netflix, and other digital media, a significant transformation in family life was observed. Digital technologies, with their positive and negative aspects, have become an ongoing challenge for parents. Parental mediation, which previously focused on supervising television—a medium relatively easy to monitor—began to face more complex issues, such as the risks of cyberbullying, interactions with strangers, and dependence on video games and smartphones (Wong, 2011).

Currently, parental mediation encompasses a broader range of practices, including promoting critical thinking about digital media use and encouraging healthy habits in the virtual environment. This practice is not limited to establishing screen time limits but also involves building a constant and collaborative dialogue with children, addressing both the benefits and risks of the digital world. Effective mediation contributes to the healthy development of children and adolescents, fostering autonomy, critical thinking, and safety. It is a fundamental approach to ensuring that children benefit from the advantages of digital technologies responsibly and safely while protecting themselves from the associated risks (Suárez-Álvarez et al., 2022).

Challenges and Risks for Children and Adolescents in the Digital World

Internet access and the time dedicated to the digital environment have become continuously growing contemporary trends, showing no signs of slowing down, driven by ongoing social and technological transformations. In Brazil, according to the *Survey on the Use of Information and Communication Technologies in Brazilian Households 2023*, conducted by the Internet Management Committee in Brazil (2023), approximately 95% of children and adolescents have some form of Internet access, highlighting the widespread nature of this phenomenon.

The evolution of digital technologies has exhibited exponential growth in recent years, making the comprehensive tracking of all innovations challenging due to the speed at which they emerge. This technological advancement, coupled with the broad accessibility of digital devices to children and adolescents, poses significant

Table 7.1 Risks of Internet use by children and adolescents

Risk	Description
Exposure to inappropriate content	Children and adolescents may unintentionally encounter harmful or explicit content online, such as violence, pornography, or hate speech. This exposure can influence violent behaviors and alter perceptions of social norms
Cyberbullying	The anonymity of the internet facilitates an increase in cases of cyberbullying, where children and adolescents become targets of harassment by peers. Consequences include emotional distress, anxiety, and, in extreme cases, depressive symptoms
Online strangers	Children and adolescents may be targeted by online predators who exploit their vulnerability to obtain personal information or lure them into unsafe interactions, posing risks to their safety
Privacy risks	A lack of understanding about privacy settings and the impact of sharing personal information can lead children and adolescents to expose sensitive data, making them vulnerable to identity theft or unwanted interactions
Technology dependence	Excessive use of the internet and digital devices can result in compulsive behaviors, impairing social interaction, physical health, and academic performance. Additionally, it can promote a sedentary lifestyle and associated health issues

challenges for mediating the consumption of online information (Bozzola et al., 2022; Odgers & Jensen, 2020a, 2020b).

The generational context plays a fundamental role in understanding children's relationships with digital technologies. Interfaces requiring simple actions, such as tapping and dragging objects on touch-screen devices, facilitate the early and intuitive integration of children into this digital universe (Edwards et al., 2018). However, while children demonstrate quick manual skills for operating electronic devices, they face limitations arising from their cognitive development, particularly concerning the understanding of abstract concepts like privacy and online exposure. This gap increases their vulnerability to risks and dangers in the digital environment (Brom et al., 2023; Dittus et al., 2023; Hu et al., 2022; Jang & Ko, 2023; Ricci et al., 2022; Savoia et al., 2021; Sina et al., 2023) (Table 7.1).

Given the technological advancements and the inherent risks of the digital environment, parental mediation emerges as an essential element to minimize potential harm and promote well-being practices in the use of digital media (Vannucci et al., 2020). Continuous supervision, combined with structured dialogue and training in digital education for parents, educators, and young people, becomes indispensable for fostering a safer and more responsible digital environment (Dittus et al., 2023; Hu et al., 2022; Jang & Ko, 2023; Ricci et al., 2022; Savoia et al., 2021; Sina et al., 2023).

Guidelines on Responsible and Safe Use of Digital Media

The phenomena associated with the use of digital technologies have shown accelerated growth, keeping pace with global technological advancements. In the context of childhood, evidence suggests that, until the age of 8, television was the predominant medium. However, this pattern has been changing due to the popularization of streaming platforms such as Netflix and YouTube (American Academy of Pediatrics (AAP), 2016). In the case of adolescents, a study conducted in the United States identified that approximately 95% have access to smartphones and use at least one social media platform daily. Furthermore, the data indicated that half of the participants classified their use as constant, while the other half reported accessing them several times throughout the day (Anderson et al., 2023).

The rapid development of digital technologies has driven the increased use of these media, resulting in various physiological, cognitive, behavioral, social, and cultural implications. The literature documents numerous benefits associated with the use of digital media, such as exposure to new ideas, opportunities for community connection, academic collaboration in online projects, facilitation of interactions between geographically distant family members and friends, and therapeutic support in virtual groups (AAP, 2016; Hoge et al., 2017).

On the other hand, excessive use of these technologies is associated with significant risks. Among the most frequent impacts are obesity, often linked to sedentary behavior (World Health Organization (WHO), 2020), changes in sleep patterns (Bruni et al., 2015), and communication difficulties related to predominant interaction in digital environments (Holtz & Appel, 2011). Additionally, although causal relationships have not yet been established, the literature suggests possible associations between excessive use of digital media and the emergence of conditions such as anxiety and depression. Evidence suggests that these issues may be related to factors such as avoidance behaviors of in-person interactions, deficits in emotional regulation skills due to using media as a form of distraction, anxiety stemming from the need to be constantly connected, and negative experiences, such as cyberbullying (Hoge et al., 2017).

Based on the various aspects mentioned, several guidelines have been developed to assist healthcare professionals in guiding parental practices aimed at promoting the healthy and safe use of digital media by children and adolescents:

- **Information on risks and benefits**: Before discussing parenting practices, it is essential for parents to properly understand the risks and benefits of digital media use, thus avoiding polarized perspectives on the topic (AAP, 2016).
- **Screen time limit for children under 5 years**: For children in this age group, it is recommended that screen time does not exceed 1 h per day to ensure they have sufficient time for play and other activities essential to their development (AAP, 2016; Coyne et al., 2017; WHO, 2020).
- **Screen time limit for children over 5 years**: For children and adolescents over 5 years of age, in accordance with recommendations on sleep and physical

activity, no more than 2 h of uninterrupted screen time should be allowed (Canadian Society for Exercise Physiology (CSEP), 2016; Guerrero et al., 2019).

- **Monitoring digital media use**: Parents should be encouraged to monitor their children's screen time, ensuring it does not interfere with physical activity or quality sleep. It is also important for parents to be aware of how their own digital media use may impact family dynamics, as parental digital behavior is a significant predictor of children's media habits (AAP, 2016; Arumugam et al., 2021; Chassiakos et al., 2016; Coyne et al., 2017; Oh et al., 2022).
- **Role of digital media in family dynamics**: Professionals should be mindful of the role digital media plays in family dynamics (Coyne et al., 2017).
- **Family media use plan**: It is recommended that parents, with the help of specialized professionals, create a "Family Media Use Plan," establishing healthy and appropriate rules and strategies tailored to the specific needs of each family regarding digital media use (AAP, 2016; Chassiakos et al., 2016; Hoge et al., 2017).
- **Use of devices during sleep**: It is recommended that children and adolescents not sleep with digital devices (AAP, 2016).
- **Use of digital media during schoolwork**: It is important not to encourage the use of digital media for entertainment during homework to avoid distractions and ensure focus on academic activities (AAP, 2016).
- **Family time without digital media**: Parents should be encouraged to establish rules for family time without digital media use, promoting physical activities, positive parental interactions (such as conversations and play), and facilitating social interactions with peers (AAP, 2016; Arumugam et al., 2021).

Supervision Strategies in Online Activities and Promoting Reflective Dialogue on Virtual Content

Considering the influence of parental habits on children's use of digital media, it is essential for parents to reflect on their own behaviors before establishing rules or initiating discussions on the topic (Chassiakos et al., 2016; Coyne et al., 2017; Zhu et al., 2022). In certain contexts, excessive media use by parents may lead to a reduction in verbal and nonverbal interactions with their children, as well as potentially increasing family conflicts (Chassiakos et al., 2016).

It is important to highlight that rules limited only to screen time are insufficient; it is crucial to also consider the content accessed, particularly with regard to the healthy and safe use of digital media. Digital content should encourage learning, creativity, expression, and imagination, rather than merely serving as a functional communication medium (Arumugam et al., 2021). Furthermore, it is necessary to ensure that children are not exposed to age-inappropriate content (Arumugam et al., 2021; Coyne et al., 2017).

Content supervision should involve joint viewing and use of digital media between parents and children, with a focus on discussing the materials consumed. Promoting dialogues about the accessed content, ethics in social media, online safety, and appropriate and respectful conduct in the digital environment, in addition to encouraging children to ask questions about what they have seen, is a relevant practice in parental mediation of digital media use. This approach can help prevent negative cognitive, behavioral, and social consequences in children's development. Supervision, joint viewing/usage, and discussions about content should be integrated into the family media use plan, which should be developed according to the family dynamics and the characteristics of the children (Arumugam et al., 2021; Chassiakos et al., 2016; Coyne et al., 2017; Hoge et al., 2017).

Parental Mediation Strategies

To mediate the use of media by children and adolescents, it is essential to create an environment that fosters open and constructive discussions, covering various topics, including the thoughts and feelings of family members. Households that promote active participation in decision-making, valuing diverse perspectives even in situations of disagreement, tend to develop interpersonal skills such as assertive communication, constructive conflict resolution, and the establishment of healthy relationships. These factors, in turn, facilitate the adoption of more effective mediation strategies (Schrodt et al., 2008).

When discussing the use of digital media, it is crucial to consider the perspectives of children and adolescents, acknowledging their concerns regarding the consequences of exposure. It is equally important to avoid blaming them for interacting with inappropriate content, as this may occur unintentionally or under peer influence. Reactions based on guilt or fear can hinder the willingness to share these experiences with caregivers. Therefore, in addition to setting restrictions, it is essential to promote an environment that encourages dialogue and critical analysis (Johnson & Francis, 2022; Livingstone et al., 2014).

Once a conducive environment for discussions about digital media is established, the next step is to define mediation strategies. These strategies should be implemented consistently, respectfully, and in a balanced manner. Key actions include establishing rules, using parental control tools, monitoring online activities, and, equally important, encouraging autonomy and critical thinking in the use of digital media. These approaches can be integrated into both active and restrictive methods, depending on the needs and family context (Johnson & Francis, 2022; Livingstone et al., 2014) por (Chen et al., 2023; Koning et al., 2018; Livingstone et al., 2014; Lukavská et al., 2022; Steinfeld, 2021).

One of the restrictive practices frequently used in the digital realm is the establishment of well-defined rules, a task that becomes more challenging with technological advancement (Fam et al., 2022). This strategy aims to reduce screen time, promoting engagement in activities such as studying, physical exercise, adequate rest, and face-to-face social interactions, all of which should be encouraged by caregivers (APA, 2023; Sociedade Brasileira de Pediatria (SBP), 2024). However, although this approach contributes to raising awareness about digital risks, it is insufficient to reduce online risk behaviors. Furthermore, restricting the use of digital media does not foster essential skills, such as self-regulation and problem-solving in the virtual environment (Steinfeld, 2021).

Monitoring online activities represents a more restrictive strategy, in which caregivers supervise the content accessed by young individuals. However, it is crucial that this supervision occurs within an environment of communication and trust, avoiding making adolescents feel invaded, as this could compromise the effectiveness of mediation (Chen et al., 2023; Koning et al., 2018; Steinfeld, 2021). From another perspective, maintaining secrets may be a form of adaptation to the relationship with caregivers. When frequent and related to the activities or feelings of young individuals, secrets may signal a desire to preserve autonomy in response to the perception of privacy invasion (Dietvorst et al., 2017).

Parental control tools, typically recommended for younger children, include features that restrict and monitor access to content, limit usage time, track location via mobile devices, and record interactions such as messages sent (Steinfeld, 2021). However, it is important to highlight that, although reducing screen time is important, this measure alone does not ensure reduced involvement in problematic digital media behaviors (Fam et al., 2022).

Mediation should be adjusted according to the age, development, social context, and individual needs of young individuals. An effective model combines active and restrictive strategies, protecting children and adolescents from online risks while promoting autonomy and critical thinking through open dialogue and well-established boundaries (Chen et al., 2023; Koning et al., 2018; Livingstone et al., 2014; Lukavská et al., 2022; Steinfeld, 2021).

Regarding age groups, more restrictive strategies tend to be effective for children, while active approaches are more appropriate for adolescents (Fam et al., 2022). For children, it is recommended to avoid screen time until the age of 2 and to limit screen time to 1 h per day between 2 and 5 years old, always under supervision. For children aged 6 to 10 years, the time can be extended to up to 2 h daily, while maintaining active supervision (SBP, 2024). During adolescence, the asynchronous development of brain structures, especially the early maturation of the limbic system in relation to the prefrontal cortex, contributes to increased impulsivity and susceptibility to digital rewards, such as "likes" (Cerniglia et al., 2017; Ernst et al., 2006; Ernst, 2014; Somerville & Casey, 2010). Therefore, monitoring should be more frequent in early adolescence, with screen time limited to 2 or 3 h per day between ages 11 and 18 (SBP, 2024).

Other practices include creating "technology-free zones" during family interactions, such as during meals, and limiting screen use before bedtime to improve sleep quality (APA, 2023; Office of the Surgeon General (OSG), 2023; SBP, 2024). Furthermore, caregivers should serve as role models, reflecting on their own digital use and demonstrating consistency between their practices and the expectations they set (OSG, 2023).

Matsuda et al. (2023) conducted a qualitative study with preadolescents and found that the main guidance provided by parents consisted of rules to prevent certain behaviors, often without adequate explanations. Instructions like "don't do that because it's wrong" or "this will harm you" can be ineffective if not accompanied by detailed descriptions of the potential consequences of behavior and appropriate alternatives. Additionally, punishing adolescents for telling the truth—such as when reporting that they experimented with an illicit substance and as a consequence being punished—does not reduce the likelihood of relapse in substance use, but diminishes the willingness to share information with parents about their behaviors.

In contrast, Liu et al. (2019) observed positive associations between effective communication with parents and the satisfaction of children's psychological needs, which in turn were negatively associated with problematic Internet use. The study demonstrated that adequate communication can foster feelings of understanding, acceptance, and affection from parents. Providing support and addressing children's psychological needs can, therefore, strengthen family communication and reduce excessive use of social media.

Resources and Tools for Online Education in Parental Mediation

Various resources can assist caregivers in parental mediation, including specialized websites and blogs that provide information and practical guidance, educational booklets, and guides (e.g., such as publications from the United Nations Children's Fund [UNICEF]). *SaferNet Brazil* (https://new.safernet.org.br/) is a reference in digital security, offering educational materials aimed at children and their caregivers. Similarly, the *Child Mind Institute* (https://childmindai.com/) addresses the impact of excessive screen use on children's mental health, providing guides with practical strategies for managing the issue. The use of parental control apps is another frequently recommended strategy. Tools such as *Google Family Link*, *Qustodio*, and *Kaspersky Safe Kids* allow caregivers to monitor online activities, set screen time limits, and restrict access to inappropriate content. In addition to promoting safety, these apps can help foster the adoption of balanced habits in the digital environment.

Assessment Instruments

The search for standardized scales to assess parental communication has significantly increased in scientific research. In this context, Zapf et al. (2023) conducted a systematic review to identify existing instruments for evaluating the quality of parental communication from the children's perspective, considering psychometric properties and theoretical foundations. The most commonly used scale was the *Parent–Adolescent Communication Scale* (PACS), available in nine languages. Although it demonstrates good internal consistency, the authors note that its conceptual and theoretical basis is not fully defined, and psychometric information is limited, such as the lack of specification regarding the discriminant validity of the construct. Furthermore, the researchers emphasize that the broad scope of the communication concept complicates its standardization.

Recently, Beyens et al. (2024) developed the *Parent–Adolescent Communication about Adolescents' Social Media Use Scale* (PACAS), with the aim of measuring four main aspects: parental inquiry, adolescent disclosure, adolescent secrecy, and parental knowledge about adolescents' online behavior. The instrument is directed at children and includes questions such as the frequency with which they are questioned by parents about social media use, the information shared with parents about online activities, the frequency with which they conceal these activities, and how much parents know about their children's digital behavior. After two validation phases, the scale demonstrated good internal validity; however, its application in Brazil is currently unfeasible due to the lack of adaptations for the local context.

Despite the limitation of standardized scales, several authors have developed materials aimed at characterizing and guiding parents on family communication. Alvarenga et al. (2016) analyzed constructs from developmental psychology through the lens of behavior analysis, aiming to review concepts and improve interventions. In this context, they defined parenting styles as a set of practices involving nonverbal communication, hierarchy, decision-making, and the intensity and frequency of affectionate expressions. Additionally, they operationalized two central concepts: *responsiveness*, which encompasses physical contact, support, cooperation, and encouragement as positive reinforcers for children's behaviors that foster family communication and healthy development, and *demandingness*, which involves monitoring, establishing well-defined and consistent rules, defining values, and presenting the consequences of children's behaviors.

Reflections on the Role of Parental Mediation in the Development of Digital Citizenship

Parental mediation in the development of digital citizenship has become an increasingly important topic, particularly in a context where children and adolescents are becoming more immersed in the digital environment. The role of parents goes beyond simply protecting against the inherent risks of the online world, encompassing the development of skills for conscious and responsible technology use. This process begins with promoting critical thinking, an essential competence for navigating the complex interactions between the benefits and risks associated with social media. Encouraging young people to question the information they consume and to discern reliable sources from misinformation strengthens their informational literacy, preparing them for a more informed and responsible digital citizenship (Huang et al., 2023; Liu et al., 2023; Nielsen et al., 2019; Si & Lee, 2023; Tao et al., 2022; Zhao et al., 2024).

Informational literacy has proven to be a determining factor in the formation of responsible digital citizens, as the ability to identify false information and assess the credibility of sources is essential, especially at a time when misinformation circulates widely on digital platforms. Studies indicate a positive correlation between critical thinking skills and informational literacy, suggesting that the more critical young people are about the content they consume, the better prepared they will be to exercise responsible digital citizenship. In this context, parents play a central role, educating their children on how to verify the truthfulness of information and the importance of consulting reliable sources, promoting the ability to discern what is true and relevant (Huang et al., 2023; Liu et al., 2023; Nielsen et al., 2019; Si & Lee, 2023; Tao et al., 2022; Zhao et al., 2024).

Promoting values such as ethics, respect, and responsibility is a fundamental component of parental mediation in building digital citizenship. Education focused on digital citizenship helps children and adolescents understand the consequences of their actions in the online environment, fostering the development of ethical attitudes in digital interactions. As emphasized by Pujianti et al. (2024), digital education stresses respectful and ethical practices, key aspects in creating a healthy online environment. By integrating concepts such as empathy, privacy, and responsibility in technology use, parents not only protect their children but also empower them to adopt ethical and respectful behaviors, reducing harmful behaviors such as cyberbullying and the spread of misinformation (Malik, 2024).

Preparing children and adolescents to become critical and active digital citizens should be considered a priority in both schools and family environments. This involves promoting digital literacy, which goes beyond the simple use of technologies, encompassing the ability to act critically, responsibly, and ethically in the online space. According to Lu and Gu (2024), self-efficacy in the Internet is an important indicator of digital citizenship, as it contributes to increasing young people's confidence in their ability to interact safely and efficiently on digital platforms.

Finally, preparing young people for digital citizenship involves not only developing technical skills but also encouraging ethical commitment and active participation in democracy. Teaching good digital conduct practices, such as promoting respectful communication in the online environment, and raising awareness about the legal and moral implications of actions in the digital space are fundamental steps in the formation of responsible digital citizens (Lomachinska & Volynets, 2023). By empowering their children to engage in global and local issues through social media, parents and educators contribute to the formation of a generation that is more engaged and aware of its role in the digital world (Hughes et al., 2024).

However, it is necessary to recognize that, despite the directed initiatives, inequalities in access to technology can create substantial disparities in educational opportunities and the development of digital citizenship. The lack of adequate resources may hinder the acquisition of essential competencies for the safe and ethical use of digital platforms. Therefore, it is essential that educational and social policies be structured to ensure that all young people have the tools and support needed to become critical and responsible digital citizens.

References

Alvarenga, P. A., Weber, L. N. D., & Bolsoni-Silva, A. T. (2016). Cuidados parentais e desenvolvimento socioemocional na infância e na adolescência: Uma perspectiva analítico-comportamental. *Revista Brasileira de Terapia Comportamental e Cognitiva, 18*(1), 4–21.

American Academy of Pediatrics (AAP) Council on Communications and Media. (2016). Media use in school-aged children and adolescents. *Pediatrics, 138*(5), e20162592. https://doi.org/10.1542/peds.2016-2592

American Psychological Association (APA). (2023). *Health advisory on social media use in adolescence*. [Online report]. Retrieved from https://www.apa.org/topics/social-media-internet/health-advisory-adolescent-social-media-use.pdf

Anderson, M., Faverio, M., & Gottfried, J. (2023). *Teens, social media and technology 2023*. Pew Research Center. Retrieved from https://www.pewresearch.org

Ariès, P. (1981). *História social da criança e da família* (2nd ed.). LTC.

Arumugam, C. T., Said, M. A., & Nik Farid, N. D. (2021). Screen-based media and young children: Review and recommendations. *Malaysian Family Physician, 16*(2), 7–13. https://doi.org/10.51866/rv1143

Barkin, S., et al. (2006). Parental media mediation styles for children aged 2 to 11 years. *Archives of Pediatrics & Adolescent Medicine, 160*(4), 395–401. https://doi.org/10.1001/archpedi.160.4.395

Beyens, I., Keijsers, L., & Valkenburg, P. M. (2024). Development, validity, and reliability of the parent-adolescent communication about adolescents' social media use scale (PACAS). *Journal of Children and Media, 18*(2), 159–177. https://doi.org/10.1080/17482798.2023.2299828

Bozzola, E., Spina, G., Agostiniani, R., Barni, S., Russo, R., Scarpato, E., Di Mauro, A., Di Stefano, A. V., Caruso, C., Corsello, G., & Staiano, A. (2022). The use of social media in children and adolescents: Scoping review on the potential risks. *International Journal of Environmental Research and Public Health, 19*(16), 9960. https://doi.org/10.3390/ijerph19169960

Brom, C., Yaghobová, A., Drobná, A., et al. (2023). 'The internet is in the satellites!': A systematic review of 3–15-year-olds' conceptions about the internet. *Education and Information Technologies, 28*, 14639–14668. https://doi.org/10.1007/s10639-023-11775-9

Bruni, O., Sette, S., Fontanesi, L., Baiocco, R., Laghi, F., & Baumgartner, E. (2015). Technology use and sleep quality in preadolescence and adolescence. *Journal of Clinical Sleep Medicine, 11*(12), 1433–1441. https://doi.org/10.5664/jcsm.5282

Canadian Society for Exercise Physiology (CSEP). (2016). *Canadian 24-hour movement guidelines for children and youth: An integration of physical activity, sedentary behaviour, and sleep*. CSEP. Retrieved from https://www.csep.ca/guidelines

Cerniglia, L., Zoratto, F., Cimino, S., Laviola, G., Ammaniti, M., & Adriani, W. (2017). Internet addiction in adolescence: Neurobiological, psychosocial and clinical issues. *Neuroscience and Biobehavioral Reviews, 76*(Pt A), 174–184. https://doi.org/10.1016/j.neubiorev.2016.12.024

Chang, F.-C., et al. (2015). The relationship between parental mediation and internet addiction among adolescents, and the association with cyberbullying and depression. *Comprehensive Psychiatry, 57*, 21–28. https://doi.org/10.1016/j.comppsych.2014.11.013

Chassiakos, Y. L. R., & AAP Council on Communications and Media. (2016). Children and adolescents and digital media. *Pediatrics, 138*(5). https://doi.org/10.1542/peds.2016-2593

Chen, L., Liu, X., & Tang, H. (2023). The interactive effects of parental mediation strategies in preventing cyberbullying on social media. *Psychology Research and Behavior Management, 16*, 1009–1022. https://doi.org/10.2147/PRBM.S431039

Chou, H.-L., Liu, Y.-L., & Chou, C. (2019). Privacy behavior profiles of underage Facebook users. *Computers & Education, 128*, 473–485. https://doi.org/10.1016/j.compedu.2018.08.019

Comstock, G. A. (1978). *Television and human behavior*. Columbia University Press.

Coyne, S. M., et al. (2011). Game on… girls: Associations between co-playing video games and adolescent behavioral and family outcomes. *Journal of Adolescent Health, 49*(2), 163–168. https://doi.org/10.1016/j.jadohealth.2010.11.249

Coyne, S. M., Radesky, J., Collier, K. M., Gentile, D. A., Linder, J. R., Nathanson, A. I., Rasmussen, E. E., Reich, S. M., & Rogers, J. (2017). Parenting and digital media. *Pediatrics, 140*(Suppl. 2), S112–S116. https://doi.org/10.1542/peds.2016-1758N

Desmond, R. J., et al. (1985). Family mediation patterns and television viewing. *Human Communication Research, 11*(4), 461–480. https://doi.org/10.1111/j.1468-2958.1985.tb00056.x

Dietvorst, E., Hiemstra, M., Hillegers, M. H. J., & Keijsers, L. (2017). Adolescent perceptions of parental privacy invasion and adolescent secrecy: An illustration of Simpson's paradox. *Child Development, 89*(6), 2081–2090. https://doi.org/10.1111/cdev.13002

Dittus, P. J., Li, J., Verlenden, J. V., Wilkins, N. J., Carman-McClanahan, M. N., Cavalier, Y., Mercado, M. C., Welder, L. E., Roehler, D. R., & Ethier, K. A. (2023). Parental monitoring and risk behaviors and experiences among high school students—youth risk behavior survey, United States, 2021. *MMWR Supplements, 72*(1), 37–44. https://doi.org/10.15585/mmwr.su7201a5

Edwards, S., Nolan, A., Henderson, M., Mantilla, A., Plowman, L., & Skouteris, H. (2018). Young children's everyday concepts of the internet: A platform for cyber-safety education in the early years. *British Journal of Educational Technology, 49*(1), 45–55. https://doi.org/10.1111/bjet.12529

Ernst, M. (2014). The triadic model perspective for the study of adolescent motivated behavior. *Brain and Cognition, 89*, 104–111. https://doi.org/10.1016/j.bandc.2014.01.006

Ernst, M., Pine, D. S., & Hardin, M. (2006). Triadic model of the neurobiology of motivated behavior in adolescence. *Psychological Medicine, 36*(3), 299–312. https://doi.org/10.1017/S0033291705005891

Fam, J. Y., Männikkö, N., Juhari, R., & Kääriäinen, M. (2022). Is parental mediation negatively associated with problematic media use among children and adolescents? A systematic review and meta-analysis. *Canadian Journal of Behavioural Science/Revue Canadienne Des Sciences Du Comportement, 55*(2), 81–94. https://doi.org/10.1037/cbs0000320

Grossman, E. (1998). La adolescencia cruzando los siglos. *Adolescencia Latinoamericana, 1*, 68–74.

Guerrero, M. D., Barnes, J. D., Walsh, J. J., Tremblay, M. S., & Chaput, J. P. (2019). 24-hour movement behaviors and impulsivity. *Pediatrics, 144*(3), e20190187. https://doi.org/10.1542/peds.2019-0187

Hoge, E., Bickham, D., & Cantor, J. (2017). Digital media, anxiety, and depression in children. *Pediatrics, 140*(Suppl. 2), S76–S80. https://doi.org/10.1542/peds.2016-1758G

Holtz, P., & Appel, M. (2011). Internet use and video gaming predict problem behavior in early adolescence. *Journal of Adolescence, 34*(1), 49–58. https://doi.org/10.1016/j.adolescence.2010.02.004

Hu, W., Mao, Y., Huang, K., & Sun, Y. (2022). Does internet entertainment reduce the cognitive ability of children? Evidence from the China education panel survey. *Behavioral Science, 12*(10), 364. https://doi.org/10.3390/bs12100364

Huang, S., Lai, X., Li, Y., Wang, W., Zhao, X., Dai, X., Wang, H., & Wang, Y. (2023). Does parental media mediation make a difference for adolescents? Evidence from an empirical cohort study of parent-adolescent dyads. *Heliyon, 9*(4), e14897. https://doi.org/10.1016/j.heliyon.2023.e14897

Hughes, J., Robb, J. A., & Gadanidis, M. (2024). Educating for a just world: Empowering K–12 students as global democratic digital citizens. *Journal of Digital Life and Learning, 3*(2), 69. https://doi.org/10.51357/jdll.v3i2.240

Jang, Y., & Ko, B. (2023). Online safety for children and youth under the 4Cs framework–A focus on digital policies in Australia, Canada, and the UK. *Children (Basel, Switzerland), 10*(8), 1415. https://doi.org/10.3390/children10081415

Johnson, N. F., & Francis, Z. (2022). Positive family relationships in a digital age: Hearing the voice of young people. *Children & Society, 36*(5), 933–948. https://doi.org/10.1111/chso.12548

Koning, I. M., et al. (2018). Bidirectional effects of internet-specific parenting practices and compulsive social media and internet game use. *Journal of Behavioral Addictions, 7*(3), 624–632. https://doi.org/10.1556/2006.7.2018.68

Lee, S. (2012). Parental restrictive mediation of children's internet use: Effective for what and for whom? *New Media & Society, 15*(4), 466. https://doi.org/10.1177/1461444812452412

Liu, Q., et al. (2019). Perceived parent–adolescent communication and pathological internet use among Chinese adolescents: A moderated mediation model. *Journal of Child and Family Studies, 28*(6), 1571–1580.

Liu, J., Wu, L., Sun, X., Bai, X., & Duan, C. (2023). Active parental mediation and adolescent problematic internet use: The mediating role of parent-child relationships and hiding online behavior. *Behavioral Science, 13*(8), 679. https://doi.org/10.3390/bs13080679

Livingstone, S., & Helsper, E. J. (2008). Parental mediation of children's internet use. *Journal of Broadcasting & Electronic Media, 52*(4), 581–599. https://doi.org/10.1080/08838150802437396

Livingstone, S., Kirwil, L., Ponte, C., & Staksrud, E. (2014). In their own words: What bothers children online? *European Journal of Communication, 29*(3), 271–288. https://doi.org/10.1177/0267323114521045

Livingstone, S., et al. (2017). Maximizing opportunities and minimizing risks for children online: The role of digital skills in emerging strategies of parental mediation. *Journal of Communication, 67*(1), 82–105. https://doi.org/10.1111/jcom.12277

Lomachinska, I., & Volynets, I. (2023). Global landmarks of digital citizenship in the conditions of today's globalization challenges. *Osvìtologìčnij diskurs, 45*(2). https://doi.org/10.28925/2312-5829.2024.2.6

Lu, C., & Gu, M. (2024). A systematic review and meta-analysis of factors and outcomes of digital citizenship among adolescents. *Asia Pacific Journal of Education*, 1–16. https://doi.org/10.1080/02188791.2023.2296352

Lukavská, K., et al. (2022). The associations of adolescent problematic internet use with parenting: A meta-analysis. *Addictive Behaviors, 135*, 107423.

Malik, K. (2024). Integrating digital citizenship education in the contemporary educational ecosystem. In *Advances in education and educational studies* (pp. 215–229). https://doi.org/10.1201/9781032713366-25

Matsuda, Y., et al. (2023). Parent-child communication about substance use, puberty, sex, and social media use among Hispanic parents and pre-adolescent children. *PLoS One, 18*(11), e0295303.

Modecki, K. L., Goldberg, R. E., Wisniewski, P., & Orben, A. (2022). What is digital parenting? A systematic review of past measurement and blueprint for the future. *Perspectives on Psychological Science: A Journal of the Association for Psychological Science, 17*(6), 1673–1691. https://doi.org/10.1177/17456916211072458

Mollborn, S., & Lawrence, E. (2018). Family, peer, and school influences on children's developing health lifestyles. *Journal of Health and Social Behavior, 59*(1), 133–150. https://doi.org/10.1177/0022146517750637

Navarro, R., et al. (2013). The role of internet use and parental mediation on cyberbullying victimization among Spanish children from rural public schools. *European Journal of Psychology of Education, 28*, 725–745. https://doi.org/10.1007/s10212-012-0137-2

Nielsen, P., Favez, N., Liddle, H., & Rigter, H. (2019). Linking parental mediation practices to adolescents' problematic online screen use: A systematic literature review. *Journal of Behavioral Addictions, 8*(4), 649–663. https://doi.org/10.1556/2006.8.2019.61

Nikken, P., & Schols, M. (2015). How and why parents guide the media use of young children. *Journal of Child and Family Studies, 24*(11), 3423–3435. https://doi.org/10.1007/s10826-015-0144-4

Odgers, C. L., & Jensen, M. R. (2020a). Adolescent development and growing divides in the digital age. *Dialogues in Clinical Neuroscience, 22*(2), 143–149. https://doi.org/10.31887/DCNS.2020.22.2/codgers

Odgers, C. L., & Jensen, M. R. (2020b). Annual research review: Adolescent mental health in the digital age: Facts, fears, and future directions. *Journal of Child Psychology and Psychiatry, and Allied Disciplines, 61*(3), 336–348. https://doi.org/10.1111/jcpp.13190

Office of the Surgeon General (OSG). (2023). *Social Media and youth mental health: The U.S. Surgeon General's Advisory*. US Department of Health and Human Services.

Oh, C., Carducci, B., Vaivada, T., & Bhutta, Z. A. (2022). Interventions to promote physical activity and healthy digital media use in children and adolescents: A systematic review. *Pediatrics, 149*(Suppl. 6), e2021053852I. https://doi.org/10.1542/peds.2021-053852I

Phillips, D. A., & Lowenstein, A. E. (2011). Early care, education, and child development. *Annual Review of Psychology, 62*, 483–500. https://doi.org/10.1146/annurev.psych.031809.130707

Pujianti, A., Dornauli, K., Malau, B. R., & Ulandari, U. (2024). Membangun budaya positif berinternet berbasis etika dan kewarganegaraan serta meningkatkan kesadaran masyarakat di era digital. *Uranus, 2*(2), 61. https://doi.org/10.61132/uranus.v2i2.128

Ricci, R. C., Paulo, A. S. C., Freitas, A. K. P. B., Ribeiro, I. C., Pires, L. S. A., Facina, M. E. L., Cabral, M. B., Parduci, N. V., Spegiorin, R. C., Bogado, S. S. G., Chociay Junior, S., Carachesti, T. N., & Larroque, M. M. (2022). Impacts of technology on children's health: A systematic review. *Revista paulista de pediatria: orgao oficial da Sociedade de Pediatria de Sao Paulo, 41*, e2020504. https://doi.org/10.1590/1984-0462/2023/41/2020504

Saputri, N. A., & Wulandari, H. (2024). Parental problems in early children's education in the digital era. *Inovasi Kurikulum, 21*(1), 287–302.

Savoia, E., Harriman, N. W., Su, M., Cote, T., & Shortland, N. (2021). Adolescents' exposure to online risks: Gender disparities and vulnerabilities related to online behaviors. *International Journal of Environmental Research and Public Health, 18*(11), 5786. https://doi.org/10.3390/ijerph18115786

Schoen-Ferreira, T. H., Aznar-Farias, M., & de Silvares, E. F. M. (2010). Adolescência através dos séculos. *Psicologia: Teoria e Pesquisa, 26*(2), 227–234. https://doi.org/10.1590/S0102-37722010000200004

Schrodt, P., Witt, P. L., & Messersmith, A. S. (2008). A meta-analytical review of family communication patterns and their associations with information processing, behavioral, and psychosocial outcomes. *Communication Monographs, 75*(3), 248–269. https://doi.org/10.1080/03637750802256318

Shin, W., & Ismail, N. (2014). Exploring the role of parents and peers in young adolescents' risk taking on social networking sites. *Cyberpsychology, Behavior, and Social Networking, 17*(9), 578. https://doi.org/10.1089/cyber.2014.00

Si, E., & Lee, G. (2023). Moderating effects of digital citizenship on problematic digital Media use and children's happiness: A cross-sectional study. *The Journal of School Health, 93*(6), 485–493. https://doi.org/10.1111/josh.13275

Sina, E., Buck, C., Ahrens, W., Coumans, J. M. J., Eiben, G., Formisano, A., Lissner, L., Mazur, A., Michels, N., Molnar, D., Moreno, L. A., Pala, V., Pohlabeln, H., Reisch, L., Tornaritis, M., Veidebaum, T., Hebestreit, A., & I. Family Consortium. (2023). Digital media exposure and cognitive functioning in European children and adolescents of the I. Family study. *Scientific Reports, 13*(1), 18855. https://doi.org/10.1038/s41598-023-45944-0

Sociedade Brasileira de Pediatria (SBP). (2024, August 13). *#Menos telas #Mais saúde: Atualização 2024 (N° 163)*. Sociedade Brasileira de Pediatria.

Somerville, L. H., & Casey, B. J. (2010). Developmental neurobiology of cognitive control and motivational systems. *Current Opinion in Neurobiology, 20*(2), 236–241. https://doi.org/10.1016/j.conb.2010.01.006

Steinfeld, N. (2021). Parental mediation of adolescent internet use: Combining strategies to promote awareness, autonomy, and self-regulation in preparing youth for life on the web. *Education and Information Technologies, 26*(2), 1897–1920. https://doi.org/10.1007/s10639-020-10342-w

Suárez-Álvarez, R., Vázquez-Barrio, T., & Frutos-Torres, B. (2022). Parental digital mediation according to the age of minors: From restraint and control to active mediation. *Social Sciences, 11*(4), 178. https://doi.org/10.3390/socsci11040178

Tao, S., Reichert, F., Law, N., & Rao, N. (2022). Digital technology use and cyberbullying among primary school children: Digital literacy and parental mediation as moderators. *Cyberpsychology, Behavior and Social Networking, 25*(9), 571–579. https://doi.org/10.1089/cyber.2022.0012

Vannucci, A., et al. (2020). Social media use and risky behaviors in adolescents: A meta-analysis. *Journal of Adolescence, 79*, 258–274.

Wong, Y. C. (2011). Cyber-parenting: Internet benefits, risks, and parenting issues. *Journal of Technology in Human Services, 28*(4), 252–273. https://doi.org/10.1080/15228835.2011.562629

World Health Organization (WHO). (2020). *Diretrizes sobre atividade física, comportamento sedentário e sono para crianças com menos de 5 anos de idade*. Organização Mundial da Saúde. Retrieved from https://apps.who.int/iris/handle/10665/311663

Zapf, H., Boettcher, J., Haukeland, Y., Orm, S., Coslar, S., Wiegand-Grefe, S., & Fjermestad, K. (2023). A systematic review of parent-child communication measures: Instruments and their psychometric properties. *Clinical Child and Family Psychology Review, 26*(1), 121–142. https://doi.org/10.1007/s10567-022-00414-3

Zhao, Z., Zhu, L., Liao, J., Xia, J., & Pu, X. (2024). Parental mediation, digital media usage, and health literacy: An exploration among Chinese elementary school students. In *Health communication* (pp. 1–13). https://doi.org/10.1080/10410236.2024.2387389. Advance online publication.

Zhu, Y., Deng, L., & Wan, K. (2022). The association between parent-child relationship and problematic internet use among English- and Chinese-language studies: A meta-analysis. *Frontiers in Psychology, 13*, 847225. https://doi.org/10.3389/fpsyg.2022.847225

Chapter 8
The Gamblification of Video Games: A Case Study on Loot Boxes

Maya C. Thulin, Lindsey A. Snaychuk, Jenna L. Vieira, Sophie G. Coelho, and Hyoun S. Kim

Introduction

Video games are one of the most popular forms of entertainment, with over 2 billion individuals playing video games worldwide (Clement, 2024). Increasingly, video games feature loot boxes, which are digital items common in many popular video games. Loot boxes fall under the umbrella of microtransactions: virtual items containing bonus content for a game (e.g., in-game currency, expansion packs; Gibson et al., 2023). Though most microtransactions are inexpensive, combined they result in billions in revenue for video game companies (King et al., 2020). A loot box (often taking the form of a box/crate/chest), once acquired by the player, contains a random and unknown assortment of other digital items which can be used in the video game, such as virtual currency or character outfits (Xiao et al., 2024b). Opening a loot box is typically paired with sound effects and animations, creating an immersive experience for the player (Mills et al., 2024). Players will oftentimes be gifted loot boxes to mark an achievement in a game, or they can be purchased using either real-world money or virtual currency (Xiao et al., 2024b). The "value" of the items contained in a loot box varies, and there is the potential for players to receive rare items (Xiao et al., 2024b). One important characteristic of loot boxes is that their prize is random. While many of the prizes a player will receive in a loot box are commonplace and hold little value, the possibility remains that the player will receive an item that is rare and/or desirable (Xiao et al., 2024b). For many

M. C. Thulin · L. A. Snaychuk · J. L. Vieira · H. S. Kim (✉)
Toronto Metropolitan University, Toronto, ON, Canada
e-mail: mthulin@torontomu.ca; lindsey.snaychuk@torontomu.ca; jlvieira@torontomu.ca; andrewhs.kim@torontomu.ca

S. G. Coelho
York University, Toronto, ON, Canada
e-mail: scoelho@yorku.ca

A. L. M. Andrade (ed.), *Digital Addictions*,
https://doi.org/10.1007/978-3-031-87986-9_8

games, the odds of acquiring a rare item are not clearly stated (Cordes et al., 2024). It is the random mechanics of loot boxes paired with ability to purchase them with real money that have led to the suggestion that loot boxes (especially when purchased with real money) constitutes a form of gambling (Larche et al., 2021).

Popularity of Loot Boxes

Loot boxes were introduced in Korea in 2003, with the first loot box-like system believed to be the Gachapon ticket in MapleStory, a free-to-play game (Lemmens, 2022). However, loot boxes were not widely available worldwide until 2008–2010, first appearing in the video game FIFA Ultimate Team under the name of player packs (Decamp & Daly, 2023; Lemmens, 2022). Through their inclusion in several popular games (i.e., Team Fortress 2, Mass Effect 3), loot boxes rose to prominence in 2012. By 2017–2018, loot boxes had become widespread, drawing international attention from academics, the general public, regulators, and lawmakers. For example, government officials in Australia, America, and Europe publicly raised concerns about loot boxes, in particular, their impact on youth, and introduced legislation aiming to protect video game consumers. This concern has not stopped the expansion of loot boxes, and by 2020, the majority of the most popular games for iPhone (59%) and Android (58%) contained loot boxes (Zendle et al., 2020a, 2020b).

Indeed, loot boxes have become popular among gamers worldwide and are now available in some of the most popular video games, such as Fortnite, Overwatch, and Halo (Clement, 2024). The popularity of loot boxes has only continued to rise, with revenue from loot boxes expected to exceed $20 billion USD by 2025—an increase from $15 billion USD in 2020 (Juniper Research, 2021). Indeed, a study of American eighth grade students (13–14 years) and 11th grade students (16–17 years) found that 35% of eighth grade video game players had purchased loot boxes in 2018, with the prevalence rising to 41% in 2022 (DeCamp & Daly, 2023). Of note, this increase in prevalence was not as large in 11th grade students, with 29% of these older video game players purchasing loot boxes in 2018 and 30% in 2022 (DeCamp & Daly, 2023). Loot boxes are popular among adolescents, as well as readily available. When examining video games containing loot boxes, over 90% were rated suitable for ages 12+ years (Zendle et al., 2020a, 2020b). However, loot boxes are not only appealing to adolescents. A study of 6600 Spanish adolescents and young adults found that 32% of young adults (age 18–30) had purchased loot boxes in the past 12 months (González-Cabrera et al., 2022). The popularity of loot boxes with adolescents and young adults is one reason why loot boxes have been scrutinized for their potential similarities with gambling with concerns that they may act as a "gateway" to real money gambling in this vulnerable population.

Are Loot Boxes Gambling?

A key concern that has been raised is whether loot boxes are a form of gambling in disguise (Xiao et al., 2022a). One reason for this is that several structural characteristics (i.e., inherent features) of loot boxes appear to overlap with those of gambling, an activity whose risks and addictive potential are widely recognized (Wilson et al., 2024). Loot boxes feature random reward mechanisms whereby the specific contents (i.e., "loot") an individual will receive from a box are unknown prior to opening and are determined entirely by chance (Nielsen & Grabarczyk, 2019). Smaller rewards that are perceived as less valuable (e.g., a common weapon) tend to be more commonly obtained than rarer rewards (e.g., a legendary weapon that can only be obtained via loot boxes or special in-game events) (Larche et al., 2021). This closely resembles the unpredictable nature of gambling and the tendency for riskier activities, such as slot machines, to distribute losses and small wins much more commonly than large wins (Larche et al., 2021). Drawing additional parallels to slot machines is the tendency for audiovisual displays (e.g., a spinning wheel, bright colors, loud music) to accompany the presentation of loot box outcomes, which can facilitate increases in arousal as well as the experience of reward, thereby potentially encouraging further loot box purchasing (Larche et al., 2021) just as they influence the continuation of gambling (Spetch et al., 2020). In some video games such as *DOTA 2*, players are shown "near misses"—in other words, the rarer rewards they could have won alongside their actual obtained reward (Zendle et al., 2019). Near misses are also commonly featured in gambling (e.g., obtaining the pattern cherry-cherry-lemon on a slot machine when cherry-cherry-cherry would have produced a win; Pisklak et al., 2020) and have been identified as motivators of excessive and uncontrollable gambling because they lead individuals to believe that they are close to a win (Clark et al., 2009).

The overwhelming similarities between loot box mechanics and those of gambling have led to international debates regarding the extent to which loot boxes should be conceptualized, and thus regulated, as a form of gambling (Xiao et al., 2022b). In recent years, several countries have made efforts to protect consumers from the potential risks associated with loot boxes through the introduction of laws and regulations (for a comprehensive review, see Xiao, 2023). Some have taken the approach of enforcing existing gambling and consumer protection laws to loot boxes. Perhaps most notably, in 2018, the Belgian gambling regulator concluded that loot boxes containing rewards of both monetary and non-monetary value constitute illegal forms of gambling (Xiao, 2023). Despite this conclusion, Xiao (2023) notes that a substantial number of iPhone games offered by the Belgian Apple App Store continue to sell loot boxes, suggesting that enforcement of outright bans on loot boxes is challenging to enforce. Other countries such as Taiwan, South Korea, and China have implemented laws that require gaming companies to disclose the percentage probability of winning each loot box reward, with noncompliance being punishable by imprisonment in South Korea (Xiao, 2023). However, evidence has indicated that although most video game players in China reported having seen probability disclosures, most also reported that their spending on loot boxes did not change as a result (Xiao, 2023).

Other countries have taken approaches such as requiring gaming companies to include age ratings and warning labels on games that contain loot boxes (e.g., Australia, Germany), changing the definition of gambling to include loot boxes (e.g., Finland, Brazil), and applying existing European Union consumer protection law to loot boxes (e.g., Italy, the Netherlands), each with mixed success in terms of enforcement (Xiao, 2023). Regulatory efforts will likely be dynamic and ongoing as empirical evidence continues to develop regarding the links between loot box engagement and gambling, as subsequently detailed.

Associations of Loot Box Purchasing with Gambling and Problem Gambling

Debate about whether loot boxes should be conceptualized as a form of gambling has prompted growing research attention toward whether individuals who purchase loot boxes also report greater or more problematic engagement in other forms of gambling. Several cross-sectional studies have now examined associations of loot box purchasing with gambling and problem gambling (Gibson et al., 2022; Kim et al., 2023; Montiel et al., 2022; Spicer et al., 2022). Although these studies have varied in their operationalizations of loot box purchasing (e.g., any versus no loot box purchasing, total expenditure on loot box purchasing), gambling (e.g., any versus no gambling, gambling frequency, gambling expenditure), and problem gambling (e.g., categorical problem gambling status, continuous problem gambling severity level), nearly all have established that purchasing loot boxes is associated with a greater likelihood of or more severe gambling and problem gambling (Gibson et al., 2022; Kim et al., 2023; Montiel et al., 2022; Spicer et al., 2022), with moderate meta-analytic effect sizes (Garea et al., 2021; Spicer et al., 2022).

One explanation for the association of loot box purchasing with gambling and problem gambling is that loot box purchasing represents a "gateway" to gambling behaviors due to parallels between loot boxes and real-world gambling, for example, in their structural characteristics (e.g., variable ratio reinforcement schedule; Drummond & Sauer, 2018) and in the arousal and reward responses elicited during engagement (Larche et al., 2021). Alternatively, purchasing loot boxes may appeal most to individuals exhibiting greater gambling engagement and problems, perhaps given their exposure to wagering real money on chance-based outcomes of uncertain value. Further, it is possible that associations of loot box purchasing with gambling and problem gambling reflect an effect of selection rather than exposure—that is, that the effects of confounding or "third" variables predispose individuals to both loot box purchasing and gambling (Kim & King, 2020). However, recent data support the persistence of associations of loot box purchasing with gambling and problem gambling, even while controlling for their common risk factors, such as impulsivity, emotion dysregulation, depressive and anxiety symptoms, and adverse childhood experiences (Coelho et al., 2023).

More recently, select longitudinal studies have sought to clarify the directionality of associations of loot box purchasing with gambling and problem gambling and the extent to which purchasing loot boxes causes gambling initiation and problem gambling escalation. Brooks and Clark (2023) assessed loot box expenditure, risky loot box engagement, and gambling participation at two time points in a sample of young adults reporting engagement with video gaming, recruited from the United States, the United Kingdom, and Canada. Among participants who did not report gambling at baseline, greater baseline loot box expenditure and risky loot box engagement each predicted an increased likelihood of gambling initiation and higher gambling expenditure at follow-up. Further, among participants who reported gambling, but not loot box purchasing, at baseline, elevated baseline gambling-related cognitive distortions (but not other gambling-related variables, such as problem gambling severity and gambling expenditure) predicted greater loot box expenditure at follow-up. González-Cabrera et al. (2023) similarly examined prospective associations of loot box purchasing with online gambling behaviors among adolescents in Spain, observing associations of reporting any loot box purchasing at baseline with an increased likelihood of reporting online gambling 6 months later, and with an increased likelihood of reporting problem online gambling 6 months later among female (but not male) participants. Taken together, these studies provide empirical support for the "gateway" hypothesis wherein individuals migrate from loot box purchasing to gambling and problem gambling, and there is preliminary evidence for the reverse wherein gambling predicts subsequent elevations in loot box engagement. However, further longitudinal research, especially that involving three or more assessments, is needed to replicate these findings and delineate bidirectional relations between loot box purchasing and problem gambling. Further, experimental research is needed to establish a causal role of loot box purchasing in the progression of gambling and problem gambling.

Recent Studies

In addition to examining associations of loot box purchasing with gambling and problem gambling, more recent research has focused on two key themes: (1) understanding the potential harms posed by loot boxes and (2) examining characteristics that may predispose individuals to purchase loot boxes.

Harms Posed by Loot Boxes

In order to investigate the harms associated with loot boxes, researchers need to be able to measure these harms. Although there is not a specific measure that assesses harms caused by loot boxes, Brooks and Clark (2019) created the Risky Loot Box Index (RLBI), which includes several items that provide insights into potential harms of loot boxes. Specifically, the RLBI contains five items, with questions examining preoccupation with loot boxes, neglecting obligations to collect loot boxes, and continued engagement with loot boxes after failing to receive a valuable prize (e.g., "I have bought more loot boxes after failing to receive valuable items"). In the initial validation study, scores on the RLBI were correlated with measures of gambling behavior, risk-taking, and gambling-related cognitive distortions, providing preliminary support for the validity of the RLBI. Since its development, further research has examined the psychometric properties of the RLBI. For example, Primi et al. (2024) conducted an item response theory analysis of the RLBI in an adolescent sample, finding acceptable item-level properties and that the RLBI was adequately informative and invariant across gender.

Problem gambling is the most common outcome studied in relation to loot box purchasing, with problem gambling leading to significant psychological, financial, and interpersonal harms. With the relationship between loot box engagement and problem gambling consistently found throughout studies, more recent research has focused on strengthening support for this relationship. For example, researchers have questioned whether study participants who engage with loot boxes respond to problem gambling questions in reference to their loot box use (Sidloski et al., 2022). If this were the case, then loot box users scoring high on measures of problem gambling would actually be indicating that their loot box use was problematic, rather than that they were engaging in problematic gambling. Xiao et al. (2024c) further tested this theory and found that, even after experimentally manipulating the survey measures of problem gambling, the association between loot box purchasing and problem gambling severity remained, strengthening support for this relationship.

Furthermore, loot boxes have been linked to harms unrelated to gambling. A study by Drummond et al. (2022) examined levels of psychological distress (i.e., levels of anxiety, depression, and overall mental distress) in individuals who had purchased loot boxes compared to those who had not purchased loot boxes. Individuals who had purchased loot boxes were at a moderately higher risk of experiencing severe psychological distress, and this relationship remained even after controlling for demographic characteristics (i.e., age, gender) as well as meeting the cutoff of problem gambling. Loot boxes have also been linked to other psychological and financial harms, such as post-purchasing regret and excessive spending (Ash et al., 2022; Garea et al., 2023). These results suggest that purchasing loot boxes may be associated with psychological harm, over and above the consistent association with problem gambling.

In addition to identifying harms posed by loot boxes, researchers have also begun to study how these harms may be minimized. Macey et al. (2022) established a working group of experts in the field who were then subjected to presentations relevant to loot box harms (i.e., presentations from individuals with lived experience with problematic gambling and gaming; a games industry representative, etc.). Following these presentations, the working group identified possible actions to minimize loot box harms. Recommendations included regulation to increase transparency, bolstering research through funding and data provided by game companies, raising awareness of potential harms posed by loot boxes, and modifying the structures of video games to protect players (i.e., clearly displaying the amount spent in a game, preventing minors from making unauthorized purchases; Macey et al., 2022). Further research is needed to identify the feasibility and usefulness of these recommended actions.

Who Purchases Loot Boxes?

Given the research linking loot box purchasing to potential harms (i.e., problems arising from problematic gambling, psychological harms), it is imperative to examine who is more likely to purchase loot boxes, in order to understand who may be at higher risk of these harms. Large-scale studies have begun to elucidate some of the demographic factors that are correlated with loot box engagement. Indeed, a study of over 16,000 individuals who play video games in the United Kingdom compared gamers who have purchased loot boxes to those who have not purchased loot boxes. Participants who were male, younger, unemployed, and not university-educated were more likely to report purchasing loot boxes (Close et al., 2022). Additionally, individuals who purchase loot boxes may be more likely to have friends who also purchase loot boxes, play video games on more devices, play a wide variety of video games, and experience problematic gaming and/or problematic gambling symptoms (for a review, see Yokomitsu et al., 2021). Psychological characteristics, such as gambling-related cognitive distortions (i.e., irrational beliefs about gambling, such as believing that one can control the outcome of an uncontrollable event, e.g., a slot machine), and positive attitudes towards gambling/loot boxes have also been associated with a greater likelihood of risky engagement with loot boxes (Yokomitsu et al., 2021).

Directions for Future Research

Since loot boxes became popular in the 2010s, they have been extensively researched, providing valuable insights to the similarities between loot boxes and traditional forms of gambling, the relationship between loot boxes and problem gambling, and characteristics of those who purchase loot boxes. Nonetheless, there remain opportunities for future research. These include further investigation into (1) the mechanisms underlying transitions from loot box purchasing to gambling, (2) more objective measures of loot box expenditure, and (3) cross-cultural data on loot box engagement and related harms.

The Loot Box Gambling Link

Loot boxes have caused concern for many due to their similarity to gambling. However, whether loot boxes act as a gateway to more traditional forms of gambling (i.e., slot machines, casino table games, etc.) remains unknown. A cross-sectional study, where participants are only assessed once, by Spicer et al. (2022) surveyed over 1000 participants who reported both purchasing loot boxes and gambling. This study found that close to 20% of participants self-reported that there was a link between their loot box purchasing and their gambling (Spicer et al., 2022). Complicating these findings, there was a similar amount of participants who reported purchasing loot boxes before starting to gamble as there were who endorsed the opposite (i.e., they were already engaging in gambling before they started purchasing loot boxes). This makes it difficult to form an opinion on whether purchasing loot boxes influenced individuals to start gambling, or vice versa. Longitudinal research is needed to understand the mechanisms underlying the relationship between gambling and loot boxes. For example, a study involving individuals who report purchasing loot boxes, collecting survey data from these participants every 3 months for 1 year to examine how many of these participants start gambling. Participants who start gambling could be compared to those who were gambling at the baseline survey, seeing how these two groups differ from each other. Studying the same participants at multiple timepoints would provide further information on the transition from purchasing loot boxes to gambling, thus clarifying previous cross-sectional studies.

Objective Data

Research on loot box expenditure has often used self-report measures (i.e., a participant will be asked "how much money did you spend on loot boxes in the past 12 months?"; Carey et al., 2022; Garrett et al., 2022). While this is usually considered adequate, more objective data on loot box expenditure could increase confidence in the accuracy of a study's findings. This could be achieved through having participants upload anonymized receipts of their loot box transactions in a given timeframe, or through collaboration with gaming companies. Gambling operators have previously collaborated with researchers, granting access to their gambling sites' behavioral tracking data (Auer & Griffiths, 2022). Behavioral tracking data from operators can provide objective measures of key variables such as the number of players in a specific time period, average expenditure, and average time spent gaming. This would reduce the effort required from study participants to estimate their responses to survey questions, as well as increase confidence in the accuracy of study data.

Another way to collect data less susceptible to self-report-related biases is through Ecological Momentary Assessment (EMA). EMA involves repeatedly collecting data in real time (Shiffman et al., 2008), often through the use of smartphones. In the context of loot boxes, participants could be asked multiple times per day, for a set period of time, about their loot box engagement. This approach aims to minimize recall bias (i.e., the inaccurate recollection of an event) and provides data on contextual factors related to loot box engagement (e.g., whether individuals are more likely to purchase loot boxes while drinking alcohol).

Cross-Cultural Data

Loot boxes are popular worldwide. However, relatively few studies have studied loot boxes in different countries to see any factors which may differ between countries. Cross-cultural data is important for the generalizability of study results. For example, results drawn from data in an individualistic culture may not generalize to individuals in a collectivistic culture. This is particularly important regarding associations between loot boxes and gambling. Limited research has begun to investigate loot boxes in a non-Western context, with a recent study by Xiao et al. (2024a) replicating the relationship between higher loot box spending and greater problem gambling in Mainland China. However, there are countries (i.e., South Korea) where loot boxes are available in video games, but gambling is prohibited. Research linking loot box engagement to problem gambling may not be generalizable to these countries, though further research is needed to clarify. Furthermore, countries where gambling is prohibited may provide insight into non-gambling-related harms of loot boxes—if gambling is unavailable, there may be limited harms linked to loot boxes, or a greater incidence of harms of a different form (i.e., psychological, financial).

Conclusions

Though they were originally created as a novel feature of video games in the early 2000s, loot boxes have since become a global phenomenon, contributing significantly to industry revenue over the last several decades. Yet, loot boxes are subject to criticism by experts who highlight their similarities to gambling. Because of these similarities, evidence consistently links the loot boxes to problem gambling and other harms, which highlights the potential risk. Research also suggests that loot boxes may serve as a gateway to gambling, though more longitudinal research is needed to clarify this relationship. Further, loot boxes are also associated with other harms including financial loss and psychological distress.

In response to the harms associated with loot boxes, many regulatory efforts (e.g., increasing transparency, bans) have been implemented cross-nationally to mitigate risk. However, enforcement of such efforts remains challenging. Therefore, as the popularity and profitability of loot boxes continue to grow, it is essential for policy makers to continue addressing concerns around harm. Future research should aim to collect objective, longitudinal data across diverse populations to better understand the trajectories of individuals who use loot boxes to inform the development of targeted interventions that target risk and associated harm.

References

Ash, J., Gordon, R., & Mills, S. (2022). *Between gaming and gambling: Children, young people, and paid reward systems in digital Games* (p. 28). Newcastle University. https://www.gaming-gamblingresearch.org.uk/wp-content/uploads/2022/10/ESRC-BGG-Final-Report-2022.pdf

Auer, M., & Griffiths, M. D. (2022). Gambling before and during the COVID-19 pandemic among online casino gamblers: An empirical study using behavioral tracking data. *International Journal of Mental Health and Addiction, 20*(3), 1722–1732. https://doi.org/10.1007/s11469-020-00462-2

Brooks, G. A., & Clark, L. (2019). Associations between loot box use, problematic gaming and gambling, and gambling-related cognitions. *Addictive Behaviors, 96*, 26–34. https://doi.org/10.1016/j.addbeh.2019.04.009

Brooks, G. A., & Clark, L. (2023). The gamblers of the future? Migration from loot boxes to gambling in a longitudinal study of young adults. *Computers in Human Behavior, 141*, 107605. https://doi.org/10.1016/j.chb.2022.107605

Carey, P. A. K., Delfabbro, P., & King, D. (2022). An evaluation of gaming-related harms in relation to gaming disorder and loot box involvement. *International Journal of Mental Health and Addiction, 20*(5), 2906–2921. https://doi.org/10.1007/s11469-021-00556-5

Clark, L., Lawrence, A. J., Astley-Jones, F., & Gray, N. (2009). Gambling near-misses enhance motivation to gamble and recruit win-related brain circuitry. *Neuron, 61*(3), 481–490. https://doi.org/10.1016/j.neuron.2008.12.031

Clement, J. (2024, June 3). *Video gaming worldwide—Statistics & Facts*. Statista. https://www.statista.com/topics/1680/gaming/#topicOverview

Close, J., Spicer, S. G., Nicklin, L. L., Lloyd, J., & Lloyd, H. (2022). Loot box engagement: Relationships with educational attainment, employment status and earnings in a cohort of 16 000 United Kingdom gamers. *Addiction, 117*(8), 2338–2345. https://doi.org/10.1111/add.15837

Coelho, S. G., Keough, M. T., Hodgins, D. C., Shead, N. W., Parmar, P. K., & Kim, H. S. (2023). Loot box purchasing is associated with gambling and problem gambling when controlling for known psychological risk factors of gambling. *Addiction Research & Theory, 31*(4), 260–269. https://doi.org/10.1080/16066359.2022.2141717

Cordes, S., Dertwinkel-Kalt, M., & Werner, T. (2024). What drives demand for loot boxes? An experimental study. *Journal of Economic Behavior & Organization, 228*, 106755. https://doi.org/10.1016/j.jebo.2024.106755

DeCamp, W., & Daly, K. (2023). Loot box consumption by adolescents pre- and post- pandemic lockdown. *PeerJ, 11*, e15287. https://doi.org/10.7717/peerj.15287

Drummond, A., & Sauer, J. D. (2018). Video game loot boxes are psychologically akin to gambling. *Nature Human Behaviour, 2*(8), 530–532. https://doi.org/10.1038/s41562-018-0360-1

Drummond, A., Hall, L. C., & Sauer, J. D. (2022). Surprisingly high prevalence rates of severe psychological distress among consumers who purchase loot boxes in video games. *Scientific Reports, 12*, 16128. https://doi.org/10.1038/s41598-022-20549-1

Garea, S. S., Drummond, A., Sauer, J. D., Hall, L. C., & Williams, M. N. (2021). Meta-analysis of the relationship between problem gambling, excessive gaming and loot box spending. *International Gambling Studies, 21*(3), 460–479. https://doi.org/10.1080/14459795.2021.1914705

Garea, S. S., Sauer, J. D., Hall, L. C., Williams, M. N., & Drummond, A. (2023). The potential relationship between loot box spending, problem gambling, and obsessive-compulsive gamers. *Journal of Behavioral Addictions, 12*(3), 733–743. https://doi.org/10.1556/2006.2023.00038

Garrett, E. P., Sauer, J. D., Drummond, A., & Lowe-Calverley, E. (2022). Problem gambling and income as predictors of loot box spending. *International Gambling Studies, 22*(3), 432–443. https://doi.org/10.1080/14459795.2022.2029528

Gibson, E., Griffiths, M. D., Calado, F., & Harris, A. (2022). The relationship between videogame micro-transactions and problem gaming and gambling: A systematic review. *Computers in Human Behavior, 131*, 107219. https://doi.org/10.1016/j.chb.2022.107219

Gibson, E., Griffiths, M. D., Calado, F., & Harris, A. (2023). Videogame player experiences with micro-transactions: An interpretative phenomenological analysis. *Computers in Human Behavior, 145*, 107766. https://doi.org/10.1016/j.chb.2023.107766

González-Cabrera, J., Basterra-González, A., Montiel, I., Calvete, E., Pontes, H. M., & Machimbarrena, J. M. (2022). Loot boxes in Spanish adolescents and young adults: Relationship with internet gaming disorder and online gambling disorder. *Computers in Human Behavior, 126*, 107012. https://doi.org/10.1016/j.chb.2021.107012

González-Cabrera, J., Basterra-González, A., Ortega-Barón, J., Caba-Machado, V., Díaz-López, A., Pontes, H. M., & Machimbarrena, J. M. (2023). Loot box purchases and their relationship with internet gaming disorder and online gambling disorder in adolescents: A prospective study. *Computers in Human Behavior, 143*, 107685. https://doi.org/10.1016/j.chb.2023.107685

Juniper Research. (2021, March 9). *Video game loot boxes to generate over $20 billion in revenue by 2025*. Juniper Research. https://www.juniperresearch.com/press/video-game-loot-boxes-to-generate-over-20-billion/

Kim, H. S., & King, D. L. (2020). Gambling-gaming convergence: New developments and future directions. *International Gambling Studies, 20*(3), 373–379. https://doi.org/10.1080/14459795.2020.1822905

Kim, H. S., Leslie, R. D., Stewart, S. H., King, D. L., Demetrovics, Z., Andrade, A. L. M., Choi, J.-S., Tavares, H., Almeida, B., & Hodgins, D. C. (2023). A scoping review of the association between loot boxes, esports, skin betting, and token wagering with gambling and video gaming behaviors. *Journal of Behavioral Addictions, 12*(2), 309–351. https://doi.org/10.1556/2006.2023.00013

King, D. L., Russell, A. M. T., Delfabbro, P. H., & Polisena, D. (2020). *Fortnite* microtransaction spending was associated with peers' purchasing behaviors but not gaming disorder symptoms. *Addictive Behaviors, 104*, 106311. https://doi.org/10.1016/j.addbeh.2020.106311

Larche, C. J., Chini, K., Lee, C., Dixon, M. J., & Fernandes, M. (2021). Rare loot box rewards trigger larger arousal and reward responses, and greater urge to open more loot boxes. *Journal of Gambling Studies, 37*(1), 141–163. https://doi.org/10.1007/s10899-019-09913-5

Lemmens, J. S. (2022). Play or pay to win: Loot boxes and gaming disorder in FIFA ultimate team. *Telematics and Informatics Reports, 8*, 100023. https://doi.org/10.1016/j.teler.2022.100023

Macey, J., Cantell, M., Tossavainen, T., Karjala, A., & Castrén, S. (2022). How can the potential harms of loot boxes be minimised?: Proposals for understanding and addressing issues at a national level. *Journal of Behavioral Addictions, 11*(2), 256–266. https://doi.org/10.1556/2006.2022.00016

Mills, S., Ash, J., & Gordon, R. (2024). Children and young people's experiences and understandings of gambling-style systems in digital games: Loot boxes, popular culture, and changing childhoods. *Annals of the American Association of Geographers, 114*(1), 200–217. https://doi.org/10.1080/24694452.2023.2248293

Montiel, I., Basterra-González, A., Machimbarrena, J. M., Ortega-Barón, J., & González-Cabrera, J. (2022). Loot box engagement: A scoping review of primary studies on prevalence and association with problematic gaming and gambling. *PLoS One, 17*(1), e0263177. https://doi.org/10.1371/journal.pone.0263177

Nielsen, R. K. L., & Grabarczyk, P. (2019). Are loot boxes gambling? Random reward mechanisms in video games. *Transactions of the Digital Games Research Association, 4*(3), 171. https://doi.org/10.26503/todigra.v4i3.104

Pisklak, J. M., Yong, J. J. H., & Spetch, M. L. (2020). The near-miss effect in slot machines: A review and experimental analysis over half a century later. *Journal of Gambling Studies, 36*(2), 611–632. https://doi.org/10.1007/s10899-019-09891-8

Primi, C., Sanson, F., & Donati, M. A. (2024). Measuring risky loot box use: An item response theory analysis of the risky loot box index among adolescents. *Psychology of Addictive Behaviors, 38*(5), 637–648. https://doi.org/10.1037/adb0001009

Shiffman, S., Stone, A. A., & Hufford, M. R. (2008). Ecological momentary assessment. *Annual Review of Clinical Psychology, 4*, 1–32. https://doi.org/10.1146/annurev.clinpsy.3.022806.091415

Sidloski, B., Brooks, G. A., Zhang, K., & Clark, L. (2022). Exploring the association between loot boxes and problem gambling: Are video gamers referring to loot boxes when they complete gambling screening tools? *Addictive Behaviors, 131*, 107318. https://doi.org/10.1016/j.addbeh.2022.107318

Spetch, M. L., Madan, C. R., Liu, Y. S., & Ludvig, E. A. (2020). Effects of winning cues and relative payout on choice between simulated slot machines. *Addiction, 115*(9), 1719–1727. https://doi.org/10.1111/add.15010

Spicer, S. G., Nicklin, L. L., Uther, M., Lloyd, J., Lloyd, H., & Close, J. (2022). Loot boxes, problem gambling and problem video gaming: A systematic review and meta-synthesis. *New Media & Society, 24*(4), 1001–1022. https://doi.org/10.1177/14614448211027175

Wilson, C., Butler, N., Quigg, Z., & Sumnall, H. (2024). Associations between loot box purchasing and gambling behaviours, financial problems, and low mental wellbeing in a household sample from a British Island, a cross-sectional study. *Journal of Public Health*, 1–9. https://doi.org/10.1007/s10389-024-02355-3

Xiao, L. Y. (2023). *Loot box state of play 2023: Law, regulation, policy, and enforcement around the world (Working Paper No. 110)*. Stanford-Vienna Transatlantic Technology Law Forum. https://law.stanford.edu/publications/no-110-loot-box-state-of-play-2023-law-regulation-policy-and-enforcement-around-the-world/

Xiao, L. Y., Henderson, L. L., & Newall, P. W. S. (2022a). Loot boxes are more prevalent in United Kingdom video games than previously considered: Updating Zendle et al. (2020). *Addiction, 117*(9), 2553–2555. https://doi.org/10.1111/add.15829

Xiao, L. Y., Henderson, L. L., Nielsen, R. K. L., & Newall, P. W. S. (2022b). Regulating gambling-like video game loot boxes: A public health framework comparing industry self-regulation, existing national legal approaches, and other potential approaches. *Current Addiction Reports, 9*, 163–178. https://doi.org/10.1007/s40429-022-00424-9

Xiao, L. Y., Fraser, T. C., Nielsen, R. K. L., & Newall, P. W. S. (2024a). Loot boxes, gambling-related risk factors, and mental health in mainland China: A large-scale survey. *Addictive Behaviors, 148*, 107860. https://doi.org/10.1016/j.addbeh.2023.107860

Xiao, L. Y., Henderson, L. L., Nielsen, R. K. L., Grabarczyk, P., & Newall, P. W. S. (2024b). Loot boxes: Gambling-like mechanics in video games. In N. Lee (Ed.), *Encyclopedia of computer graphics and games* (pp. 1075–1081). Springer. https://doi.org/10.1007/978-3-031-23161-2_459

Xiao, L. Y., Newall, P., & James, R. J. E. (2024c). To screen, or not to screen: An experimental comparison of two methods for correlating video game loot box expenditure and problem gambling severity. *Computers in Human Behavior, 151*, 108019. https://doi.org/10.1016/j.chb.2023.108019

Yokomitsu, K., Irie, T., Shinkawa, H., & Tanaka, M. (2021). Characteristics of gamers who purchase loot box: A systematic literature review. *Current Addiction Reports, 8*(4), 481–493. https://doi.org/10.1007/s40429-021-00386-4

Zendle, D., Meyer, R., & Over, H. (2019). Adolescents and loot boxes: Links with problem gambling and motivations for purchase. *Royal Society Open Science, 6*(6), 190049. https://doi.org/10.1098/rsos.190049

Zendle, D., Meyer, R., & Ballou, N. (2020a). The changing face of desktop video game monetisation: An exploration of exposure to loot boxes, pay to win, and cosmetic microtransactions in the most-played steam games of 2010-2019. *PLoS One, 15*(5), e0232780. https://doi.org/10.1371/journal.pone.0232780

Zendle, D., Meyer, R., Cairns, P., Waters, S., & Ballou, N. (2020b). The prevalence of loot boxes in mobile and desktop games. *Addiction, 115*(9), 1768–1772. https://doi.org/10.1111/add.14973

Chapter 9
From Virtual to Real: Considerations on Life Purpose and Media Use in Adolescents

Juliano Porto de Cerqueira Leite and Letícia Lovato Dellazzana-Zanon

Introduction

Life purpose and behavioral dependencies related to digital media use are topics of growing relevance in today's world. We live in a society where digitalization permeates various aspects of daily life, significantly impacting adolescents, who are major consumers of technology. On the other hand, the concept of life purpose, defined as a stable intention directed beyond oneself and imbued with personal meaning, has been associated with positive development and mental health (Bronk, 2014; Damon, 2008). Analyzing the interactions between these two phenomena is crucial to understanding the challenges and opportunities for promoting well-being in an increasingly digital world.

The emergence of digital dependencies, including excessive use of social media, online gaming, and other forms of digital entertainment, has been linked to psychological issues such as anxiety, depression, and social isolation (Kuss & Griffiths, 2011; Martins et al., 2021) and lower well-being (Twenge, 2019). Adolescents are more susceptible to these problems due to developmental characteristics of this life stage, such as the search for belonging, the need for validation, and identity exploration (Twenge & Campbell, 2018). This chapter seeks to explore how the development of life purpose can serve as a protective factor against excessive digital media use in adolescents, presenting concepts, evidence, and suggestions to foster a balance between healthy technology use and personal growth.

J. P. de Cerqueira Leite · L. L. Dellazzana-Zanon (✉)
Pontifical Catholic University of Campinas, Campinas, Brazil
e-mail: juliano.pcl1@puccampinas.edu.br; leticia.zanon@puc-campinas.edu.br

A. L. M. Andrade (ed.), *Digital Addictions*,
https://doi.org/10.1007/978-3-031-87986-9_9

Life Purpose in Adolescence

Life purpose is a multidimensional construct that integrates intention, engagement, and prosocial motivation, as defined by Damon et al. (2003). It extends beyond personal goals, involving a commitment to actions that transcend individual interests and contribute to society. During adolescence, the formation of life purpose is particularly relevant as it is closely tied to identity development and the establishment of core values for adulthood (Bronk, 2014; Silva & Danza, 2022). Reflection and identification of personal and social values enhance the capacity to face the challenges typical of this developmental stage (Dellazzana-Zanon et al., 2020).

Having a life purpose is considered essential for healthy life development (Dellazzana-Zanon & Freitas, 2016). Adolescents who develop a life purpose demonstrate greater self-regulation, resilience in the face of adversity, and engagement in activities that promote collective well-being (Hill et al., 2016). Additionally, life purpose has been associated with higher levels of life satisfaction, mental health, and academic performance (Burrow & Rainone, 2017). These benefits highlight the organizing role of purpose in structuring life goals, encompassing both short- and long-term objectives.

Although the development of life purpose is an individual process, it can be facilitated by educational and social interventions (e.g., Pereira & Dellazzana-Zanon, 2021). Environments that provide opportunities to explore interests, along with emotional and social support, foster the emergence of meaningful purposes (Malin et al., 2017). A recent study demonstrated that awareness of purpose and prosocial purpose are predictors of self-esteem among high school students, underscoring the importance of educational programs that help adolescents identify how their life purpose can positively impact society (Sharma et al., 2023).

Another important aspect to consider is the context: studies on adolescents' life projects indicate that the environment in which they are embedded plays a significant role in how these projects are developed (e.g., Dellazzana-Zanon et al., 2021; Sumner et al., 2018). Schools, families, and communities thus play a fundamental role in facilitating this process, especially in contexts of social vulnerability. Such support can guide adolescents beyond superficial contexts or narratives centered solely on individual survival, fostering intentional maturity and a deeper sense of belonging (Reilly & Mariano, 2021).

However, the practical implementation of life purpose also faces challenges, particularly when adolescents are exposed to environments that do not encourage deep reflection on interests and values. The competition for time and attention generated by digital media presents an additional obstacle. In this context, the promotion of life purpose emerges as a strategy to rebalance priorities and create a stronger sense of direction in young people's lives (Schaefer et al., 2013).

Digital Media Use in Adolescence

The use of media by adolescents can generate both benefits and challenges (Uhls et al., 2017). Although not necessarily linked to substance-related dependencies, behavioral addictions related to digital media use exhibit characteristics similar to other types of addictions, such as impaired control, compulsive behavior, and negative impacts on daily life (Kuss & Griffiths, 2011). Social media, video streaming, and online gaming are among the most common forms of problematic media use, especially among adolescents, with negative implications for mental health, including anxiety, depression, and social isolation (Cantero et al., 2024; Twenge & Campbell, 2018). Adolescents are particularly vulnerable due to the immaturity of their self-regulation systems and the digitized social context, which amplifies their need for belonging and validation.

A central feature of digital media is its ability to provide immediate rewards, such as likes, shares, and gaming achievements, which stimulate the brain's reward system and contribute to compulsive use (Crone & Konijn, 2018). This mechanism, combined with social pressure to remain constantly connected, makes voluntary disconnection difficult and reinforces dependency patterns (Burrow & Rainone, 2017). Additionally, exposure to inappropriate content and the opportunity to display and receive validation through peer approval for risky behaviors may lead some adolescents to make poor decisions regarding what to share on social media (Uhls et al., 2017).

Research indicates that excessive digital media use may also be associated with individual and social vulnerabilities, exacerbating preexisting psychopathological conditions (Cantero et al., 2024). For instance, studies on individuals diagnosed with eating disorders show that prolonged exposure to social media reinforces idealized thinness standards, intensifying dysfunctional behaviors and compromising mental health (Moraes et al., 2021). These effects are not limited to digital platforms themselves but reflect their interaction with personal and social factors, creating a cycle that is difficult to break (Moraes et al., 2021). This evidence underscores the importance of understanding these processes to develop strategies that help adolescents balance technology use with their psychological well-being.

In light of this scenario, it is crucial to understand how interventions can support young people in navigating the digital environment healthily. Strategies that promote digital literacy, balance between online and offline activities, and the strengthening of socioemotional skills are essential (Twenge & Campbell, 2018). Furthermore, the development of a life purpose can serve as an anchor, directing adolescents' energy and time toward more meaningful activities that are less dependent on digital stimuli.

Opportunities in the Digital World for Life Purpose Development

Although excessive use of digital media can present significant challenges for adolescent development, the digital world, when used consciously and in balance, offers opportunities for identity discovery and development (Uhls et al., 2017). Digital platforms expand access to information, connections, and experiences that can inspire and guide young people in exploring their interests and defining meaningful goals, which in turn has the potential to contribute to the construction of life purpose. According to Bronk (2014), purpose is partly constructed through exposure to different perspectives and contexts, something the Internet facilitates in an unparalleled way.

The digital world allows adolescents to explore causes, communities, and initiatives that resonate with their values and interests. Social media, for example, can serve as spaces for engagement in social movements, volunteer campaigns, and discussions about global issues. These experiences can foster the prosocial dimension of life purpose, helping young people link their individual actions to a broader societal impact. Platforms like YouTube, TikTok, and Instagram, when used appropriately, also allow adolescents to share their ideas and projects, receive positive feedback, and build support networks.

Furthermore, the Internet democratizes access to information about careers, courses, and opportunities that might otherwise be out of reach in in-person contexts. Young people from various socioeconomic backgrounds can access free educational resources, such as online courses and inspiring lectures, which help them visualize future possibilities and build meaningful trajectories (Twenge & Campbell, 2018). Self-directed learning, facilitated by digital tools, can contribute to the development of autonomy and the alignment between personal interests and life purpose.

The digital world also plays a crucial role in shaping adolescents' identities. Interaction with diverse cultures and experiences stimulates reflection on values and personal goals, enhancing young people's ability to define their place in the world. In general, digital technologies, when used in a balanced way, can be powerful allies in human connectivity (Cantero et al., 2024), acting as catalysts for self-knowledge and meaningful engagement, thereby strengthening the development of life purpose (Malin et al., 2017).

Life Purpose and Digital Dependencies: Possible Associations

The absence of life purpose is often linked to feelings of existential emptiness, boredom, and disconnection from the surrounding environment (Edwards & Holden, 2001). For many adolescents, especially those facing practical life challenges, such as economic, relational, or emotional difficulties, the digital world presents an appealing alternative (Nesi, 2020). In this space, it is possible to create a parallel reality where the challenges of real life are temporarily forgotten (Przybylski et al., 2012). Digital platforms, such as social media and online games, offer a form of escapism, providing instant rewards, simulated social interactions, and the opportunity to play roles that the adolescent may not be able to assume in their daily life (Kuss & Griffiths, 2011).

This escapism mechanism is intensified in contexts of psychological suffering or social vulnerability. Adolescents experiencing family crises, bullying, school issues, or disorders such as anxiety and depression are particularly prone to seeking refuge in virtual environments (Kircaburun et al., 2019). These digital spaces, often designed to capture the user's attention, offer a sense of control and comfort lacking in the tangible reality (King & Delfabbro, 2018). However, while they temporarily alleviate suffering, these virtual environments can perpetuate a cycle of dependence. Excessive immersion prevents the adolescent from facing real challenges, promoting alienation and distancing from activities necessary for the development of life purpose (Kircaburun et al., 2019).

On the other hand, adolescents with a clear purpose are less likely to engage in excessive behaviors and more inclined to seek social interactions and activities aligned with their goals (Burrow & Hill, 2011). Therefore, it can be argued that being engaged in the construction of a life purpose can act as a protective factor against digital dependencies, as a greater sense of direction and meaning would reduce the attraction to digital activities. Developing a purpose requires individuals to explore their interests, skills, and values, as well as engage in activities that promote personal and social growth (Damon, 2008). Adolescents who spend excessive hours connected to digital media often neglect these activities. Rather than investing in experiences that could help them understand their place in the world, they are trapped in a cycle of immediate reward, drifting away from reality and their future responsibilities.

Life purpose is not merely a philosophical matter but also a practical one; it involves setting goals, learning skills, and building relationships that sustain a healthy transition to adulthood (Damon, 2008). Without this preparation, adolescents who live immersed in virtual realities may face adulthood without the necessary structure to handle its demands. Ultimately, digital dependence, as a defense mechanism against the difficulties of practical life, distances young people from developing a sense of purpose that could help them face and overcome these same difficulties.

Therefore, it is essential to understand how problematic use of the digital world can reinforce patterns of escapism and alienation, creating significant barriers to purpose development. This points to the need for interventions that not only limit excessive technology use but also help adolescents confront real-life challenges and invest time in activities that promote their personal and social growth. Educational programs that integrate life purpose development with digital literacy have shown promising results (Rohandi et al., 2023). Through a combination of self-knowledge, goal-setting, and practical strategies for managing online time, these programs help young people find a healthy balance between the digital world and personal development.

Implications for Interventions and Education

The promotion of life purpose in adolescents has significant implications for educational interventions and support programs aimed at balancing technology use and well-being. Considering that life purpose serves as a motivational guide, helping young people direct their actions toward long-term goals (Damon, 2008), this concept can be integrated into school curricula through activities that encourage reflection on values, interests, and aspirations. In this way, education can encourage students to explore their purposes both inside and outside the classroom (Moran, 2023). Besides schools, families also play a central role in this process: by offering guidance and opportunities for adolescents to think about and develop their life projects, parents can contribute significantly to the process (Leite & Dellazzana-Zanon, 2021).

Studies suggest that purpose-based interventions can improve self-regulation and school engagement (Malin et al., 2017; Yeager & Bundick, 2009), which, in turn, may reduce the negative impacts of excessive digital media use. For example, extracurricular activities promoting community engagement and creative projects have proven effective in helping young people explore deeper meanings and develop personal and social goals (Damon, 2004; Malin et al., 2017). Additionally, developing socioemotional skills, such as empathy, resilience, and critical thinking, is key to mitigating the risks associated with problematic digital technology use (Silva & Silva, 2017). These skills not only promote well-being but also help adolescents more critically evaluate digital interactions, reducing dependence and enhancing their ability to choose activities aligned with their purposes.

Conclusion

This chapter explores the relationship between purpose in life and the use of digital media during adolescence, highlighting both the challenges and opportunities inherent in this context. Purpose in life, essential for positive development, provides direction and resilience, key elements for building a solid identity and successfully transitioning into adulthood. Excessive use of technology can hinder this process, impeding self-awareness and making it difficult to establish long-term goals, which are fundamental to adolescent maturation. However, when used in a balanced way, digital tools can facilitate the discovery of purpose, connecting young people to social causes, communities, and sources of knowledge that stimulate their values and aspirations.

The development of purpose in life during adolescence is closely linked to identity, self-regulation, and resilience, which in turn contributes to overall well-being and social engagement. Various studies show that adolescents with a clear sense of purpose report higher life satisfaction, better academic performance, and better mental health. In this regard, educational and social interventions that encourage the exploration of interests and provide emotional support play a crucial role, especially in contexts of vulnerability. However, environments that do not promote deep reflection on adolescents' interests and values, coupled with the competition for attention generated by digital media, pose a significant challenge to purpose development.

Although the use of digital media presents risks, it also offers valuable opportunities for the development of purpose in life. The Internet democratizes access to information and broadens interaction with different cultures and perspectives, enabling adolescents to explore their interests and define personal causes and values. Digital platforms can serve as spaces for engagement in social initiatives and provide resources for self-directed learning, promoting autonomy and alignment with life goals. When used consciously, the digital environment can act as a catalyst for self-awareness and human connectivity, strengthening the development of purpose in life.

Finally, the chapter emphasizes the importance of educational interventions that promote a healthy balance between technology use and purpose development. Programs that integrate reflections on values, interests, and goals into the school curriculum are essential to mitigate the negative effects of digital media. Extracurricular activities and the development of socio-emotional skills, such as empathy and resilience, have been shown to effectively reduce digital dependence and guide adolescents toward more meaningful personal growth aligned with their purposes.

References

Bronk, K. C. (2014). *Purpose in life: A critical component of optimal youth development*. Springer. https://doi.org/10.1007/978-94-007-7491-9

Burrow, A. L., & Hill, P. L. (2011). Purpose as a form of identity capital for positive youth adjustment. *Developmental Psychology, 47*(4), 1196–1206. https://doi.org/10.1037/a0023818

Burrow, A. L., & Rainone, N. (2017). How many likes did I get? Purpose moderates links between positive social media feedback and self-esteem. *Journal of Experimental Social Psychology, 69*, 232–236. https://doi.org/10.1016/j.jesp.2016.09.005

Cantero, J. B., Meurer, M. F. M., & Vogt, R. L. (2024). A influência das redes sociais na adolescência: uma análise da perspectiva dos pais de adolescentes. *Revista Contemporânea, 4*(12), 1–23. https://doi.org/10.56083/RCV4N12-122

Crone, E. A., & Konijn, E. A. (2018). Media use and brain development during adolescence. *Nature Communications, 9*(1), 588. https://doi.org/10.1038/s41467-018-03126-x

Damon, W. (2004). What is positive youth development? *The Annals of the American Academy of Political and Social Science, 591*(1), 13–24. https://doi.org/10.1177/0002716203260092

Damon, W. (2008). *The path to purpose: How young people find their calling in life*. Free Press.

Damon, W., Menon, J., & Bronk, K. C. (2003). The development of purpose during adolescence. *Applied Developmental Science, 7*(3), 119–128. https://doi.org/10.1207/S1532480XADS0703_2

Dellazzana-Zanon, L. L., & Freitas, L. B. L. (2016). Uma Revisão de Literatura sobre a Definição de Projeto de Vida na Adolescência. *Interação em Psicologia, 19*(2), 1. https://doi.org/10.5380/psi.v19i2.35218

Dellazzana-Zanon, L. L., Araujo, M. F., Vieira, G. P., & Freitas, L. B. L. (2020). O papel do projeto de vida no desenvolvimento de adolescentes. In E. S. Ferrão, S. R. F. Enumo, & M. B. M. Linhares (Eds.), *Infância esegurança: Interdisciplinaridade na proteção do desenvolvimento sadio infantojuvenil* (Vol. 2, pp. 151–172). Editora CRV.

Dellazzana-Zanon, L. L., Zanon, C., Tudge, J. R. H., & Freitas, L. B. L. (2021). Life purpose and sibling care in adolescence: Possible associations. *Estudos De Psicologia (Campinas), 38*, e200038. https://doi.org/10.1590/1982-0275202138e200038

Edwards, J. R., & Holden, R. R. (2001). Coping, meaning in life, and suicidal manifestations: Examining gender differences. *Journal of Clinical Psychology, 57*(12), 1517–1534. https://doi.org/10.1002/jclp.1120

Hill, P. L., Burrow, A. L., Brandenberger, J. W., Lapsley, D. K., & Quaranto, J. C. (2016). Purpose orientations and developmental outcomes in emerging adulthood. *Journal of Applied Developmental Psychology, 42*, 60–70. https://doi.org/10.1016/j.appdev.2015.11.001

King, D. L., & Delfabbro, P. H. (2018). Predatory monetization schemes in video games (e.g., 'loot boxes') and internet gaming disorder. *Addiction, 113*(11), 1967–1969. https://doi.org/10.1111/add.14286

Kircaburun, K., Alhabash, S., Tosuntaş, Ş. B., & Griffiths, M. D. (2019). Uses and gratifications of problematic social media use among university students: A simultaneous examination of the big five of personality traits, social media platforms, and social media use motives. *International Journal of Mental Health and Addiction, 17*(1), 136–153. https://doi.org/10.1007/s11469-018-9940-6

Kuss, D. J., & Griffiths, M. D. (2011). Online social networking and addiction—A review of the psychological literature. *International Journal of Environmental Research and Public Health, 8*(9), 3528–3552. https://doi.org/10.3390/ijerph8093528

Leite, J. P. C., & Dellazzana-Zanon, L. L. (2021). *Promovendo projetos de vida na adolescência: Cartilha para adolescentes, pais e professores*. PUC-Campinas. Trabalho gráfico de Luisa Porto, & Ângela Lovato Dellazzana. Recuperado em 30 de dezembro de 2024, de. https://www.puc-campinas.edu.br/wp-content/uploads/2021/04/cartilha_leticia-1.pdf

Malin, H., Reilly, T. S., Quinn, B., & Moran, S. (2017). Adolescent purpose development: Exploring empathy, discovering roles, shifting priorities, and creating pathways. *Journal of Research on Adolescence, 27*(2), 309–323. https://doi.org/10.1111/jora.12288

Martins, G. D. G., Caricati, V. V., Barbugli, B. C., Ribeiro, C. M. S., Lobato, F. B. H., Scatena, A., Lessa, R. T., De Micheli, D., & Andrade, A. L. M. (2021). The biopsychosocial impact of abusive use of digital media. In D. De Micheli & A. L. M. Andrade (Eds.), *Drugs and human behavior: Biopsychosocial aspects of psychotropic substances use* (pp. 459–468). Springer. https://doi.org/10.1007/978-3-030-55330-7

Moraes, R. B., Santos, M. N., & Leonidas, C. (2021). Repercussões do acesso às redes sociais em pessoas com diagnóstico de anorexia nervosa. *Psicologia & Sociedade, 33*(4), 1178–1199. https://doi.org/10.1590/1807-0310/2021v33n4p150782

Moran, S. (2023). Educating the youth to develop life purpose: An eco-systemic approach. *Revista de Investigación Educativa, 41*(1), 15–31. https://doi.org/10.6018/rie.539521

Nesi, J. (2020). The impact of social media on youth mental health: Challenges and opportunities. *North Carolina Medical Journal, 81*(2), 116–121. https://doi.org/10.18043/ncm.81.2.116

Pereira, P., & Dellazzana-Zanon, L. L. (2021). Programa de intervenção para promoção de projetos de vida de adolescentes. *Revista de Educação PUC-Campinas, 26*, e215296. https://doi.org/10.24220/2318-0870v26e2021a5296

Przybylski, A. K., Weinstein, N., Murayama, K., Lynch, M. F., & Ryan, R. M. (2012). The ideal self at play: The appeal of video games that let you be all you can be. *Psychological Science, 23*(1), 69–76. https://doi.org/10.1177/0956797611418676

Reilly, T. S., & Mariano, J. M. (2021). Fostering mature purpose beyond the classroom: Considering family and other institutions in agentic purpose commitment. *Estudos De Psicologia (Campinas), 38*, e210115. https://doi.org/10.1590/1982-0275202138e210115

Rohandi, M. M. A., Permana, R. M. T., & Pratiwi, R. E. (2023). Enhancing digital literacy through instructional videos and social media engagement. *Mimbar, 39*(2), 251–257. https://doi.org/10.29313/mimbar.v39i2.2983
Schaefer, S. M., Morozink Boylan, J., van Reekum, C. M., Lapate, R. C., Norris, C. J., Ryff, C. D., & Davidson, R. J. (2013). Purpose in life predicts better emotional recovery from negative stimuli. *PLoS One, 8*(11), e80329. https://doi.org/10.1371/journal.pone.0080329
Sharma, A., Gupta, P., & Chopra, R. (2023). Adolescent purpose and its impact on self-esteem in educational settings. *Journal of Educational Psychology, 115*(3), 456–469. https://doi.org/10.1037/edu0001234
Silva, M. A. M. D., & Danza, H. C. (2022). Projeto de vida e identidade: Articulações e implicações para a educação. *Educação em Revista, 38*, e35845. https://doi.org/10.1590/0102-469835845
Silva, J., & Silva, L. (2017). Competências socioemocionais: Uma abordagem crítica para a educação do século XXI. *Educação & Realidade, 42*(4), 1327–1347. https://doi.org/10.1590/1982-0275201742421126
Sumner, R., Burrow, A. L., & Hill, P. L. (2018). The development of purpose in life among adolescents who experience marginalization: Potential opportunities and obstacles. *American Psychologist, 73*(6), 740–752. https://doi.org/10.1037/amp0000249
Twenge, J. M. (2019). More time on technology, less happiness? Associations between digital-media use and psychological well being. *Current Directions in Psychological Science, 28*(4), 372. https://doi.org/10.1177/0963721419838244
Twenge, J. M., & Campbell, W. K. (2018). Associations between screen time and lower psychological well-being among children and adolescents: Evidence from a population-based study. *Preventive Medicine Reports, 12*, 271–283. https://doi.org/10.1016/j.pmedr.2018.10.003
Uhls, Y. T., Ellison, N. B., & Subrahmanyam, K. (2017). Benefits and costs of social media in adolescence. *Pediatrics, 140*(Supplement_2), S67–S70. https://doi.org/10.1542/peds.2016-1758E
Yeager, D. S., & Bundick, M. J. (2009). The role of purposeful work goals in promoting meaning in life and in schoolwork during adolescence. *Journal of Adolescent Research, 24*(4), 423–452. https://doi.org/10.1177/0743558409336749

Chapter 10
Digital Addiction, Depression, and Suicide

Makilim Nunes Baptista, Vithor Rosa Franco, Bruno Bonfá-Araujo, Mateus Eduardo Romão, Giacomo Belli, Silvia Damiana Visonà, Ilaria Setti, and Serena Barello

Technology and Mental Health: Where We Stand?

The discussion on the use of technologies and games is neither new nor underexplored. The excessive use of video games, as well as "tube" television, has long been the subject of debates and scientific studies. For example, Tonge addressed as early as the 1990s that children were influenced by the type of television programs they watched, noting that children who viewed violent and aggressive programs tended to exhibit similar behaviors. Studies on the influence of television programs have generated fruitful debates (Tonge, 1990), including the establishment of age-appropriate ratings for television programs. Similarly, Friedrich-Cofer and Huston (1986) highlighted research that considered the causal relationship between violent programs and violent children, even suggesting a bidirectional influence. Currently, it is possible to know the nature of the content being viewed on various television channels (e.g., "this program contains scenes of violence, sex, and drugs"). Likewise, the use of violent video games has raised similar concerns in the scientific community (Ellis, 1990), as has the study of compulsive gamblers, including older forms of gambling such as lotteries (Burns et al., 1990).

M. N. Baptista (✉)
Pontifical Catholic University of Campinas, Campinas, Brazil

V. R. Franco
São Francisco University, Campinas, Brazil

B. Bonfá-Araujo
University of Western Ontario, London, Canada

M. E. Romão · G. Belli · S. D. Visonà · I. Setti · S. Barello
University of Pavia, Pavia, Italy
e-mail: mateuseduardo.romao01@universitadipavia.it; giacomo.belli01@universitadipavia.it; silviadamiana.visona@unipv.it; ilaria.setti@unipv.it; serena.barello@unipv.it

A. L. M. Andrade (ed.), *Digital Addictions*,
https://doi.org/10.1007/978-3-031-87986-9_10

The use of digital technologies has been increasing worldwide, and the consequences of this behavior can be both positive and negative, depending on factors such as duration of use, context, purpose, and other variables. The use of digital technologies in children, for example, seems to follow a "U-shaped" pattern, where both non-use and overuse can lead to negative consequences (Kardefelt-Winther, 2017). According to Small et al. (2020), the overuse of digital technologies may be associated with impacts on certain brain functions and behavior. Prolonged screen use tends to contribute to an increase in attentional problems, impaired emotional and social intelligence, dependency, social isolation, impaired brain development, and sleep problems, among other potential consequences. On the other hand, appropriate and contextual use of technologies and screens can bring benefits, such as improved memory, multitasking abilities, fluid intelligence, and other cognitive skills.

Meng et al. (2022), in a systematic review and meta-analysis, report that one quarter of the population may be affected by at least one subtype of digital addiction, which is more commonly found in lower-income (underdeveloped) countries, with men showing higher frequencies of both digital and gaming addictions. Based on 341 studies, the authors found a mixed prevalence of 14.22% for Internet addiction, 6.04% for gaming addiction (from 78 studies), 26.99% for smartphone addiction (from 82 studies), 17.42% for social media addiction (from 31 studies), and 8.23% for cybersex addiction (from only 6 studies).

Using bibliometric analysis and scientific mapping methods, Karakose et al. (2023) analyzed three periods between 1983 and 2022, concluding that Internet addiction, followed by social media addiction, was the most significant themes found. Issues related to mental health also emerged during this period, specifically depression, with themes associated with cognitive distortion, insomnia, loneliness, self-esteem, social support, alexithymia, as well as cyber victimization or academic performance. It is interesting to note that reviews do not always indicate a direct and/or causal association between digital technology use and poor mental health (Odgers & Jensen, 2020); however, there is a growing body of scientific evidence linking digital media with depression, anxiety, and suicide. Anxiety and depression often appear together due to a series of symptoms that co-vary in both conditions, with suicide being more strongly associated with cyberbullying (Hoge et al., 2017).

Depression, considered an extremely common diagnosis, and suicide, another frequent public health issue, are complex phenomena with broad and varied biological/genetic, social, and psychological components that cannot be explained in a reductionist manner. In this sense, it is important to clarify that the aim is not to establish a cause-and-effect relationship between digital addictions. This chapter aims to explore the relationship between digital addictions and mental health, specifically regarding depression symptoms and suicidal behavior.

Depression and Digital Addiction: Concepts and Evidence

Digital addictions, encompassing the excessive use of Internet, social media, video games, and smartphones, have emerged as significant concerns in relation to mental health. Research highlights that prolonged exposure to digital platforms is associated with a variety of negative psychological outcomes, including anxiety, depression, and social isolation (Twenge & Campbell, 2018). Studies indicate that overuse of these technologies can impair cognitive functions, emotional regulation, and sleep patterns, which may contribute to an overall decline in mental well-being (e.g., Brand et al., 2014). For instance, individuals who spend excessive time on passive social media use are at greater risk of experiencing higher levels of interest loss, concentration problems, fatigue, and loneliness, with this pattern of behavior more strongly related to depression symptoms (Aalbers et al., 2019).

Although not all research establishes a direct causal link between digital use and poor mental health, the relationship is complex and multifaceted (Ferguson, 2024). Factors such as social environment, genetic predispositions, and preexisting psychological conditions can moderate or exacerbate the impact of digital addictions. Moreover, recent evidence suggests a bidirectional relationship between digital media use and mental health problems, where mental health issues might lead to greater dependence on digital technologies, further perpetuating a cycle of negative outcomes (Aalbers et al., 2019). As digital technologies continue to become integral to daily life, understanding their mental health implications is crucial for developing effective interventions and promoting healthier usage patterns.

Depression is one of the most prevalent mental disorders that has been associated with the addictive usage of digital platforms (Aalbers et al., 2019). Specifically, excessive engagement with digital media, especially social networking sites, has been linked to heightened symptoms of depression, particularly among adolescents and young adults. The constant comparison to others' curated online personas, exposure to negative content, and cyberbullying are some of the mechanisms that can exacerbate feelings of inadequacy, loneliness, and hopelessness, which are core features of depression.

However, it should be noted the relationship between depression—and probably other mental disorders—and digital addictions is often bidirectional. While excessive use of digital platforms may contribute to the onset of depressive symptoms, individuals who are already struggling with depression may also turn to these platforms as a form of escape or coping mechanism (Ferguson, 2024). This can create a vicious cycle in which digital media use intensifies depressive symptoms, further driving the individual into prolonged, unhealthy screen time. Research has also shown that excessive use of digital technologies can disrupt sleep patterns and reduce physical activity, both of which are critical factors in maintaining mental health and mitigating depressive symptoms (Twenge & Campbell, 2018).

One salient concern on the increase of depression cases is the well-known link of this disorder with suicidal behavior (World Health Organization, 2014, 2020). Depression, particularly when untreated, is a significant risk factor for suicidal ideation, attempts, and completion. Individuals suffering from depression often experience profound feelings of hopelessness, isolation, and worthlessness, which can escalate into suicidal thoughts, especially when combined with the effects of digital addictions such as cyberbullying or social media-induced loneliness (Kowalski et al., 2014). Studies have shown that the negative emotional impact of digital interactions, particularly among vulnerable populations like adolescents, can intensify depressive symptoms and heighten the risk of suicidal behavior.

There are, of course, several theoretical models that help explain the complex connection between depression and suicide. One of such models is the Interpersonal Theory of Suicide (Van Orden et al., 2010). This model suggests that suicidal behavior arises from a combination of perceived burdensomeness and thwarted belongingness, both of which are often exacerbated by depression and worsened by digital addictions (He et al., 2024). Digital platforms can amplify these feelings by fostering social disconnection and reinforcing negative self-perceptions through constant comparison or cyberbullying. Furthermore, the prolonged use of digital technologies has been linked to emotional dysregulation, which can reduce an individual's ability to cope with stress, increasing the likelihood of suicidal ideation.

At this point, we emphasize that the relationship between mental health and digital media addiction is undeniably complex, as excessive engagement with digital technologies can both contribute to and be exacerbated by underlying psychological conditions such as depression and anxiety. The current *zeitgeist* of the field strongly suggests that the negative impact of digital addiction on mental health can create a vicious cycle where poor mental health drives increased digital use, which in turn worsens mental well-being (Ferguson, 2024; Odgers & Jensen, 2020). This interplay highlights the importance of understanding the psychological mechanisms at play, especially through the lens of Cognitive Behavioral Models of Addiction. These models offer valuable insights into how maladaptive thoughts, behaviors, and emotional patterns related to digital use can reinforce addictive tendencies and mental health problems.

Cognitive Behavioral Models of Addiction

Addiction, both related to substances and behaviors, has been widely investigated through cognitive-behavioral approaches. These provide a solid understanding of the mechanisms that underlie addictive behaviors. In the current context, digital addiction, characterized by compulsive use of electronic devices and online platforms, has become an increasing concern. This chapter analyzes the main cognitive-behavioral models used in the study of addiction, with a special emphasis on digital addiction. It examines risk factors and mechanisms that contribute to the development of this dependence.

Cognitive-behavioral therapy (CBT; Beck, 1963) for addiction is based on the idea that an interaction between cognitive, emotional, and behavioral factors sustains addictive behaviors. According to this perspective, addiction is not only the result of a biological predisposition; it is also linked to distorted cognitive processes and inappropriate behavioral responses that reinforce addictive behavior (Koob, 2013; Edwards, 2016). One of the most influential concepts in CBT is the cycle of negative reinforcement. This pattern indicates that people resort to addictive behaviors, such as excessive use of social media or online games, to escape from cognitive distortions and negative emotions, such as stress, anxiety, or boredom. The temporary sense of relief reinforces the behavior, leading to repetition and, over time, to compulsion. Furthermore, cognitive distortions, such as the belief that technology use is the only way to alleviate these feelings or that one has no control over their own behavior, perpetuate the addiction (Lopez-Fernandez et al., 2022). The cognitive-behavioral model recognizes that certain risk factors have a direct impact on a person's vulnerability to digital addiction.

Psychological factors play a fundamental role in the development of digital addictions. People with low self-esteem, challenges in emotional regulation, or who face disorders such as depression and anxiety may turn to the digital environment as a form of escapism (Karakose et al., 2023). The Internet and social networks provide instant gratification, which momentarily disguises emotional discomfort. This contributes to the previously mentioned cycle of negative reinforcement, in which the temporary reduction of distress intensifies digital use, especially in teenagers (Prikhodko et al., 2020; Behzad, 2019; Dolev-Cohen & Barak, 2013).

The design of digital platforms is strategically developed to keep the user engaged, using constant notifications, visual rewards, and rapid social interactions. This aligns with intermittent reinforcement, where unpredictable rewards (such as likes or comments) increase the likelihood of the user repeating the behavior, as the expectation of a reward is always heightened (Mujica et al., 2022). The contemporary digital environment is distinct due to its omnipresence and accessibility, facilitating the repetition of compulsive behaviors that can eventually become an addiction. Social pressure and the FoMO syndrome (fear of missing out on updates and events) are also powerful mechanisms of influence. Social networks, for example, encourage a relentless pursuit of validation and social connection, establishing a cycle where people always feel obligated to be online to avoid missing out on relevant information, events, or interactions (Anastasya et al., 2022). This recurring habit of checking one's phone constantly intensifies digital addiction, as the fear of disconnecting results in excessive use.

In the neurological field, digital addiction can also be explained by changes in the brain's reward circuits. Continuous use of digital technologies stimulates the release of dopamine, a neurotransmitter associated with pleasure and the sense of reward. The constant flow of dopamine motivates the search for instant gratification, leading people to seek more online stimuli, even if this interferes with their daily activities (Sussman et al., 2018). Cognitive-behavioral models provide a valuable framework for understanding the development and maintenance of digital addiction. The cycle of negative reinforcement, stimulus control, and cognitive distortions are fundamental elements that help explain how psychological, social, and neurological factors can impact compulsive behavior in the digital environment. Understanding these mechanisms is essential to creating effective interventions that aim not only to interrupt addictive behavior but also to promote lasting cognitive and behavioral change.

Digital addiction, though often underestimated in comparison to substance addictions, can significantly affect the neurobiological functioning and overall health of individuals. Excessive and continuous use of digital devices alters the structure and functioning of the brain, in addition to having important impacts on physical and psychological well-being (Wacks & Weinstein, 2021; Hoehe & Thibaut, 2020). In this context, understanding the neurobiological effects and their impacts on overall health is fundamental to addressing this growing dependence. It causes changes in the brain like those observed in behavioral and substance addictions. The human brain is extremely sensitive to instant rewards, and digital interactions provide exactly a continuous cycle of gratifying stimuli through social networks, video games, and other forms of online media (Dziura et al., 2023).

One of the most evident neurobiological effects of digital addiction is related to the brain's reward system, particularly with the mesolimbic circuit, which includes the nucleus accumbens and the prefrontal cortex. Dopamine is released whenever a person interacts with stimulating digital content, such as likes on posts, instant messages, or victories in online games (Saberi, 2019; Persson & Persson, 2023). The continuous activation of the reward system provides positive reinforcement, causing the individual to seek more stimuli to replicate the sensation of pleasure, resulting in compulsive and prolonged use. Over time, the brain may become accustomed to these stimuli, causing the user to need more time online or more intense digital stimuli to reach the same level of satisfaction. This can create a cycle of dependence similar to what happens in chemical addictions. Excessive exposure to digital technology can compromise the functioning of the prefrontal cortex, the brain area responsible for impulse control, decision-making, and emotional regulation (Wang et al., 2021; Dossi & Pesce, 2023). Research indicates that excessive use of digital devices can reduce the ability to control impulses and make rational decisions, making it difficult for individuals to manage their online time and resist the temptation to check their devices constantly (Dossi & Pesce, 2023). The reduction of prefrontal cortex function is also linked to an increase in impulsivity and a diminished ability to plan and prioritize activities. Individuals with digital addiction may, therefore, display more impulsive behaviors and disregard the negative consequences of their compulsive use of technology. This further intensifies the addiction cycle (Patil et al., 2021).

In the context of digital addiction, neural plasticity may act to the detriment of the individual. Repetitive and compulsive use of technologies strengthens certain neural connections related to addictive behavior, making it even harder to break this cycle. The continuous repetition of behavioral patterns, reinforced by constant digital rewards, can shape neural circuits and create deep and automatic habits. Over time, these structural changes in the brain make digital detoxification more difficult and make recovery an even greater challenge. Beyond neurobiological effects, digital addiction can also have significant consequences for overall health, impacting people's physical, emotional, and social well-being (Reichert et al., 2021).

Unfortunately, at the state of the art, little is known regarding the neurobiology of Internet addiction. This condition may involve neurotrophic factors and neurobiological mechanisms of many neurotransmitters (e.g., the metabolism of dopamine, serotonin, opioids, and some other neurotransmitters that impact executive functioning, salience attribution, reward processing, habit development, and substance use disorders) (Montag et al., 2016; Carpita et al., 2021). Using neuroimaging methods, several changes in the brain linked to Internet addiction were identified (Meshi et al., 2015; Park et al., 2017; Weinstein et al., 2017), such as (1) a reduction of the density of gray matter (particularly in the motor area, prefrontal and orbitofrontal layers); (2) an increase of the function of reward-dependent brains areas; (3) an increase of glucose metabolism, especially in brain regions related to impulsivity or reward; and (4) an increase of dopamine secretion. Coherently to those findings, the Internet addiction problem is connected to symptoms such as anxiety, aggression, hostility, impulsivity, drug abuse, low self-esteem, and hostility (Hahn & Kim, 2014).

From a psychological perspective, digital addiction has been linked to an increase in the occurrence of anxiety and depression. Excessive time on social networks can heighten feelings of inadequacy and social isolation, as people tend to constantly compare themselves with others (Karakose et al., 2023). The relentless pursuit of validation on social networks, coupled with the fear of exclusion or FoMO syndrome, generates a cycle of anxiety that can negatively impact mental health. Technology addiction can lead to a decrease in emotional well-being, as time spent online often replaces face-to-face social interactions and leisure activities that usually provide a sense of accomplishment and connection. The reduction of these face-to-face interactions can increase feelings of loneliness and social disconnection, worsening symptoms of depression and anxiety (Tsang et al., 2022).

Among the 16 studies analyzed by Andrade et al. (2024), a positive association was observed between gaming disorder and impulsivity measures, as well as self-reported impulsive behaviors. Gaming disorder was related to high-risk tendencies, high sensitivity to rewards, reduced inhibitory control, and low self-control among players. Souza and Da Cunha (2019) analyzed 27 studies, and the results confirmed that there are relationships between technological dependence and the psychological health of adolescents and young people. It was also observed that virtual social networks can intensify social problems, causing significant impacts on people's lives, such as anxiety, depression, and addiction.

For children and adolescents, the impact of digital addiction is especially concerning. During these critical phases of development, excessive use of technology can impair the acquisition of social and cognitive skills. Young people who spend much of their time in digital environments may face challenges in developing interpersonal communication skills, which can affect their social relationships and ability to resolve conflicts in a healthy way (Hooker, 2016). Additionally, there is evidence that excessive use of digital devices impairs concentration and attention capacity. Constantly switching tasks between different apps, social networks, and digital stimuli can reduce the ability to focus on longer and more challenging activities, such as studying or working (Mendoza et al., 2018).

The neurobiological effects and the impacts of digital addiction on overall health demonstrate the complexity of this phenomenon. The changes in brain reward circuits, the weakening of impulse control, and the neural adaptations that reinforce compulsive behaviors are fundamental elements in maintaining digital addiction. Moreover, the adverse effects on physical, emotional, and cognitive health highlight the importance of a multidisciplinary approach to prevent and treat this emerging dependence. Becoming aware of these effects is essential to implementing effective interventions that aim to minimize the damage caused by excessive exposure to digital technologies.

No research conclusively explains the neurology of Internet addiction, due to its complexity and potential for brain circuit overlap with other signal pathways, such as the aggressive one, that are frequently connected to Internet addiction. Additionally, diagnosing Internet addiction may be challenging, due to the possible connection with other psychiatric disorders (such as affective disorder, substance use disorder, depression, bipolar I disorder, general anxiety disorder, personality disorder, suicidal ideation, and obsessive-compulsive disorder). The literature on Internet addiction is mostly related to small samples of patients or cross-sectional studies and therefore reveals a certain degree of evidence weakness. Further research is necessary to fully comprehend the phenomenon of Internet addiction and all of its neurobiological and clinical implications, especially with longitudinal studies. Furthermore, in the DSM-5, this condition did not have sufficient evidence to justify the inclusion of Internet addiction in the diagnostic category of nonsubstance addictions (APA, 2014). Different from other types of addictions (such as drug abuse and gambling), the recognition of online addictions will enable clinicians to tackle new challenges. In this regard, it is becoming increasingly clear that we are living in a digital age and that life cannot exist without the Internet, since nowadays people use the Internet for social and cultural as well as professional reasons.

Digital Addictions: Prevention and Intervention

As digital technologies become more integrated into daily life, the prevalence of digital addictions has increased, requiring effective prevention and intervention strategies. Addressing digital addictions is crucial not only to reduce associated mental health risks but also to promote healthier engagement with technology. Digital addiction can worsen existing risk factors and contribute to the emergence of new ones. The compulsive use of digital platforms often leads to social isolation, sleep disturbances, and increased exposure to cyberbullying, all of which are risk factors for mental health disorders such as depression and anxiety. The overstimulation of the brain's reward system through constant digital engagement can create neurochemical imbalances, reinforcing addictive behaviors and impairing cognitive functions like attention and impulse control (Brand et al., 2014). Additionally, excessive screen time can displace activities that are protective for mental health, such as physical exercise, face-to-face social interactions, and sufficient sleep, thereby increasing vulnerability to psychological distress (Twenge & Campbell, 2018).

Preventing digital addictions requires a multifaceted approach that includes digital education and control of screen time. Digital literacy programs can empower individuals, especially young people, to use technology responsibly by fostering critical thinking about online content and awareness of the potential risks associated with excessive use (Livingstone et al., 2017). Educational interventions promote healthy digital habits, such as setting boundaries for screen time and encouraging participation in offline activities. Strategies for controlling screen time involve implementing guidelines and tools to monitor and limit the duration of digital device usage. Parental supervision, along with technological solutions such as app timers and screen time tracking, can help reduce excessive use among children and adolescents (Hill et al., 2016). Encouraging a balanced lifestyle that integrates physical activity, social interaction, and digital engagement is essential for prevention efforts.

Therapeutic Interventions: Cognitive-Behavioral Therapy and Psychopharmacological Approaches

Cognitive-behavioral therapy (CBT) is recognized as an effective intervention for treating digital addictions (Zajac et al., 2020). CBT focuses on modifying maladaptive thoughts and behaviors associated with excessive digital use by enhancing self-control and coping strategies (Young, 2011). Through techniques such as cognitive restructuring and behavioral modification, individuals learn to recognize triggers for their addictive behaviors and develop healthier patterns of technology use (King et al., 2012). Psychopharmacological approaches may also be considered, especially when digital addiction co-occurs with other mental health disorders. Medications such as selective serotonin reuptake inhibitors (SSRIs) can be used to address underlying psychiatric conditions that may contribute to or result from digital addiction (Dell'Osso et al., 2006). However, pharmacotherapy should be combined with psychotherapy for comprehensive treatment.

Public policies play a pivotal role in the prevention and intervention of digital addictions. Regulatory measures can be implemented to ensure that digital platforms adopt designs that minimize addictive features, such as excessive notifications and autoplay functions (Montag et al., 2019). Policymakers can enforce age-appropriate content regulations and promote transparency regarding how user data is used to tailor content that may encourage prolonged engagement. Mental health policies should incorporate guidelines for digital well-being, supporting initiatives that fund research, education, and access to treatment services for digital addiction (World Health Organization, 2020). Collaboration among governments, health organizations, and technology companies is essential to create an environment prioritizing user well-being over engagement metrics.

Final Remarks

This chapter examines the complex interplay between digital addiction, depression, and suicide, emphasizing the significant impact of excessive digital technology use on mental health. While digital platforms offer cognitive and social benefits, excessive engagement can lead to negative outcomes such as attentional problems, social isolation, and sleep disturbances. Various forms of digital addiction, including Internet, gaming, smartphone, and social media addiction, are prevalent globally and closely linked to mental health issues like depression and suicidal behavior. These associations are fueled by factors such as social comparison, cyberbullying, and exposure to negative content, creating a bidirectional relationship where depression and digital addiction perpetuate one another. Neurobiological impacts, such as changes in neural plasticity and the brain's reward system, further reinforce compulsive technology use, contributing to heightened anxiety, impaired cognitive function, and diminished impulse control. Psychological vulnerabilities, including low self-esteem, impulsivity, and social anxiety, combined with addictive design features like intermittent reinforcement and the fear of missing out (FoMO), exacerbate these risks.

Our discussion highlights the need for a balanced approach to digital technology use, advocating for prevention and intervention strategies to mitigate its risks. Digital literacy, screen time control, and therapeutic interventions such as cognitive-behavioral therapy (CBT) are emphasized, alongside regulatory policies to address the broader societal impact. Public awareness campaigns and education programs can help individuals cultivate healthier digital habits, prioritize offline activities, and foster meaningful face-to-face interactions. By nurturing a culture of mindful technology use and promoting resilience among vulnerable groups like adolescents, society can better navigate the challenges posed by digital addiction. As digital technologies continue to evolve, ongoing vigilance and multidisciplinary approaches will be essential in safeguarding mental health and encouraging purposeful engagement with digital platforms.

References

Aalbers, G., McNally, R. J., Heeren, A., De Wit, S., & Fried, E. I. (2019). Social media and depression symptoms: A network perspective. *Journal of Experimental Psychology: General, 148*(8), 1454–1462. https://psycnet.apa.org/buy/2018-61357-001

American Psychiatric Association—APA. (2014). *Diagnostic and statistical manual of mental disorders (DSM-5)*. American Psychiatric Association.

Anastasya, Y., Hadiah, C., Amalia, I., & Suzanna, E. (2022). Correlation between fear of missing out and internet addiction in students. *International Journal of Islamic Educational Psychology, 3*, 36. https://doi.org/10.18196/ijiep.v3i1.14038

Andrade, A. L. M., Lobato, F. B. H., Stange, N., Scatena, A., Oliveira, W. A., Kim, H. S., & Lopes, F. M. (2024). The association between gaming disorder and impulsivity: A systematic review. *Estudos De Psicologia (Campinas), 41*, e220032. https://doi.org/10.1590/1982-0275202441e220032

Beck, A. T. (1963). Thinking and depression. Idiosyncratic content and cognitive distortions. *Archives of General Psychiatry, 9*, 324–333. https://doi.org/10.1001/archpsyc.1963.01720160014002

Behzad, S. (2019). Reward System Components in Addictive Disorders. *Open Access Journal of Addiction & Psychology, 2*(2). OAJAP.MS.ID.000535.

Brand, M., Young, K. S., & Laier, C. (2014). Prefrontal control and internet addiction: A theoretical model and review of neuropsychological and neuroimaging findings. *Frontiers in Human Neuroscience, 8*, 375. https://doi.org/10.3389/fnhum.2014.00375

Burns, A. C., Gillett, P. L., Rubinstein, M., & Gentry, J. W. (1990). An exploratory study of lottery playing, gambling addiction and links to compulsive consumption. *Advances in Consumer Research, 17*(1), 1.

Carpita, B., Muti, D., Nardi, B., Benedetti, F., Cappelli, A., Cremone, I. M., Carmassi, C., & Dell'Osso, L. (2021). Biochemical correlates of video game use: From physiology to pathology. A narrative review. *Life (Basel), 11*(8), 775. https://doi.org/10.3390/life11080775. PMID: 34440519; PMCID: PMC8401252.

Dell'Osso, B., Altamura, A. C., Allen, A., Marazziti, D., & Hollander, E. (2006). Epidemiologic and clinical updates on impulse control disorders: A critical review. *European Archives of Psychiatry and Clinical Neuroscience, 256*, 464–475. https://doi.org/10.1007/s00406-006-0668-0

Dolev-Cohen, M., & Barak, A. (2013). Adolescents' use of instant messaging as a means of emotional relief. *Computers in Human Behavior, 29*, 58–63. https://doi.org/10.1016/j.chb.2012.07.016

Dossi, N., & Pesce, R. C. (2023). Neural mechanisms of the reward system and the cognitive control system in internet addicts. *Science Insights, 42*(3), 867–875. https://doi.org/10.15354/si.23.re255

Dziura, S., McNaughton, K., Giacobbe, E., Yarger, H., Hickey, A., Shariq, D., & Redcay, E. (2023). Neural sensitivity to social reward predicts links between social behavior and loneliness in youth during the COVID-19 pandemic. *Developmental Psychobiology, 65*(6), e22413. https://doi.org/10.1002/dev.22413

Edwards, S. (2016). Reinforcement principles for addiction medicine; from recreational drug use to psychiatric disorder. *Progress in Brain Research, 223*, 63–76. https://doi.org/10.1016/bs.pbr.2015.07.005

Ellis, J. (1990). Computer games and aggressive behavior: A review of the literature. *Educational Technology, 30*(2), 37–40. http://www.jstor.org/stable/44425832.

Ferguson, C. J. (2024). Do social media experiments prove a link with mental health: A methodological and meta-analytic review. Psychology of Popular Media. Advance Online Publication. https://doi.org/10.1037/ppm0000541.

Friedrich-Cofer, L., & Huston, A. C. (1986). Television violence and aggression: The debate continues. *Psychological Bulletin, 100*(3), 364–371. https://doi.org/10.1037/0033-2909.100.3.364

Hahn, C., & Kim, D. J. (2014). Is there a shared neurobiology between aggression and internet addiction disorder? *Journal of Behavioral Addictions, 3*(1), 12–20. https://doi.org/10.1556/JBA.3.2014.1.2

He, X., Chen, S., Yu, Q., Yang, P., & Yang, B. (2024). Correlations between problematic internet use and suicidal behavior among Chinese adolescents: A systematic review and meta-analysis. *Frontiers in Psychiatry, 15*, 1484809. https://doi.org/10.3389/fpsyt.2024.1484809

Hill, D., Ameenuddin, N., Reid Chassiakos, Y. L., Cross, C., Hutchinson, J., Levine, A., Boyd, R., Mendelson, R., Moreno, M., & Swanson, W. S. (2016). Media and young minds. *Pediatrics, 138*(5), e20162591. https://doi.org/10.1542/peds.2016-2591

Hoehe, M., & Thibaut, F. (2020). Going digital: How technology use may influence human brains and behavior. *Dialogues in Clinical Neuroscience, 22*, 93–97. https://doi.org/10.31887/DCNS.2020.22.2/mhoehe

Hoge, E., Bickham, D., & Cantor, J. (2017). Digital media, anxiety, and depression in children. *Pediatrics, 140*(2), 76–80. https://doi.org/10.1542/peds.2016-1758G

Hooker, M. (2016). *The relationship between digital technology and the interpersonal communication skills of generation Y*. Elsevier. https://doi.org/10.2139/ssrn.3057797

Karakose, T., Yıldırım, B., Tülübaş, T., & Kardas, A. (2023). A comprehensive review on emerging trends in the dynamic evolution of digital addiction and depression. *Frontiers in Psychology, 14*, 1126815. https://doi.org/10.3389/fpsyg.2023.1126815

Kardefelt-Winther, D. (2017). How does the time children spend using digital technology impact their mental Well-being, social relationships and physical activity? An evidence-focused literature review. In *Florence: Innocenti Discussion Paper*. UNICEF Office of Research–Innocenti.

King, D. L., Delfabbro, P. H., Griffiths, M. D., & Gradisar, M. (2012). Cognitive-behavioral approaches to outpatient treatment of internet addiction in children and adolescents. *Journal of Clinical Psychology, 68*(11), 1185–1195. https://doi.org/10.1002/jclp.21918

Koob, G. (2013). Negative reinforcement in drug addiction: The darkness within. *Current Opinion in Neurobiology, 23*, 559–563. https://doi.org/10.1016/j.conb.2013.03.011

Kowalski, R. M., Giumetti, G. W., Schroeder, A. N., & Lattanner, M. R. (2014). Bullying in the digital age: A critical review and meta-analysis of cyberbullying research among youth. *Psychological Bulletin, 140*(4), 1073–1137. https://doi.org/10.1037/a0035618

Livingstone, S., Mascheroni, G., & Staksrud, E. (2017). European research on children's internet use: Assessing the past and anticipating the future. *New Media & Society, 20*(3), 1103–1122. https://doi.org/10.1177/1461444816685930

Lopez-Fernandez, O., Romo, L., Kern, L., Rousseau, A., Graziani, P., Rochat, L., Achab, S., Zullino, D., Landrø, N., Zacarés, J., Serra, E., Chóliz, M., Pontes, H., Griffiths, M., & Kuss, D. (2022). Perceptions underlying addictive technology use patterns: Insights for cognitive-Behavioural therapy. *International Journal of Environmental Research and Public Health, 19*, 544. https://doi.org/10.3390/ijerph19010544

Mendoza, J., Pody, B., Lee, S., Kim, M., & McDonough, I. (2018). The effect of cellphones on attention and learning: The influences of time, distraction, and nomophobia. *Computers in Human Behavior, 86*, 52–60. https://doi.org/10.1016/j.chb.2018.04.027

Meng, S. Q., Cheng, J. L., Li, Y. Y., Yang, X. Q., Zheng, J. W., Chang, X. W., et al. (2022). Global prevalence of digital addiction in general population: A systematic review and meta-analysis. *Clinical Psychological Review, 92*, 102128. https://doi.org/10.1016/j.cpr.2022.102128

Meshi, D., Tamir, D. I., & Heekeren, H. R. (2015). The emerging neuroscience of social media. *Trends in Cognitive Science, 19*(12), 771–782. https://doi.org/10.1016/j.tics.2015.09.004

Montag, C., Sindermann, C., Becker, B., & Panksepp, J. (2016). An affective neuroscience framework for the molecular study of internet addiction. *Frontiers in Psychology, 7*, 1906. https://doi.org/10.3389/fpsyg.2016.01906

Montag, C., Lachmann, B., Herrlich, M., & Zweig, K. (2019). Addictive features of social media/messenger platforms and freemium games against the background of psychological and economic theories. *International Journal of Environmental Research and Public Health, 16*(14), 2612. https://doi.org/10.3390/ijerph16142612

Mujica, A., Crowell, C., Villano, M., & Uddin, K. (2022). ADDICTION BY DESIGN: Some dimensions and challenges of excessive social media use. *Medical Research Archives, 10*(2), 1–29. https://doi.org/10.18103/mra.v10i2.2677

Odgers, C. L., & Jensen, M. R. (2020). Annual research review: Adolescent mental health in the digital age: Facts, fears, and future directions. *Journal of Child Psychology and Psychiatry, 61*(3), 336–348. https://doi.org/10.1111/jcpp.13190

Park, B., Han, D. H., & Roh, S. (2017). Neurobiological findings related to internet use disorders. *Psychiatry and Clinical Neuroscience, 71*(7), 467–478. https://doi.org/10.1111/pcn.12422

Patil, A. U., Madathil, D., & Huang, C. M. (2021). Age-related and individual variations in altered prefrontal and cerebellar connectivity associated with the tendency of developing internet addiction. *Human Brain Mapping, 42*(14), 4525–4537. https://doi.org/10.1002/hbm.25562

Persson, P., & Persson, A. (2023). Did you know? Dopamine, pop culture and beyond. *Acta Physiologica, 238*, e13971. https://doi.org/10.1111/apha.13971

Prikhodko, O., Cherdymova, E., Lopanova, E., Galchenko, N., Ikonnikov, A., Mechkovskaya, O., & Karamova, O. (2020). Ways of expressing emotions in social networks: Essential features, problems and features of manifestation in internet communication. *Online Journal of Communication and Media Technologies, 10*(2), e202010. https://doi.org/10.29333/ojcmt/7931

Reichert, R. A., Di Girolamo Martins, G., Da Silva, A. M. B., Scatena, A., Barbugli, B. C., De Micheli, D., & Andrade, A. L. M. (2021). *New forms of addiction: Digital media* (Vol. 43–53). Springer. https://doi.org/10.1007/978-3-030-62106-3_3

Saberi, B. (2019). Reward system components in addictive disorders. *Open Access Journal of Addiction and Psychology, 2*(2), 1–2. https://doi.org/10.33552/OAJAP.2019.02.000535

Small, G. W., Lee, J., Kaufman, A., Jalil, J., Siddarth, P., Gaddipati, H., & Bookheimer, S. Y. (2020). Brain health consequences of digital technology use. *Dialogues in Clinical Neuroscience, 22*(2), 179–187. https://doi.org/10.31887/DCNS.2020.22.2/gsmall

Souza, K., & Da Cunha, M. X. C. (2019). Impactos do uso das redes sociais virtuais na saúde mental dos adolescentes: uma revisão sistemática da literatura. *Revista Educação Psicologia e Interfaces, 3*(3), 204–2017. https://doi.org/10.37444/issn-2594-5343.v3i3.156

Sussman, C., Harper, J., Stahl, J., & Weigle, P. (2018). Internet and video game addictions: Diagnosis, epidemiology, and neurobiology. *Child and Adolescent Psychiatric Clinics of North America, 27*(2), 307–326. https://doi.org/10.1016/j.chc.2017.11.015

Tonge, B. J. (1990). The impact of television on children and clinical practice. *Australian and New Zealand Journal of Psychiatry, 24*(4), 552–560. https://doi.org/10.3109/00048679009062912

Tsang, V., Tse, D., Chu, L., Fung, H., Mai, C., & Zhang, H. (2022). The mediating role of loneliness on relations between face-to-face and virtual interactions and psychological well-being across age: A 21-day diary study. *International Journal of Behavioral Development, 46*, 500–509. https://doi.org/10.1177/01650254221132775

Twenge, J. M., & Campbell, W. K. (2018). Associations between screen time and lower psychological well-being among children and adolescents: Evidence from a population-based study. *Preventive Medicine Reports, 12*, 271–283. https://doi.org/10.1016/j.pmedr.2018.10.003

Van Orden, K. A., Witte, T. K., Cukrowicz, K. C., Braithwaite, S. R., Selby, E. A., & Joiner, T. E., Jr. (2010). The interpersonal theory of suicide. *Psychological Review, 117*(2), 575–600. https://doi.org/10.1037/a0018697

Wacks, Y., & Weinstein, A. (2021). Excessive smartphone use is associated with health problems in adolescents and Young adults. *Frontiers in Psychiatry, 12*, 669042. https://doi.org/10.3389/fpsyt.2021.669042

Wang, Y., Toyoshima, O., Kunimatsu, J., Yamada, H., & Matsumoto, M. (2021). Tonic firing mode of midbrain dopamine neurons continuously tracks reward values changing moment-by-moment. *eLife, 10*, e63166. https://doi.org/10.7554/elife.63166

Weinstein, A., Livny, A., & Weizman, A. (2017). New developments in brain research of internet and gaming disorder. *Neuroscience and Biobehavioral Reviews, 75*, 314–330. https://doi.org/10.1016/j.neubiorev.2017.01.040

World Health Organization. (2014). *Preventing suicide: A global imperative*. World Health Organization.

World Health Organization. (2020). *Guidelines on mental health promotive and preventive interventions for adolescents: Helping adolescents thrive*. World Health Organization.

Young, K. S. (2011). CBT-IA: The first treatment model for internet addiction. *Journal of Cognitive Psychotherapy, 25*(4), 304. https://doi.org/10.1891/0889-8391.25.4.304

Zajac, K., Ginley, M. K., & Chang, R. (2020). Treatments of internet gaming disorder: A systematic review of the evidence. *Expert Review of Neurotherapeutics, 20*(1), 85–93. https://doi.org/10.1080/14737175.2020.1671824

Chapter 11
Transmedia and Digital Addiction

Fernando Ferreira Semolini, Laura Soares da Silva, Amanda Severo Lins Vitta, Evelin Moreira Freires, and André Luiz Monezi Andrade

Introduction to the Concept of Transmedia

Technological advancements during the cultural globalization of the twenty-first century enabled the expansion of the internet worldwide, as well as the proliferation of electronic devices and social media (Cohen-Almagor, 2013). Within this context, cultural globalization facilitated media convergence as a process of intensifying the continuous flow of information across various media platforms (Jenkins, 2006). These changes brought significant consequences to human behavior, leading to more fragmented consumption of information and entertainment (Roncallo-Dow & Arango-Forero, 2017). As a result, greater interactivity with consumed content became a new demand, explored by the entertainment, marketing, and advertising industries. Among the strategies developed, the use of multiple platforms and narrative formats gave rise to what is now known as transmedia (Lähteenmäki, 2021).

In this context, the concept of transmedia was proposed to define a new trend in presenting narratives, information, and advertisements. Expanding beyond isolated niches of dissemination and accessibility, the practice of transmedia consists of spreading content across various media outlets (digital media, newspapers, websites, television channels) or formats (films, series, books, comics, games) that mutually complement each other and uniquely contribute to the narrative (Jenkins, 2006). This creates an ecosystem where each medium plays a collaborative role in enhancing the narrative's growth and depth (Evans, 2019).

In transmedia, the experience of complementarity across platforms creates a sense of unity, offering the audience the opportunity to engage in constant active interaction with the content (Henriques, 2018; Evans, 2019). In this sense,

F. F. Semolini · L. S. da Silva · A. S. L. Vitta · E. M. Freires · A. L. M. Andrade (✉)
Pontifical Catholic University of Campinas, Campinas, Brazil
e-mail: fernando.fs4@puccampinas.edu.br; laura.ss2@puccampinas.edu.br; amanda.slv@puccampinas.edu.br; evelin.mf@puccampinas.edu.br; andre.andrade@puc-campinas.edu.br

A. L. M. Andrade (ed.), *Digital Addictions*,
https://doi.org/10.1007/978-3-031-87986-9_11

transmedia is necessarily characterized by (1) sharing potential, which is the ability to disseminate content across various media, allowing the audience to fully experience the work in its depth; (2) multiplicity, the adaptability of the narrative, which multiplies and expands according to the audience's active participation; (3) immersion, the opportunity for the audience to immerse themselves in the narrative through events or locations that induce real experiences, as well as through the materialization of content in fan service products used in everyday life, such as clothing, objects, and accessories; (4) world-building, the creation and detailing of the environment in which the narrative takes place; (5) seriality, the use of various platforms and media to continue the narrative, such as the creation of spin-offs in different formats; (6) subjectivity, the diversity of ways in which content is narrated, avoiding narrative monism; and (7) performance, the possibility for the audience to become part of the narrative and actively participate in its construction and dissemination (Jenkins, 2009).

These characteristics demonstrate that, in the realm of entertainment, transmedia is increasingly employed to enhance audience engagement (Jenkins, 2014). An example of a successful transmedia project in this domain is the *Harry Potter* narrative by J. K. Rowling. Initially originating as physical books, it adopted transmedia strategies, being adapted into other formats such as films and games and expanding its presence in various digital media and websites (Brummitt, 2016). The universe's expansion with the new series *Fantastic Beasts* and the game *Hogwarts Legacy*, along with the creation of theme parks and merchandise, are also part of this transmedia strategy. The proliferation of virtual communities on social media, the expansion of media channels, and the promotion of constant interaction among fans on these platforms further reinforce this narrative. In this context, the transmedia characteristics present in the *Harry Potter* narrative contributed to the work's worldwide engagement. This strategy has been similarly employed by other successful entertainment narratives, such as *Star Wars* (Guynes & Hassler-Forest, 2017), *A Song of Ice and Fire* (Escurignan, 2022), and the *Marvel Universe* (Richter, 2016).

Another example is the music industry, which has also been adapting to new trends in public engagement and dissemination. While in the past, music was commonly distributed only through CDs or radio programs, today, people consume music through various platforms (Bengtsson & Edlom, 2021). In this context, Big Hit Music, with the group Bangtan Boys (BTS), serves as a transmedia success story in the music industry. Beyond the music itself, BTS incorporates multifaceted strategies across various platforms and formats that engage fans in the group's narrative, creating unique experiences with a strong emotional connection and audience participation. Through constant interaction on social media platforms such as Twitter, Instagram, YouTube, TikTok, and blogs, the group generates diverse content that complements the musical experience while reinforcing the narrative present in their songs, resulting in a broader global audience (Zuhadmono, 2021). Interactive elements in live performances, as well as insights into the daily lives of the group members, further strengthen the transmedia narrative, making fans feel like part of the project (Piccialli, 2021). These strategies are also employed by other companies in the music industry, exemplifying the use of transmedia in today's world (Brembilla, 2018).

Transmedia in Digital Media

The presence of the Internet has proven to be a determining factor in behavioral changes regarding the production and consumption of content and narratives (Garza, 2002). In this context, digital media has become an indispensable channel for current transmedia practices, as it provides the fundamental infrastructure to ensure greater connectivity between creators and users, rapid dissemination of narratives, and narrative ubiquity (Kustritz, 2018). The accessibility of social media further strengthens transmedia narratives; through smartphones, narratives can be consumed anywhere or anytime, making transmedia dissemination a daily occurrence (Tajudeen et al., 2016). On the other hand, digital media has also facilitated the work of content creators, who can share their narratives across multiple platforms in an accessible and cost-effective manner, increasing the number of independent transmedia narratives (Scolari, 2014).

The use of social media in transmedia narratives enables interactive experiences across various complementary platforms, allowing aspects of the narrative to be disseminated in diverse, unique formats (Gürel & Tığlı, 2014). For instance, short videos, texts, photos, webtoons, and audio features, optimized for each social network, encourage active audience participation through shares and discussions. They also facilitate interactions between transmedia narratives and fans by allowing users to create memes, artwork, fanfiction, and communities that enrich the narrative and engage the audience within the social network. Additionally, social media enables real-time updates and expansions of the narrative, wherein supplementary content and behind-the-scenes material are used to keep audiences active within communities (Yong, 2019).

For transmedia, online games can serve either as the primary generators of the narrative or as a media variant of another format. In this context, it has been observed that in the case of online games as primary generators of the narrative, audiences show much more interest in the gameplay itself than in the narrative (Stein, 2016). Thus, transmedia strategies tend to expand or deepen the experience of gameplay through other formats and digital media (Willett, 2016). On the other hand, in the case of online games as a media variant of other formats, transmedia narratives primarily aim to provide users with an active participatory experience within the narrative universe, contributing to the expansion of the universe, audience interactivity, and immersion through the gratification of immediate feedback when the controlled character influences and drives changes within the universe, creating the sensation of being part of the narrative (Cardozo & Mattar, 2017).

Web series, in turn, are becoming increasingly prominent in transmedia narratives as online audiovisual content gains popularity over traditional television programming (Kohli, 2020). Web series are often used to popularize narratives from other formats, such as books or games. In this context, the division of the narrative into weekly episodes allows for prolonged audience interaction and engagement. Additionally, the interaction of characters and cast members with audiences via social media and other media channels strengthens consumers' connection to the narrative. It is also common to see the creation of communities that discuss and theorize about the storyline's direction throughout the weekly episodes, creating the impression of real-time involvement (Atarama-Rojas et al., 2020).

With the rise of mobile devices, digital applications available on smartphones, tablets, and notebooks have become increasingly popular. These applications stand out in transmedia narratives by enabling personalized experiences tailored to the narrative's needs and providing exclusive content to application users (Kim & Baek, 2018).

In this way, the use of digital media in transmedia narratives significantly impacts user engagement and immersion, becoming not only mechanisms for transmedia dissemination but also primary components of the narrative itself. In this context, digital media platforms enhance users' active participation, such that their role as co-creators of the narrative strengthens emotional engagement. Furthermore, the various means of accessibility contribute to greater interactivity and immersion in transmedia through the sharing of debates, ideas, and interpretations, the creation of secondary content, and the expansion of the universe in which the narrative takes place (Jenkins, 2006). Additionally, digital media have also enabled more dynamic fragmentation of narratives, giving rise to numerous ways of expanding target audiences and personalizing interaction channels through social media, applications, websites, and online games.

Transmedia and User Engagement

One of the primary objectives of transmedia storytelling is to increase user engagement (Henriques, 2018). With this goal in mind, transmedia strategies seek to provide multifaceted experiences with unique contributions on various platforms, thus encouraging users to access each one of them, giving rise to a continuous cycle of new discoveries and interactions that motivate the audience to remain engaged in the narrative (Evans, 2019). In order to enhance engagement, this strategy increases the amount of time the user is in contact with the narrative, as they seek it out and consume it in various media. Additionally, the ubiquity of the narrative, present in almost all media accessed by the individual, reinforces the emotional connection of the audience, found in all platforms consumed in everyday life (Dahlgren & Hill, 2022).

While increasing user engagement, transmedia can also promote intensive use behaviors. By offering different means of interaction, such as active and real-time participation on social networks, missions and objectives to be accomplished in online games, exclusive content on apps, and prolonged follow-up of the narrative in web series, transmedia storytelling makes the audience become part of the narrative itself (Sutherland & Barker, 2023a). This motivation generates in individuals the feeling of being constantly rewarded for their effort, corroborating the maintenance of the behavior through greater involvement and development of loyalty towards the narrative. In turn, this cycle of continuous immersion, always positively reinforced by new interactions, potentiates patterns of intensive use behaviors of digital media such as increasing the number of daily hours consuming the narrative, prioritizing contact with digital media over other activities, and social harms resulting from this behavior (Evans, 2019).

Given the effectiveness with which transmedia engages users, it is not surprising its widespread use for marketing purposes (Vinerean & Opreana, 2021). In this context, transmedia strategies in marketing potentiate emotional engagement, through new ways of generating positive emotions in consumers from the wide range of digital media. Cognitive engagement can be mentioned, through the possibility of consumers carrying out a deeper information processing of the brand content, as well as behavioral engagement, through the incentive to active participation of the consumer in actions related to the product (Sutherland & Barker, 2023b). Such forms of engagement are enabled in transmedia marketing campaigns by brands due to the influence of factors such as personalization, as the ability to adapt personalized content according to the needs and preferences of each individual; interactivity, as the possibility of establishing interactions between consumers and the brand; narrative coherence, as the perception on the part of consumers of being faced with a cohesive narrative that extends across the various platforms; and, finally, novelty, as the creative expansion that transmedia has enabled, giving rise to new elements and innovative ways of attracting the attention of the target audience (Sutherland & Barker, 2023c).

Therefore, engagement is a priority factor in marketing actions, but it also expresses equal importance in the educational context. In this context, transmedia allows the application of pedagogical principles that are difficult to implement, such as promoting motivating experiences, connections between topics, and content personalization in order to diversify learning modes (Runchina et al., 2022). Promoting engagement in learning through transmedia expands its potential in the introduction of games and the digital universe as learning tools (Kim & Castelli, 2021). These resources can be used to engage students in the study of less attractive curricular competencies, as well as serve as a pretext for establishing interdisciplinary relationships. Such strategies are particularly explored among the child audience (González-Martínez et al., 2019). More specifically, the incorporation of transmedia strategies promotes greater involvement through dynamic and enjoyable learning structures, capturing students' attention. Interaction through diverse means also potentiates multisensory learning, in order to facilitate the processing and retention of information, factors that aid in engagement with the content. In turn, the potential to promote students' active participation expands, so that the feeling of ownership of knowledge increases engagement and emotional connection with the content (Amon, 2019). In this way, transmedia can transcend limiting factors of formal learning, promoting broad engagement resources.

However, both in the educational environment and in marketing, the use of transmedia, when not executed properly, can generate risks for audience engagement. In this sense, excessive fragmentation of content can end up confusing the individual, just as an excess of fragmented information can overload them, promoting states of generalized disinterest, saturation, or aversion to content (Liu et al., 2022; Altinpulluk et al., 2020). More specifically in the context of learning, especially among the child audience, the use of media and playful formats can divert students' focus, distorting pedagogical objectives and potentiating the search for entertainment only.

Implications for Behavioral Addictions and Mental Health

The characteristics and potential of transmedia content, which provide greater engagement, intensive use behavior, and prolonged involvement, can, however, contribute to the development of behavioral addictions. The uninterrupted search for new fragments of the story that unfold across multiple platforms, highly interactive and immersive experiences, as well as gamification with immediate reinforcing rewards can influence users' behavior, leading them to prioritize the consumption of transmedia narratives, generating a compulsive cycle. In this way, the prolonged exposure time to media and the difficulty of disconnecting from platforms can interfere with the individual's social and family context through mechanisms similar to those of digital addictions (Martins et al., 2021; Reichert et al., 2021a).

Research shows that one of the factors most positively correlated with digital addictions is the increase in screen time for users (Nakshine et al., 2022; Reichert et al., 2021b). Thus, the fragmentation of content into multiple multifaceted platforms, coupled with interactive interconnectivity between them, induces users to use digital media for longer periods to consume transmedia narratives. In this context, increased screen time reduces the subject's interpersonal adaptation capacities, increases the desire to continue consuming content (Lissak, 2018), and produces psychobiological changes associated with lower cognitive control, inhibitory control, and emotional regulation (Small et al., 2020) which corroborates the development of digital addiction behaviors (Kim et al., 2023a, 2023b).

The increase in behavioral addictions resulting from transmedia content is also influenced by gamification. In transmedia content, this process occurs through the use of game elements (competition, scoring, and reward systems) as a digital marketing strategy to increase users' deep involvement in other platforms related to the expansion of content to game formats (Andrade et al., 2024; Hamid & Kuppusamy, 2017). Additionally, gamification involves adapting games to other media, making participation and interaction on external media platforms a form of reward within the original game. In this context, the use of game mechanics, thought processes, and design elements enhances both the extrinsic and intrinsic motivation of transmedia content consumers (Castellano-Tejedor & Cencerrado, 2024). Thus, with gamification, the search for immediate rewards in the consumption of transmedia content increases the risk of users developing behavioral addictions or intensive use behaviors.

In turn, a factor that impacts the behavior of transmedia content consumers is the Fear of Missing Out (FOMO), which is the anxiety felt about not being aware of all the online information on a subject (Wegmann et al., 2017). In transmedia, each platform offers a unique experience of the narrative, so that when consuming this content, the fear of not enjoying it as a whole, or of being out of date on some aspect, induces individuals to consume content more incisively, corroborating with greater compulsivity and intensive use behaviors (Mao et al., 2023). In this way, FOMO in relation to transmedia content contributes to the development of low satisfaction with interpersonal relationships and fear of loneliness, which corroborate as risk factors for behavioral addictions (Andrade et al., 2021a).

From another perspective, associated with behavioral addictions, transmedia content can impact the mental health and social behaviors of users. Research that has addressed the influence of social networks, online games, and series points out that the intensive and compulsive consumption of this content can affect the mental health as well as the social life of individuals, especially among children and adolescents (Andrade et al., 2020; Cruz et al., 2018; Henzel & Håkansson, 2021; Eichenberg et al., 2024). Thus, the immersion and prolonged involvement provided by transmedia content corroborates with behavioral patterns associated with damage to mental, physical, and social quality of life.

In this context, research shows that the increase in screen time, induced by transmedia content, is associated with higher rates of insomnia and poor sleep due to the use of digital media during the nighttime (Lissak, 2018; Cheung et al., 2017). This time spent consuming media, along with sleep problems, is related to poor mental health and an increase in problematic behaviors (Paulich et al., 2021). More specifically, a greater presence of psychiatric comorbidities, depressive symptoms, suicidal ideation, social isolation, low emotional regulation, anxiety, stress, and digital addictions was observed (Nakshine et al., 2022; Publishers, 2024; Schou Andreassen et al., 2016; Twenge & Campbell, 2019). Such problematic behaviors in relation to the consumption of transmedia content can also produce impacts on brain functions, potentially increasing symptoms of attention deficit; lowering inhibitory control; reducing the individual's general, emotional, and social intelligence; as well as impairing neural development in children and adolescents (Andrade et al., 2021b; Twenge & Campbell, 2018).

Studies have been conducted to understand the influence of increased screen time on ADHD cases. The results of these studies indicate a positive correlation between increased screen time and ADHD risk (Liu et al., 2023), also that this relationship may be mediated by sleep problems induced by excessive screen exposure. Thus, excessive consumption of transmedia content on digital media induces a state of neural hyper-excitation and acceleration of the subject's normal rhythm, activating dopaminergic pathways and altering the structures of brain regions (Yang et al., 2022). In addition, another study suggested that screen time may be responsible for incorrect ADHD diagnoses and that reducing time spent consuming screens decreases ADHD-related behaviors (Lissak, 2018).

On the other hand, other studies highlight the positive effects that transmedia content can offer for individuals' mental health, such as strengthening online communities (Kim et al., 2023b). In this context, the engagement of online communities around transmedia narratives increases users' sense of belonging and social connection, who in turn have higher self-esteem and lower feelings of loneliness when in contact with online communities (Publishers, 2024). Active participation encourages community members to interact with each other and exchange information, potentiating the development of group identity, becoming a protective factor (Sundet & Petersen, 2020).

The engagement potential of transmedia is also used to encourage treatments or programs focused on mental health. Research has shown how strategies involving transmedia have increased the engagement and participation of users in apps for the mental health of Latina women in the United States (Soderlund et al., 2021; Heilemann et al., 2018). Similarly, other studies have demonstrated a significant reduction in symptoms of poor mental health, such as depression and anxiety, with the implementation of transmedia in therapeutic interventions (Ogbeiwi et al., 2024).

Strategies for Responsible Transmedia Consumption

The primary objective of guidelines for consuming transmedia content is to promote mental health integrity among users, as well as to respect their rights as consumers. Therefore, users, or those responsible for users in situations involving minors, should strive for conscious consumption of digital content through screen time management, careful content selection, and attention to the user's mental health.

Setting limits on the time spent consuming transmedia content aims to prevent isolation and dependence. A balance between online and offline activities is essential for maintaining individuals' mental health (Radesky, 2021). In this sense, the development of harmonious relationships between online and offline activities is associated with greater life satisfaction, a reduced sense of loneliness, and a decreased risk of digital addiction (Lin et al., 2018). Additionally, prioritizing content that promotes learning and well-being for the individual also contributes to a lower emotional impact of the content consumed by the user, promoting mental health care (Publishers, 2024).

Given the characteristic of active participation promoted by transmedia, respect within online environments, avoiding discrimination, harassment, or hate speech promotes the development of inclusive and healthy environments, with a lower chance of causing negative affects and damage to users' mental health. In this same environment of interactions, there should be caution regarding the disclosure of intimate information, always ensuring that the platforms' privacy policy is in accordance with the protection of users' data.

Critical consciousness should be developed regarding the consumption of transmedia content. Verifying the source or credibility of content is essential to avoid being misled within digital media. Attention should be paid to the commercial or ideological biases present in transmedia content. Furthermore, the context in which transmedia is created should be evaluated to better interpret and understand its objectives. Such critical consciousness regarding transmedia content serves as a protective factor against alienation and manipulation that can lead to psychological and emotional impacts, as well as dependencies.

Transmedia content creators have an ethical responsibility to ensure the veracity of the information they produce, avoiding misinformation and manipulation that could harm users (Publishers, 2024). Transmedia content should be created and disseminated, avoiding abusive strategies that induce intensive and compulsive use. Moreover, content creators should always maintain transparency regarding their objectives and conflicts of interest.

In this context, parents, educators, and health professionals play a fundamental role in guiding conscious consumption of transmedia content. They should help young people to consume the experiences offered by digital media in a healthy and balanced way (Scolari et al., 2018). Parents should monitor their children's screen time to establish a balance between online and offline activities. They should also manage their children's digital activities, providing initial guidance on the conscious consumption of digital media (Ramos et al., 2023). The importance of maintaining an open dialogue about the potential impacts of excessive screen time should be emphasized. Educators, on the other hand, must adapt to the new demands of the digital age, integrating digital literacy into school curricula as a necessary new requirement (Reddy et al., 2020). Furthermore, they should teach students to interact with transmedia content in a way that utilizes platforms constructively, always providing the necessary tools and support for the conscious and responsible use of transmedia within digital media.

In this way, parents and educators must collaborate to develop in young people the competencies required by the modern landscape of new media and communication formats within digital media. In this context, the main skills necessary to integrate into the world of transmedia are (1) the ability to use transmedia means to find solutions to problems; (2) the ability to appropriate transmedia content in carrying out daily tasks or creating new content; (3) the ability to analyze, organize, and concentrate on multitasking within the transmedia universe; (4) the ability to connect, compare, and gather diverse knowledge in digital media to achieve a goal; (5) the ability to judge and correctly evaluate the credibility of various sources and information present in digital media; (6) the ability to navigate the transmedia universe, following the flow of information from various platforms or formats involved; (7) the ability to research and synthesize information within the networking universe; and (8) the ability to traverse various online communities or platforms, knowing how to discern them and understanding the different norms and perspectives of each medium (Jenkins et al., 2009).

In turn, health professionals should always be attentive to the signs and causes of digital dependencies within transmedia content, as well as the potential social, emotional, and psychological impacts related to the excessive consumption of this content within digital media. From the understanding of this phenomenon, health professionals should establish intervention strategies with the objective of providing appropriate guidance on the consumption of transmedia content related to the physical, social, and mental well-being of users.

Challenges and Future Prospects

With the expansion of new transmedia strategies to various sectors of society, the production and consumption of such content have become the subject of discussions on ethical and regulatory issues. The main challenges surrounding this theme revolve around the high potential for manipulation of behavior, given how transmedia strategies, aiming for engagement, can exploit cognitive and emotional vulnerabilities and, consequently, induce excessive consumption, behavioral addictions, and problematic use of digital media.

In this regard, the implementation of guidelines to protect consumers against aggressive marketing practices, misinformation, and manipulation is encompassing the use of transmedia strategies for these purposes, especially when targeting children. This is also an ethical challenge that addresses the responsibility of content producers in creating transmedia content, while also seeking to resolve the existing ambiguity between factual and fictional aspects (Gambarato & Nanì, 2016; Gambarato & Heuman, 2023). The solutions discussed and proposed for these ethical challenges aim primarily to guarantee the creative freedom that transmedia has enabled, while preserving the responsibility of producers to ensure transparent practices and respect for consumer rights (Publishers, 2024).

Regarding future perspectives, the evolution of transmedia storytelling does not seem to be nearing its limit. Accompanying the growing technological evolution, transmedia can benefit from both the rise of new artificial intelligences and virtual and augmented reality (Hergenrader, 2020). Both technologies can increase the immersive nature of experiences, as well as expand the options for interactivity, personalization, and engagement in digital media.

While these innovations excite digital content producers, on the other hand, they raise social issues. The growing influence of the digital world on human behavior is reflected in the greater impact of online communities on the construction of identities and collective experiences. Thus, the interconnections between the real and virtual worlds will tend to intensify with future innovations in transmedia storytelling within digital media. This requires adaptation to new changes and reflections on the challenges that arise from them.

References

Altinpulluk, H., Kilinc, H., Firat, M. H., & Yumurtaci, O. (2020). The influence of segmented and complete educational videos on the cognitive load, satisfaction, engagement, and academic achievement levels of learners. *Journal of Computers in Education, 7*, 155–182. https://doi.org/10.1007/s40692-019-00151-7

Amon, B. T. (2019). *Transmedia narratives in education: The potentials of multisensory emotional arousal in teaching and learning contexts*. IntechOpen. https://doi.org/10.5772/intechopen.88168

Andrade, A. L. M., Scatena, A., Bedendo, A., Enumo, S. R. F., Dellazzana-Zanon, L. L., Prebianchi, H. B., Macgado, W. L., et al. (2020). Findings on the relationship between internet addiction and psychological symptoms in Brazilian adults. *International Journal of Psychology, 55*(6), 941–950. https://doi.org/10.1002/ijop.12670

Andrade, A. L. M., Scatena, A., Bedendo, A., Enumo, S. R. F., Dellazzana-Zanon, L. L., Prebianchi, H. B., & De Micheli, D. (2021a). Internet addiction among Brazilian students: Prevalence and association with emotional problems. *Universitas Psychologica, 20*, 1–15. https://doi.org/10.11144/Javeriana.upsy20.iabs

Andrade, A. L. M., Enumo, S. R. F., Passos, M. A. Z., Vellozo, E. P., Shoen, T. H., Kulik, M. A., Niskier, S. R., et al. (2021b). Problematic internet use, emotional problems and quality of life among adolescents. *Psico-USF, 26*(1), 41–51. https://doi.org/10.1590/1413-82712021260104

Andrade, A. L. M., Lobato, F. B. H., Stange, N., Scatena, A., Oliveira, W. A. D., Kim, H. S., & Lopes, F. M. (2024). The association between gaming disorder and impulsivity: A systematic review. *Estudos de Psicologia (Campinas), 41*, e220032. https://doi.org/10.1590/1982-0275202441e220032

Atarama-Rojas, T., Guerrero-Perez, E., & Gerbolini, V. (2020). Participation and transmediality: Audience influence on web series. *International Journal of Communication, 14*, 3615. https://ijoc.org/index.php/ijoc/article/view/14024/0

Bengtsson, R. L., & Edlom, J. (2021). Mapping transmedia marketing in the music industry: A methodology. *Media and Communication, 9*(3), 164–174. https://doi.org/10.17645/mac.v9i3.4064

Brembilla, P. (2018). Transmedia music: The values of music as a transmedia asset. In *The Routledge companion to transmedia studies* (pp. 82–89). Routledge.

Brummitt, C. (2016). Pottermore: Transmedia storytelling and authorship in Harry potter. *The Midwest Quarterly, 58*(1), 112. https://www.proquest.com/docview/1832925509?sourcetype=Scholarly%20Journals

Cardozo, M., & Mattar, J. (2017). *Adaptação transmídia de/para games: revisão de literatura* (Vol. 16). Simpósio Brasileiro de Jogos e Entretenimento digital (SBGAMES).

Castellano-Tejedor, C., & Cencerrado, A. (2024). Gamification for mental health and Health Psychology: Insights at the first quarter mark of the 21st century. *International Journal of Environmental Research and Public Health, 21*(8), 990. https://doi.org/10.3390/ijerph21080990

Cheung, C. H. M., Bedford, R., Saez De Urabain, I. R., Karmiloff-Smith, A., & Smith, T. J. (2017). Daily touchscreen use in infants and toddlers is associated with reduced sleep and delayed sleep onset. *Scientific Reports, 7*(46104), 1–7. https://doi.org/10.1038/srep46104

Cohen-Almagor, R. (2013). *Internet history. In moral, ethical, and social dilemmas in the age of technology: Theories and practice* (pp. 19–39). IGI Global.

Cruz, F. A. D., Scatena, A., Andrade, A. L. M., & De Micheli, D. (2018). Evaluation of internet addiction and the quality of life of Brazilian adolescents from public and private schools. *Estudos de Psicologia (Campinas), 35*(2), 193–204. https://doi.org/10.1590/1982-02752018000200008

Dahlgren, P., & Hill, A. (2022). *Media engagement*. Routledge.

Eichenberg, C., Schneider, R., & Rumpl, H. (2024). Social media addiction: Associations with attachment style, mental distress, and personality. *BMC Psychiatry, 24*, 278. https://doi.org/10.1186/s12888-024-05709-z

Escurignan, J. (2022). *TV fandom across media: Transnational fans and transmedia experience of 'Game of Thrones'*. [doctoral dissertation, University of Roehampton].

Evans, E. (2019). *Understanding engagement in transmedia culture*. Routledge.

Gambarato, R. R., & Heuman, J. (2023). Beyond fact and fiction: Cultural memory and transmedia ethics in Netflix's the crown. *European Journal of Cultural Studies, 26*(6), 803–821. https://doi.org/10.1177/13675494221128332

Gambarato, R. R., & Nanì, A. (2016). Blurring boundaries, transmedia storytelling and the ethics of C. S. Peirce. In S. Maras (Ed.), *Ethics in screenwriting. Palgrave studies in screenwriting*. Palgrave Macmillan. https://doi.org/10.1057/978-1-137-54493-3_7

Garza, G. (2002). The internet, narrative, and subjectivity. *Journal of Constructivist Psychology, 15*(3), 185–203. https://psycnet.apa.org/doi/10.1080/10720530290100433

González-Martínez, J., Esteban-Guitart, M., Rostan-Sánchez, C., Serrat Sellabona, E., & Estebanell-Minguell, M. (2019). What's up with transmedia and education? A literature review. *Digital Education Review, 36*, 207–222. https://doi.org/10.1344/der.2019.36.207-222

Gürel, E. M. E. T., & Tığlı, Ö. (2014). New world created by social media: Transmedia storytelling. *Journal of Media Critiques, 1*(1), 35–65. https://doi.org/10.17349/jmc114102

Guynes, S. A., & Hassler-Forest, D. (2017). *Star wars and the history of transmedia storytelling*. Amsterdam University Press. https://library.oapen.org/bitstream/id/4974d8b6-737a-49dd-ac4f-892f606a2a1b/637514.pdf.

Hamid, M., & Kuppusamy, M. (2017). Gamification implementation in service marketing: Literature. *Electronic Journal of Business & Management, 2*(1), 38–50.

Heilemann, M. V., Martinez, A., & Soderlund, P. D. (2018). A mental health storytelling intervention using transmedia to engage Latinas: Grounded theory analysis of Participants' perceptions of the Story's Main character. *Journal of Medical Internet Research, 20*(5), e10028. https://doi.org/10.2196/10028

Henriques, C. M. (2018). *Narrativa Transmídia e Educação para o Consumo*. Anais CIET: Horizonte.

Henzel, V., & Håkansson, A. (2021). Hooked on virtual social life. Problematic social media use and associations with mental distress and addictive disorders. *PLoS One, 16*(4), e0248406. https://doi.org/10.1371/journal.pone.0248406

Hergenrader, T. (2020). Transmedia storytelling, immersive storyworlds, and virtual reality. *Frameless, 2*(1), 5. https://repository.rit.edu/cgi/viewcontent.cgi?article=1023&context=frameless

Jenkins, H. (2006). *Convergence culture: Where old and new media collide*. New York University Press.

Jenkins, H. (2009). *Revenge of the Origami Unicorn: The remaining four principles of transmedia storytelling*. https://henryjenkins.org/blog/2009/12/revenge_of_the_origami_unicorn.html

Jenkins, H. (2014). Transmedia storytelling and entertainment: An annotated syllabus. In *Entertainment industries* (pp. 145–160). Routledge.

Jenkins, H., Purushotma, R., Weigel, M., Clinton, K., & Robison, A. J. (2009). *Confronting the challenges of participatory culture: Media education for the 21st century*. The MIT Press. https://doi.org/10.7551/mitpress/8435.001.0001

Kim, S., & Baek, T. H. (2018). Examining the antecedents and consequences of mobile app engagement. *Telematics and Informatics, 35*(1), 148–158. https://doi.org/10.1016/j.tele.2017.10.008

Kim, J., & Castelli, D. M. (2021). Effects of gamification on behavioral change in education: A meta-analysis. *International Journal of Environmental Research and Public Health, 18*(7), 3550. https://doi.org/10.3390/ijerph18073550

Kim, H. S., Leslie, R. D., Stewart, S. H., King, D. L., Demetrovics, Z., Andrade, A. L. M., Choi, J. S., Tavares, H., Almeida, B., & Hodgins, D. C. (2023a). A scoping review of the association between loot boxes, esports, skin betting, and token wagering with gambling and video gaming behaviors. *Journal of Behavioral Addictions, 12*, 309–351. https://doi.org/10.1556/2006.2023.00013

Kim, M. S., Wang, S., & Kim, S. (2023b). Effects of online fan Community interactions on well-being and sense of virtual community. *Behavioral sciences (Basel, Switzerland), 13*(11), 897. https://doi.org/10.3390/bs13110897

Kohli, C. (2020). The replacement of conventional television by streaming services. *International Journal of Research in Engineering, Science and Management, 3*(10), 59–67. https://journal.ijresm.com/index.php/ijresm/article/view/337

Kustritz, A. (2018). Transmedia serial narration: Crossroads of media, story, and time. *Media/Culture Journal, 21*(1), 1. https://doi.org/10.5204/mcj.1388

Lähteenmäki, I. (2021). Transmedia history. *Rethinking History, 25*(3), 281–306. https://doi.org/10.1080/13642529.2021.1963597

Lin, X., Su, W., & Potenza, M. N. (2018). Development of an online and offline integration hypothesis for healthy internet use: Theory and preliminary evidence. *Frontiers in Psychology, 9*, 492. https://doi.org/10.3389/fpsyg.2018.00492

Lissak, G. (2018). Adverse physiological and psychological effects of screen time on children and adolescents: Literature review and case study. *Environmental Research, 164*, 149–157. https://doi.org/10.1016/j.envres.2018.01.015

Liu, W., Huang, H., Saleem, A., & Zhao, Z. (2022). The effects of university students' fragmented reading on cognitive development in the new media age: Evidence from Chinese higher education. *PeerJ, 10*, e13861. https://doi.org/10.7717/peerj.13861

Liu, H., Chen, X., Huang, M., Yu, X., Gan, Y., Wang, J., Chen, Q., Nie, Z., & Ge, H. (2023). Screen time and childhood attention deficit hyperactivity disorder: A meta-analysis. *Reviews on Environmental Health, 39*(4), 643. https://doi.org/10.1515/reveh-2022-0262

Mao, J., Fu, G. X., & Huang, J. J. (2023). The double-edged sword effects of active social media use on loneliness: The roles of interpersonal satisfaction and fear of missing out. *Frontiers in Psychology, 14*, 1108467. https://doi.org/10.3389/fpsyg.2023.1108467

Martins, G. D. G., Caricati, V. V., Barbugli, B. C., Silva Ribeiro, C. M. D., Lobato, F. B. H., Scatena, A., & Andrade, A. L. M. (2021). The biopsychosocial impact of abusive use of digital media. In *Drugs and human behavior* (pp. 459–468). Springer.

Nakshine, V. S., Thute, P., Khatib, M. N., & Sarkar, B. (2022). Increased screen time as a cause of declining physical, psychological health, and sleep patterns: A literary review. *Cureus, 14*(10), e30051. https://doi.org/10.7759/cureus.30051

Ogbeiwi, O., Khan, W., Stott, K., Zaluczkowska, A., & Doyle, M. (2024). A systematic review of digital storytelling as psychotherapy for people with mental health needs. *Journal of Psychotherapy Integration, 34*(2), 115–132. https://doi.org/10.1037/int0000325

Paulich, K. N., Ross, J. M., Lessem, J. M., & Hewitt, J. K. (2021). Screen time and early adolescent mental health, academic, and social outcomes in 9-and 10-year-old children: Utilizing the adolescent brain cognitive development (ABCD) study. *PLoS One, 16*(9), e0256591. https://doi.org/10.1371/journal.pone.0256591

Piccialli, S. (2021). Connect, BTS: An example of innovative transmedia branding to rethink spatiality and meaning-making. *Asia Marketing Journal, 22*(4), 150. https://doi.org/10.15830/amj.2020.22.4.151

Publishers, K. (2024). Exploring the influence of online platforms on Well-being: The intersection of social media and mental health. *Public Healthcare and Ancient Science, 4*(1), 1. https://doi.org/10.5281/zenodo.10900010

Radesky, J. S. (2021). Young children's online-offline balance. *Acta Paediatrica, 110*(3), 748–749. https://doi.org/10.1111/apa.15649

Ramos, R. F. S., Scatena, A., Kim, H. S., de Oliveira, W. A., & Andrade, A. L. M. (2023). Brazilian digital warriors: Unraveling the nexus of adolescent cyber aggressors, problematic Internet & smartphone use, emotional struggles, and parental mediation. *Trends in Psychology*, 1–17. https://doi.org/10.1007/s43076-023-00338-z

Reddy, P., Sharma, B., & Chaudhary, K. (2020). Digital literacy: A review of literature. *International Journal of Technoethics (IJT), 11*(2), 65–94. https://doi.org/10.4018/IJT.20200701.oa1

Reichert, R. A., Calixto, F., Silva, A. M. B. D., Martins, G. D. G., Barbugli, B. C., Scatena, A., & Andrade, A. L. M. (2021a). Digital games, shopping, sex, and other addictions: Neuropsychological and behavioral correlates. In *Drugs and human behavior* (pp. 443–458). Springer.

Reichert, R. A., Martins, G. D. G., Silva, A. M. B. D., Scatena, A., Barbugli, B. C., Micheli, D. D., & Andrade, A. L. M. (2021b). New forms of addiction: Digital media. In *Psychology of substance abuse* (pp. 43–53). Springer.

Richter, A. (2016). The marvel cinematic universe as a transmedia narrative. *AMERICANA E-Journal of American Studies in Hungary, 12*(1), 1. https://www.americanaejournal.hu/index.php/americanaejournal/article/view/45110

Roncallo-Dow, S., & Arango-Forero, G. (2017). Introducing three dimensions of audience fragmentation. *Signo y Pensamiento, 36*(70), 74–90. https://www.redalyc.org/pdf/860/86052830004.pdf

Runchina, C., Fauth, F., & González-Martínez, J. (2022). Adolescents facing transmedia learning: Reflections on what they can do, what they think and what they feel. *Behavioral Sciences (Basel, Switzerland), 12*(4), 112. https://doi.org/10.3390/bs12040112

Schou Andreassen, C., Billieux, J., Griffiths, M. D., Kuss, D. J., Demetrovics, Z., Mazzoni, E., & Pallesen, S. (2016). The relationship between addictive use of social media and video games and symptoms of psychiatric disorders: A large-scale cross-sectional study. *Psychology of Addictive Behaviors: Journal of the Society of Psychologists in Addictive Behaviors, 30*(2), 252–262. https://doi.org/10.1037/adb0000160

Scolari, C. A. (2014). Transmedia storytelling: New ways of communicating in the digital age. *The International Journal of Multimedia & Its Applications, 6*, 69–79. https://www.accioncultural.es/media/Default%20Files/activ/2014/Adj/Anuario_ACE_2014/EN/6Storytelling_CScolari.pdf

Scolari, C. A., Masanet, M. J., Guerrero Pico, M. D. M., & Establés, M. J. (2018). Transmedia literacy in the new media ecology: Teens' transmedia skills and informal learning strategies. *Profesional De La información, 27*(4), 801–812. https://doi.org/10.3145/epi.2018.jul.09

Small, G. W., Lee, J., Kaufman, A., Jalil, J., Siddarth, P., Gaddipati, H., Moody, T. D., & Bookheimer, S. Y. (2020). Brain health consequences of digital technology use. *Dialogues in Clinical Neuroscience, 22*(2), 179–187. https://doi.org/10.31887/DCNS.2020.22.2/gsmall

Soderlund, P. D., Martinez Hollingsworth, A. S., & Heilemann, M. V. (2021). Participant engagement in a transmedia storytelling web-based app intervention for mental health of Latina women: Qualitative analysis. *JMIR Mental Health, 8*(1), e22575. https://doi.org/10.2196/22575

Stein, M. (2016). Relações entre Games e Franquias Transmídia. Até onde o mercado interfere? *Proceedings of SBGames, 2016*, 1340–1346. Retrieved from https://www.sbgames.org/sbgames2016/downloads/anais/159702.pdf

Sundet, V. S., & Petersen, L. N. (2020). Ins and outs of transmedia fandom: Motives for entering and exiting the SKAM fan community online. *Poetics, 84*, 101510. https://doi.org/10.1016/j.poetic.2020.101510

Sutherland, K. E., & Barker, R. (2023a). Audience participation and "learning" transmedia storytelling. In *Transmedia brand storytelling*. Palgrave Macmillan. https://doi.org/10.1007/978-981-99-4001-1_6

Sutherland, K. E., & Barker, R. (2023b). The creative logic of transmedia brand storytelling. In *Transmedia Brand Storytelling*. Palgrave Macmillan, Singapore. https://doi.org/10.1007/978-981-99-4001-1_3

Sutherland, K. E., & Barker, R. (2023c). Transmedia brand storytelling—Immersive campaign experiences from theory to practice. In *Transmedia brand storytelling*. Palgrave Macmillan, Singapore. https://doi.org/10.1007/978-981-99-4001-1_1

Tajudeen, F. P., Jaafar, N. I., & Sulaiman, A. (2016). Role of social media on information accessibility. *Pacific Asia Journal of the Association for Information Systems, 8*(4), 3. https://doi.org/10.17705/1pais.08402

Twenge, J. M., & Campbell, W. K. (2018). Associations between screen time and lower psychological Well-being among children and adolescents: Evidence from a population-based study. *Preventive Medicine Reports, 12*, 271–283. https://doi.org/10.1016/j.pmedr.2018.10.003

Twenge, J. M., & Campbell, W. K. (2019). Media use is linked to lower psychological Well-being: Evidence from three datasets. *The Psychiatric Quarterly, 90*(2), 311–331. https://doi.org/10.1007/s11126-019-09630-7

Vinerean, S., & Opreana, A. (2021). Measuring customer engagement in social media marketing: A higher-order model. *Journal of Theoretical and Applied Electronic Commerce Research, 16*(7), 2633–2654. https://doi.org/10.3390/jtaer16070145

Wegmann, E., Oberst, U., Stodt, B., & Brand, M. (2017). Online-specific fear of missing out and internet-use expectancies contribute to symptoms of Internetcommunication disorder. *Addictive Behaviors, 5*, 33–42. https://doi.org/10.1016/j.abrep.2017.04.001

Willett, R. (2016). Online gaming practices of preteens: Independent entertainment time and transmedia game play. *Children & Society, 30*(6), 467–477. https://doi.org/10.1111/chso.12155

Yang, A., Rolls, E. T., Dong, G., Du, J., Li, Y., Feng, J., Cheng, W., & Zhao, X. M. (2022). Longer screen time utilization is associated with the polygenic risk for attention-deficit/hyperactivity disorder with mediation by brain white matter microstructure. *eBioMedicine, 80*, 104039. https://doi.org/10.1016/j.ebiom.2022.104039

Yong, D. J. (2019). Transmedia storytelling in the age of digital media: East Asian perspectives. *International Journal of Communication, 13*, 2085. https://ijoc.org/index.php/ijoc/article/view/10003/2646

Zuhadmono, A. (2021). *Transmedia storytelling in the music industry: The case of BTS*. [Masters dissertation, Jönköping university]. https://www.diva-portal.org/smash/record.jsf?pid=diva2%3A1595883&dswid=4849

Index

A
Adolescence, 65, 68, 69, 89, 130, 154, 155, 158
Adolescents, 5–8, 10, 14, 23, 24, 26, 28, 29, 55, 56, 66–79, 89, 123–134, 140, 143, 144, 153–159, 165, 166, 169, 171, 172, 183

B
Behavioral addictions, 1–16, 23, 39, 53, 83–112, 155, 182–184, 186
Behavioral interventions, 108–109
Binge-watching (BW), 35–41

C
Clinical correlates, 83–112
Cognitive-behavioral therapy (CBT), 29, 56, 78, 96, 98, 102–106, 111, 166, 167, 171, 172
Cyberbullying, 26, 65–79, 124–127, 133, 164–166, 170, 172

D
Dependencies, 1–5, 9–12, 14, 36, 39–41, 50–52, 90, 96–98, 103, 153, 155–157, 164, 185
Depression, 7–9, 13, 26, 27, 29, 40, 54, 66, 71, 76, 77, 85, 87, 96–98, 100, 109, 111, 127, 144, 153, 155, 157, 164–167, 169, 170, 172, 184
Digital addictions, 2–15, 24, 29, 65–79, 163–172, 177–186
Digital dependencies, 8–10, 153, 156–157, 159, 185
Digital media, 1–16, 38, 39, 66, 68, 73, 78, 123–134, 153–159, 164–166, 177–186

E
Electronic games, 47–49, 53
Emotional problems, 164

F
Family relationships, 94

G
Gaming disorders, 13, 28, 40, 47–57, 169

H
Harms, 3, 5, 7–9, 12, 50, 53, 65, 85, 88, 99, 103, 105, 126, 131, 143–148, 181, 185
Hazardous gambling, 83–112

I
Internet addiction, 1, 2, 4, 6, 15, 23, 24, 26–29, 56, 164, 169, 170

L
Life purpose, 153–159
Loot boxes, 139–148

A. L. M. Andrade (ed.), *Digital Addictions*,
https://doi.org/10.1007/978-3-031-87986-9

M
Mental health, 4, 6–10, 12, 24–26, 36, 38–40, 50, 54, 55, 57, 66, 68, 69, 71, 75–78, 95, 96, 131, 153–155, 158, 163–166, 169–172, 182–184

N
Neurobiology, 50–53, 90–92, 112, 169

P
Parental mediation, 71, 123–134
Prevention, 28–30, 41, 55, 68, 78, 85, 89, 97, 99, 170–172
Problem gambling, 142–145, 147
Psychological disorders, 10, 89, 94
Psychosocial impacts, 53–55, 94

R
Risk factors, 10, 11, 28, 29, 39, 41, 52, 68–75, 77, 78, 88–90, 97, 142, 165–167, 170, 183

S
Series consumption, 37–40
Smartphone addiction, 2, 5, 6, 14, 23–30, 164
Social networks, 7, 9, 11, 65, 66, 68, 70, 71, 74, 76, 85, 124, 125, 167–169, 179, 180, 183
Sports betting, 83–112
Suicides, 164, 166, 172

T
Transmedia, 3, 177–186
Treatments, 4, 13, 23–30, 56–57, 68, 78, 84, 89, 90, 95, 96, 98, 104, 106, 108, 109, 111, 171, 184

V
Victimization, 66, 68–70, 72, 73, 75, 76, 78, 164
Video games, 3–6, 47–50, 125, 139–148, 163, 165, 168

MIX
Papier aus verantwortungsvollen Quellen
Paper from responsible sources
FSC® C105338

If you have any concerns about our products,
you can contact us on
ProductSafety@springernature.com

In case Publisher is established outside the EU,
the EU authorized representative is:
Springer Nature Customer Service Center GmbH
Europaplatz 3, 69115 Heidelberg, Germany

Printed by Libri Plureos GmbH
in Hamburg, Germany